TREATING ADDICTION

Treating Addiction

A Guide for Professionals

William R. Miller

Alyssa A. Forcehimes

Allen Zweben

Postscript by A. Thomas McLellan

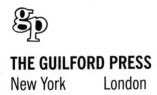

THE GUILFORD PRESS
New York   London

The authors have checked with sources believed to be reliable in their efforts to provide
information that is complete and generally in accord with the standards of practice that are
accepted at the time of publication. However, in view of the possibility of human error or
changes in behavioral, mental health, or medical sciences, neither the authors, nor the editor
and publisher, nor any other party who has been involved in the preparation or publication
of this work warrants that the information contained herein is in every respect accurate or
complete, and they are not responsible for any errors or omissions or the results obtained
from the use of such information. Readers are encouraged to confirm the information contained in this book with other sources.

Library of Congress Cataloging-in-Publication Data

Miller, William R. (William Richard)
  Treating addiction: a guide for professionals / by William R. Miller,
Alyssa Forcehimes, and Allen Zweben
      p. cm.
  Includes bibliographical references and index.
  ISBN 978-1-60918-638-8 (hardback)
  1. Substance abuse—Treatment. 2. Drug abuse—Treatment.
I. Forcehimes, Alyssa. II. Zweben, Allen, 1940– III. Title.
  RC564.M546 2011
  362.29—dc23

                                                    2011017582

To Robert G. Hall, PhD,
who in 1973 persuaded me that I ought to learn something
about addiction treatment

W. R. M.

To my sister,
who showed me that lasting change from addiction
can and does occur

A. A. F.

To my wife, Aviva,
who has always been there for me

A. Z.

About the Authors

William R. Miller, PhD, is Emeritus Distinguished Professor of Psychology and Psychiatry at the University of New Mexico in Albuquerque. Throughout his career he has developed and evaluated various methods for addiction treatment, including motivational interviewing, behavior therapies, and pharmacotherapies. More generally interested in the psychology of change, Dr. Miller has also focused on the interface of spirituality and psychotherapy. Having authored more than 40 books and 400 professional and scientific articles and chapters, Dr. Miller is listed by the Institute for Scientific Information as one of the world's most cited scientists.

Alyssa A. Forcehimes, PhD, is a clinical psychologist on the faculty of Psychiatry at the University of New Mexico Health Sciences Center. She coordinates the Southwest Node of the National Institute on Drug Abuse Clinical Trials Network, which is located at the University's Center on Alcoholism, Substance Abuse, and Addictions. Dr. Forcehimes's research focuses on processes of motivation for change and on effective methods for disseminating and teaching evidence-based behavioral treatments for addiction to mental health, substance abuse, and health care providers.

Allen Zweben, PhD, is Professor and Associate Dean for Research and Academic Affairs at the Columbia University School of Social Work in New York. Dr. Zweben has been a principal investigator on numerous federally and privately funded behavioral and medication trials, including two landmark studies funded by the National Institute on Alcohol Abuse and Alcoholism: Project MATCH, a patient–treatment matching study, and the COMBINE study, a project examining the efficacy of combining pharmacotherapy and psychotherapy interventions for alcohol problems.

Acknowledgments

For me, this book represents a retrospective of what I have learned during 37 years of work in addiction treatment and research. There is no way to adequately thank the hundreds of colleagues, students, research staff, and clients who have helped me to learn along the way, but I do want to name just a few. First of all, there is Robert G. Hall, named in the dedication. He invited a totally green summer intern into the world of addiction treatment and set me on a path that would fascinate me throughout my career. I have had the privilege of sharing the hard work of conducting many clinical research projects and discussing their implications with several long-standing colleagues, among them Drs. Reid Hester, Dick Longabaugh, Bob Meyers, Terri Moyers, Steve Rollnick, Scott Tonigan, Paula Wilbourne, and Carolina Yahne. I owe so much to two of the finest administrative assistants anyone could have, Dee Ann Quintana and Delilah Yao, who looked after me through two lively and impossibly busy decades. The last two decades of my academic career were continuously and generously funded by grants from the National Institute on Alcohol Abuse and Alcoholism and the National Institute on Drug Abuse. I spent my entire professional career at the University of New Mexico (UNM), and I can't imagine a better place to have worked. The amazing staff of UNM's Center on Alcoholism, Substance Abuse, and Addictions (CASAA) were a fine community of friends and colleagues without whom I could not have undertaken half of what I've managed to squeeze into these years. After working with 20 publishing companies throughout my career, I have settled into a happy relationship with The Guilford Press, appreciating the unusual quality of attention to detail, editing, and collaboration with authors that is reflected again in this book. Finally, I am ever grateful to my wife of 39 years, Kathy Jackson, and to our family for giving and sharing with me a life outside the frenzied world of treating addictions.

—W. R. M.

Writing a book of this size is a complex process that draws not only on the knowledge of its authors, but also on the specialized expertise of colleagues and the moral support of friends and loved ones. I deeply thank the following people, each of whom helped me in a variety of ways: my sister—whose personal experience of recovery from addiction inspired my career—and three mentors—coauthor William R. Miller, who saw the writer in me and has continued to nurture and develop that skill, and Dr. Scott Tonigan and Dr. Michael Bogenschutz, for guiding my early career development. I would also like to thank the staff with whom I work at CASAA. They are an outstanding group of scientists, program coordinators, and administrators, and I feel lucky to be affiliated with a center committed to excellent research on the treatment of addiction. Finally, I would like to thank my family—the one I came from, full of people who have loved me unconditionally and supported me throughout my life, and the one I was fortunate enough to gain through marriage and have the happiness of going home to each night. I am especially grateful to my husband, Augustine Chavez, for sharing our first year of marriage during which I was wedded, in part, to my work on this book, and for his encouragement, knowledge, and love along the way.

—A. A. F.

I am grateful to Dr. David Ockert and Armin Baier, who provided me with valuable feedback on pharmacological adjuncts. Their comments were based on having extensive knowledge and experience using pharmacotherapies in a specialty treatment setting. I am also appreciative of the help given to me by Jessica Troiano, who assisted with gathering references and other materials related to producing this book.

—A. Z.

Preface

Those of us who work in health and social services are bound to encounter substance use disorders, no matter what our specialty or setting is. The average North American has about a 15% chance of developing an addictive disorder in the course of his or her lifetime, and at any given time the prevalence rate of substance use disorders is about 8% of the population (Kessler et al., 2005; Somers, Goldner, Waraich, & Hsu, 2004). In health care and social service populations the percentage is higher still (Rose, Brondino, & Barnack, 2009; Weisner, 2002), and many more people are directly affected by a loved one with alcohol and/or drug problems. If you treat people for health, mental health, or social problems, you will see quite a few of them with addictions.

Yet, many professionals receive relatively little training or encouragement to treat this common family of problems. Though some professionals specialize in addiction treatment, little time is typically devoted to this field in generalist training for social work, psychology, counseling, medicine, and nursing. The lack of training is unfortunate because, as we discuss in the opening chapter, alcohol and drug addictions are intertwined with many other behavioral health and medical problems, and those working in health and social service settings are well positioned to identify and address them. The primary obstacle has been a lack of specific preparation to do so.

We have written this book for both generalists and specialists to provide an up-to-date foundation for helping people with addictive disorders. Together we have had nearly a century of experience in this field, in clinical psychology (W. R. M. and A. A. F.) and social work (A. Z.), and we have had the privilege to work with many dedicated counselors, nurses, physicians, and other professionals over the years who help people escape from addictive behaviors. It is rewarding work and, whether you are a generalist or an addiction specialist, we hope this book will help you gain the knowledge, confidence, and passion to address this common and significant disorder among those you serve.

Throughout this book we have sought to ground our recommendations in the best science available. "Evidence-based treatment" has become a strong emphasis in this field, and as we write this more than half of U.S. states already require the use of evidence-based practices in order to receive reimbursement for addiction treatment (Miller, Zweben, & Johnson, 2005). There is a long and fascinating history of evidence-based treatment, with more than a thousand published clinical trials of addiction treatment methods. New research appears at a dizzying rate, and we have had the privilege of being able to keep up with and translate it for clinicians whose days are filled with providing treatment. Some findings that we present may be surprising or even disturbing. They certainly were to us when we initially encountered them, sometimes as unexpected findings in our own clinical research. We cite both new and old research throughout the book; many important studies and findings were published in the latter half of the 20th century. The National Institute on Drug Abuse Clinical Trials Network alone has conducted more than 30 multisite trials since 2000. Blessed with such a large science base in addiction treatment, we owe it to those we serve to make good use of it.

That science base also includes many studies showing that *relationship* matters; it makes a difference not just what treatment is delivered, but *who* provides it and *how*. The importance of a therapist's approach is not unique to this field, but it seems to be particularly crucial to success in treating addictions, which have been so stigmatized. It makes a difference when a therapist practices with profound respect, loving compassion, and accurate empathy; some believe the quality of the relationship is the most important and powerful aspect of treatment. Thus, you will find an emphasis on relationship and style interwoven throughout this book.

What we wish to offer you, then, is an up-to-date professional resource that combines both clinical and scientific perspectives. We hope this book will be helpful to professionals who are already treating addictive disorders and for people who are just learning how to treat addictions. We also encourage health professionals more generally to think of addictions as falling within their scope of work and have kept this in mind in our writing. In addiction treatment, it makes a difference what you do and how you do it, and it is far easier to develop evidence-based practice from the outset than to change already established habits.

A WORD ABOUT WORDS

In writing this book, we had to make many decisions about terminology. The addiction field has been replete with stigmatizing and moralistic language like "clean" and "dirty." Since 1980, the American Psychiatric Association in its *Diagnostic and Statistical Manual* has recommended that diagnostic terms be used to describe disorders ("depression") rather than people ("depressives"). Although language that describes disorders is now the professional norm in most of behavioral health, in the addiction field it is still common to hear labels being applied to people (e.g., "abuser," "addict," "alcoholic"). Terminology makes a difference. In a recent survey, health professionals were much more likely to blame and recommend punishment when a person was described as a "substance abuser" rather than as "having a substance use disorder" (Kelly & Westerhoff, 2010). This detail was the only change in the case description, and yet it yielded significantly more negative perceptions and recommendations. Throughout this book we have been careful to describe conditions rather than labeling people.

A wide variety of terms are applied to people who are under professional care, among them "patient," "client," "resident," "participant," "consumer," and, at a Navajo treatment center in New Mexico, "relative." Because most treatment for substance use disorders is provided in nonmedical settings, we have most often used "clients" or "people" as the generic term and "patients" when the context is medical.

Similarly, people who provide treatment for substance use disorders encompass a wide range of professions and titles. We have used "counselor," "clinician," and "practitioner" as generics for people who provide care.

In describing conditions, we have adhered to the current, albeit somewhat awkward, terms "substance use disorder" as well as "alcohol/drug problems" or "alcohol and other drug problems," the latter being the traditional reminder that ethyl alcohol is itself a drug. As a shorthand generic, we have preferred the term "addiction," which is the title of the oldest scientific journal in the field. We use the term to refer to the full continuum of substance use disorders, much as Jellinek (1960) used the term "alcoholism," and we refer to more severe forms as "dependence" (see Chapter 2).

Another decision that we made in writing is to avoid using the word "relapse," even though it is popular and widely used. Our reasoning is that "relapse" communicates that there are only two possible states: using problematically or not using at all. Ironically, use of the term "relapse" itself implies and promotes what Marlatt has described as the "abstinence violation effect" and thus can become a self-fulfilling prophecy (Marlatt & Donovan, 2005). "Relapse" also has rather pejorative overtones and is not typically used in describing other chronic health conditions. A person with diabetes who comes into the emergency room in hypoglycemic shock is not typically said to have relapsed. Neither is a person with a recurrence of problems related to asthma or heart disease. What language, then, might one use instead? Euphemisms still retain the assumption of a binary on-or-off state, whereas treatment outcomes tend to be much more variable (Miller, 1996b; Miller, Walters, & Bennett, 2001). The clearest solution, we believe, is simply to describe the *behavior* (e.g., drinking, drug use) without adding moralistic baggage. This is the approach we have taken, using "relapse" when necessary to describe the concept. In lieu of "relapse prevention," we focus positively on maintaining change (see Chapter 19). It is a challenging discipline to write in this way, precisely because it involves shedding some old habits and assumptions.

Contents

A variety of screening and assessment measures relevant to addiction treatment are available on the book's Companion Web page (follow the link from *www.guilford.com/p/miller11*). For clinicians' use and convenience, they are provided in downloadable form with the authors' permission.

PART I

An Invitation to Addiction Treatment

W hy would you choose to treat addictions as a part of your professional career? For many who specialize in this area it comes down to a matter of the heart, a special caring and commitment for those whose lives have been torn apart by alcohol and other drugs. Decades ago, just about the only people treating addictions were those who had a personal commitment to alleviating this particular form of human suffering, often by virtue of their own recovery. The need today is much broader than specialists can address. Professionals who work in any sector of health and social services are bound to encounter many people with alcohol/drug problems and are ideally situated to help them. This book offers an integrated approach, with particular emphasis on the practical things you need to know and do. Chapter 1 offers a rationale for learning about and treating addictions. Chapter 2 clarifies some key terminology in this field, including diagnostic concepts. Because it is also important for the clinician to know something about how drugs of abuse work in the human body, Chapter 3 offers some basics of psychopharmacology.

Why Treat Addiction?

There are several good reasons why treating addictions should be of vital concern, not just for specialists in this area, but to all professionals who work in health care, behavioral health, and social services (Miller & Weisner, 2002). One of these is how common addiction problems are. In the United States, for example, current alcohol use disorders alone are diagnosable in about 7% of the general adult population (Secretary of Health and Human Services, 2000). An overlapping 15% of the population remains addicted to nicotine (Hughes, Helzer, & Lindberg, 2006), and about 2% meet diagnostic criteria for an illicit drug use disorder (Compton, Thomas, Stinson, & Grant, 2007). Still others have significant problems with addictive behaviors that do not involve a drug, such as pathological gambling, which afflicts up to 5% of the population, particularly in areas with a high concentration of legalized gaming (Petry & Armentano, 1999). Thus the sheer prevalence of these problems and the suffering they cause to the afflicted and those around them are reason enough to attend to them.

A second reason is that addictions are closely intertwined with the problems that bring people into the offices of medical, mental health, social service, and correctional workers. In most populations seen by such professionals, the prevalence of substance use disorders can be much higher than in the general population. If 1 out of every 12 people in the general population has an alcohol/drug problem (without even counting their family members and others they affect), the proportion is greater still among health care and mental health patients, as high as 20 to 50% depending

> Aware of it or not, most health and social service professionals are already treating the sequelae of addictions without directly addressing a significant source of the problems.

3

on the setting (Weisner, 2002). Thus, aware of it or not, most health and social service professionals are already treating the sequelae of addictions without directly addressing a significant source of the problems.

Why not just refer people with addictions to specialist programs? There is a role, of course, for specialist treatment of addictions, particularly when it is closely integrated with other needed services. Yet there is a downside to regarding clients' disorders as separable, to be treated by different specialists. A majority of people with alcohol or other drug dependence also have concomitant mental and/or physical disorders that need attention. The presence of concomitant disorders complicates the treatment of addictions, and vice versa. Furthermore, if addictions are chronic conditions, there is wisdom in continuous care and not just acute specialist treatment. People often get lost in the referral process, and there are well-known problems with the coordination of care when various parts of the person are being treated in separate services (Shavelson, 2001). For all these reasons, there is a trend toward integrating the treatment of addictions within a larger spectrum of health and social services.

By the time people accept specialist addiction treatment (or are compelled to do so), their problems have often reached a severe level. Often they had been seen earlier in health care, mental health, social service, or legal and correctional systems for conditions directly or indirectly related to their substance use. Yet their alcohol/drug problems were either not recognized or not addressed effectively at these times. It is clearly possible to recognize and treat alcohol/drug problems in more general practice settings. It may even be *easier* to treat them there because people tend to turn up in health care and social services at earlier stages of problem development, long before they may accept referral to a specialist addiction treatment program.

Perhaps the most persuasive reason for addressing addictions, however, is the one that attracted and has held each of us in this field over the years: *addictions are highly treatable*, and a variety of effective treatment methods are available. When people who have developed alcohol/drug dependence recover, they *really* get better. You don't need subtle psychological measures to see the change. They look better. They feel better. Their family and social functioning tends to improve. They are healthier and happier. They fare better at work, school, and play. And, contrary to public opinion, most of them do recover. With the array of effective treatments now available, it is rewarding indeed to treat addictions in practice. Furthermore, substance use disorders—particularly tobacco and alcohol—are by far the leading preventable cause of death in the Western world. Treating addictions is quite literally a matter of life and death.

> Treating addictions is quite literally a matter of life and death.

WHY *NOT* TREAT ADDICTIONS?

So why, then, have so many professionals chosen not to address this very common, life-threatening, and highly treatable class of disorders that are so intertwined with other problems? The answer lies, in part, in several misconceptions.

First, some practitioners believe treating addictions requires a mysterious and highly specialized expertise that is entirely separate from their own. In fact, as will become clear in the chapters that follow, the psychosocial treatment methods with strongest evidence of efficacy are often familiar to behavioral health professionals who treat other disorders, and are commonly part of the ordinary training and practice of many professionals: client-centered listening skills, behavior therapies, relationship counseling, good case management, and motivational

> The psychosocial treatment methods with strongest evidence of efficacy are often familiar to behavioral health professionals who treat other disorders.

interviewing. Effective medications are available to aid in treatment and long-term management of these chronic conditions. The major professional health disciplines have already contributed and will continue to contribute much in understanding and treating addictions (e.g., Miller & Brown, 1997). To be sure, there are some facts and particular skills you need to know when addressing alcohol/drug problems. Providing that background is one primary purpose of this book.

A second challenge is time. Counselors and psychotherapists may have 50-minute hours, but health care appointments are often brief, with many other tasks to be accomplished. Those who work in contexts such as primary health care, family medicine, and dentistry may understandably see substance use disorders as "not my job"—falling outside the realm of possibility within time constraints. Yet many other chronic conditions are followed and treated within the scope of routine care, and it's possible to do what you can within the time that you have. Medical professionals may have only a few minutes to address substance use concerns, but it is clear that even this amount of time when used well can make a difference (see Chapter 9). Similarly, those who work in mental health or probation services have other issues to address and may view addictions as beyond their professional responsibility or expertise, but alcohol/drug problems are intertwined with mental health and correctional concerns.

A third possible obstacle is the belief that in order to be effective in treating addictions, one must be in recovery oneself. Although a substantial minority of professionals who treat addictions are themselves in recovery, ample evidence indicates that therapeutic effectiveness is simply unrelated to one's own history of addiction. Those who are in recovery are neither more nor less effective than other professionals in treating addictions, even when delivering 12-step-related treatments (Project MATCH Research Group, 1998d). Rather, effectiveness is related to other factors of therapeutic style (see Chapter 4).

Then there is, for some, a social stigma associated with addictive disorders, sometimes linked to pessimism (among the public, professionals, and clients themselves) about the possibility of change (Moyers & Miller, 1993; Schomerus, Corrigan, et al., 2011; Schomerus, Lucht, et al., 2011). This was exacerbated by writings in the mid-20th century suggesting that people with substance dependence are pathological liars, sociopaths, and highly defended by chronic immature defense mechanisms. We also see moralizing and blaming related to the perception that these disorders are self-inflicted (overlooking that other chronic health problems are also closely linked to personal behavior and lifestyle). In truth, people with substance use disorders represent a full spectrum of personality, socioeconomic status, intelligence, and character. Research provides no support for the belief that these individuals differ from others in overusing certain defenses, and they surely have no corner on dishonesty. One reason we, the authors, have

---

BOX 1.1. Personal Reflection: Why Addictions?

What draws people into the field of addiction treatment? Often it is firsthand experience, and that was certainly the case for me. I departed for college at the same time my younger sister entered an inpatient substance abuse treatment program. The anxious feeling of being on my own for the first time was compounded by the heartache of knowing that my sister was also living away from home and struggling to overcome addiction. When I visited her a few months into treatment, I saw in her a profoundly changed life: her values had shifted and she had found peace with herself.

But *how* did she change, I wondered? When I asked my sister this question, she shrugged and responded that it was hard to explain—something just happened. No one, including my sister, seemed overly concerned with exploring this question, with understanding why. They were content to simply appreciate the results of this change. But I remained curious: What had caused this significant and sudden change that allowed her to overcome addiction?

In my clinical work now, as I hear each client's story and watch changes occur throughout our work together, I continue to wonder how it is that people change. How can I work with people most effectively to help them enact and maintain change? Why is it that some clients like my sister do change profoundly, while others do not, at least during the time in which our lives intersect? It's a privilege to be a companion and witness to such important life changes, and fascinating to continue pondering questions like these along the way.

—A. A. F.

remained in this field is that we have genuinely enjoyed treating people who are struggling with addictions, and also working with their loved ones. It is rewarding, lifesaving work.

AN INTEGRATIVE APPROACH

The approach we describe in this book is integrative in at least four ways. As the chapters to follow reveal, this approach is (1) comprehensive and evidence-based, (2) multidisciplinary, (3) holistic, and (4) collaborative.

Comprehensive and Evidence-Based

Our integrated approach is first of all grounded in available clinical science. Professional and public opinions abound regarding addictions. Such opinions, including our own, have often proved inaccurate when carefully examined in well-designed scientific research. In this book we have sought as much as possible to differentiate opinion from science, and given primary emphasis to the substantial base of scientific evidence that is now available to guide practice.

The approach we describe is also comprehensive in that it places treatment within a larger context of scientific knowledge about the nature of addictions, motivation for change, assessment and diagnosis, mutual help groups, case management, and prevention (McCrady & Epstein, 1999; Miller & Carroll, 2006). We address the full spectrum of addiction treatment, from crucial aspects of the first contact to long-term maintenance, as befits the management of a complex and often chronic condition.

Multidisciplinary

Second, we draw upon a range of professional perspectives including those from counseling and family therapy, medicine and nursing, pastoral care, psychology, and social work. In an ideal world, treatment might be delivered by a collaborative team of professionals representing these differing areas of professional expertise. In reality, treatment often relies upon a single or primary therapist whose role includes providing or serving as liaison with this range of services.

Holistic

Third, we seek in our integrated approach to consider the whole person: biological, psychological, social, and spiritual. Some think of going to a specialist for treatment of addiction, much as one goes to a dentist for care of one's teeth. Yet addictions involve and affect the whole person and those around him or her. They are biological *and* psychological *and* social *and* spiritual. By nature of disciplinary training, you may be prepared to deal best with one of these dimensions. Those who treat addictions, however, will meet all of these aspects of the person, and treatment will not be optimally effective if it is limited to only one of them.

Collaborative Care

Finally, we advocate the integration and coordination of addiction care with the broader range of health and social services. Sequestering addiction treatment in isolated programs has served in some ways to sustain stigma and discourage treatment. We favor involving a broad range of professionals in direct care for people with alcohol/drug problems. In truth, most health and social service professionals are already seeing people with addiction problems, though they may be unaware of it or regard such problems as someone else's concern. In complex disorders like addictions, where attention is needed in so many spheres, care can begin with almost any area.

Taken together, the 23 chapters of this book represent pieces of a puzzle, the building blocks of an integrative approach to addiction treatment. They describe a system of care that is comprehensive, evidence-based, multidisciplinary, holistic, and collaborative. That's a tall order for us in writing this book, and for you in practice. Taking the attitude of "My way or the highway" and offering only one brand of treatment is much simpler, but does a disservice to clients in failing to make use of the vast amount that has been learned about how to help people with addictions. An integrative approach is a challenging goal, a direction in which you can keep growing throughout your professional career. That has certainly been our continuing experience, and we are grateful for this opportunity to pass on, for your consideration, what we have learned along the way.

KEY POINTS

- Substance use disorders are prevalent in the general population, and even more so among people seen in health care, social service, and correctional settings.

- Substance use disorders are highly treatable. A majority of affected people recover.

- An encouraging armamentarium of effective, evidence-based treatment methods is available, no one of which is best for everyone with addiction problems.

- People with alcohol/drug problems commonly have other significant psychological, medical, and social problems, and coordinated treatment of these problems is needed.

- Treating addictions should be a normal part of general health care and social service systems and not limited to specialist programs.

REFLECTION QUESTIONS

Of the people you normally serve (or anticipate serving), what percentage would you estimate have alcohol or other drug problems?

What most encourages or motivates you to work with people whose lives are affected by addiction, and with their family members?

In your community, where are people with alcohol/drug problems most likely to turn up seeking help or services? (Hint: It's not in addiction treatment programs.)

CHAPTER 2

What Is Addiction?

Just about everyone has some notion of what addiction is. The website *www.dictionary.com* offers this general definition: "The condition of being habitually or compulsively occupied with or involved in something." This definition concisely reflects three aspects of the term that are found in most popular conceptions of addiction: (1) it is something done regularly, repeatedly, habitually; (2) there is a compulsive quality to it that seems at least partly beyond the individual's conscious control; and (3) it does not necessarily involve a drug, although that is the most common association.

In everyday speech, people are said to be "addicted" when they relentlessly pursue any sensation or activity, be it sex, gambling, alcohol or other drugs, work, food, shopping, or love. Peele (2000) argued that the concept of addiction has expanded to describe so many behaviors that it has almost lost its meaning. Something becomes an addiction when it increasingly dominates a person's life and, as a result, harms or detracts from other aspects of life. In this broad colloquial sense, addiction is not unusual.

For purposes of science and health care, however, a more precise meaning is needed. This meaning is usually expressed in the form of a *diagnosis* that is defined by a particular pattern of signs and symptoms. Diagnostic criteria are typically developed by consensus within a professional organization such as the World Health Organization, which is responsible for the International Classification of Diseases (ICD). The American Psychiatric Association's *Diagnostic and Statistical Manual of Mental Disorders* (DSM) has been the standard for classification by behavioral health professionals in North America. The DSM is revised every decade or so, which means that the names and criteria for diagnosing addictions have evolved over time.

UNDERSTANDING DIAGNOSES

A formal classification system such as the ICD or DSM is a way to help health professionals mean the same thing when making diagnoses. It is a bit like the biological taxonomy of life forms classified by genus and species. Such classification systems tend to become larger and more complex over time as new species and subspecies are recognized, and this has certainly happened with the DSM. What was once a single diagnosis of "alcoholism" or "drug addiction" has been differentiated into dozens of more specific categories.

It is also true that formal diagnoses often differ from popular conceptions. For example, schizophrenia is often mistakenly associated with a "split personality." When most people think of depression, they envision someone who is sad. One might imagine a woman in a housecoat, bent over on the couch with shoulders hunched and her head in her hands, weeping. These are the images used in television programming and commercials for prescription medications. Actual clinical presentations often vary widely and can depart substantially from popular stereotypes. For instance, sadness is only one possible dimension that can be present or absent in a diagnosis of depression. Common conceptions of schizophrenia focus on positive symptoms such as hallucinations and delusions rather than negative symptoms such as catatonic behavior and flat affect. Part of the skill of a behavioral health diagnostician is recognizing the variability as well as the commonality of individual clinical pictures.

The same is true with addiction, which involves multiple dimensions that are variously present or absent in an individual. Popular conceptions often focus on certain manifestations. One might imagine a disheveled man slumped on a sidewalk, surrounded by cans and bottles, having lost his family, job, and home. Classic stereotypes also tend to involve the most severe levels of use and consequences.

For professional purposes within this book, we use *addiction* as the most generic term for substance use disorders (as well as other addictive behaviors), encompassing a broad range of severity. Addiction is not currently a diagnosis in itself. As discussed in this chapter, diagnoses have become more differentiated and precise. *Addiction* is, however, the title of the oldest scientific journal of this field which covers a range of interrelated clinical problems. As an umbrella concept, addiction encompasses a wide variety of individual presentations such as:

- A 37-year-old man who drinks heavily enough most nights to still be legally intoxicated the next morning, and whose wife is threatening to leave him because of his drinking, but who appears to be in good physical health, has a good job, and has never suffered obvious negative social consequences.

- A skeletal 22-year-old who steals and trades sex to support a daily habit injecting methamphetamine.
- A successful businesswoman who began taking her daughter's prescribed methylphenidate periodically as a way to be alert and accomplish more during the day, then started needing higher doses, buying stimulants illegally and using them more regularly.
- A college student who drinks 8–12 beers three or four nights a week to feel "buzzed" and has a drink the next morning to calm his nerves.
- A 50-year-old woman who goes to the casino daily to play the quarter slot machines for 6 hours while her husband is at work and has built up $40,000 in credit card debt.
- A single parent who smokes two packs of cigarettes daily and has unsuccessfully tried several times to quit.

In short, people with addiction look and act in many different ways.

This is one reason why questionnaires that purport to detect the presence or absence of addiction are problematic. Such "dipstick" tests were once popular, an easy list of questions that would yield a plus or minus sign to tell whether the person had "a problem." Brief screening questions are useful to indicate whether more evaluation is called for, but do not themselves make a diagnosis (see Chapter 5). For now, we focus on how to think more broadly about addiction and its causes.

SEVEN DIMENSIONS OF ADDICTION

There are at least seven dimensions of addiction that, though interrelated, are also surprisingly independent of each other. All of them occur along a continuum, and knowing where an individual is on one particular dimension does not reliably tell you his or her location on the others. This is one reason why definitions and diagnostic criteria for addiction are so challenging.

Use

A first dimension to consider is the extent and pattern of the person's use of psychoactive substances. This is most often described in terms of quantity (how much?), frequency (how often?), and variability (steady vs. periodic patterns of use). Other addictive behaviors such as gambling can, of course, be measured along the same dimensions.

How do quantity, frequency, and variability differ?

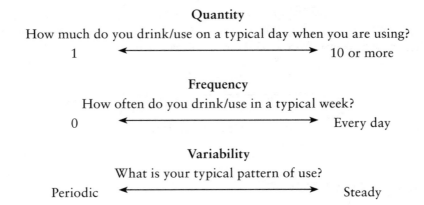

Quantity

How much do you drink/use on a typical day when you are using?

1   ←——————————————→   10 or more

Frequency

How often do you drink/use in a typical week?

0   ←——————————————→   Every day

Variability

What is your typical pattern of use?

Periodic   ←——————————————→   Steady

Problems

Just knowing how much a person is using does not in itself tell you about its effects on the person's life (though there certainly is a relationship). A second dimension to consider is the extent to which alcohol/drug use has resulted in adverse consequences for the individual and those around him or her. The term "problem drinking" historically refers to using alcohol in a way that causes negative psychosocial consequences (Cahalan, 1970). These might include, for example, problems in work, school, family and other relationships, mood, finances, and legal problems.

What kind of consequences is the person experiencing? What areas specifically?

None   ←——————————————→   Many

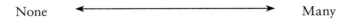

Physical Adaptation

One characteristic of many psychoactive drugs is that the body adapts as a person uses them. One such adaptation is drug *tolerance*: a reduction in the effect of a particular dose of the drug. Over time a person may require increasingly larger doses to experience the same high as before (chronic tolerance), or even to feel "normal." Having even one drink diminishes the additive impact of the next one (acute tolerance). Another way in which the body adapts over time is *physiological dependence*. With some drugs, the body becomes accustomed to their presence and adjusts normal functioning accordingly. Then when the drug is withdrawn, there is a physical rebound effect that is usually unpleasant, and opposite to the effects of intoxication. Alcohol intoxication depresses many physical functions, whereas alcohol withdrawal involves heightened arousal and sensitivity to stimuli (ranging in intensity from a hangover to severe and life-threatening withdrawal syndrome). Conversely, stimulant intoxication increases physical arousal whereas withdrawal from stimulants involves a depressing rebound.

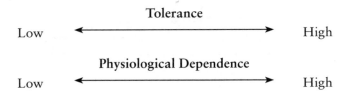

Tolerance

Low   ←——————————————————→   High

Physiological Dependence

Low   ←——————————————————→   High

Behavioral Dependence

| Physical adaptation to a drug is not the only form of dependence. | Physical adaptation to a drug is not only form of dependence. A more general pattern of behavioral dependence is that the drug gradually assumes a more central place in the person's life, displacing |

other activities, relationships, and social roles that once had greater priority (American Psychiatric Association, 1994; Edwards & Gross, 1976). Increasing amounts of the person's time, energy, and resources are devoted to obtaining, using, and recovering from the effects of the drug. People can also come to rely on a drug for certain coping functions. If the use of a drug is the only or primary way that someone has to cope with a particular feeling or situation, the person is psychologically dependent on the drug for that purpose (see Chapter 7).

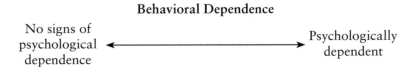

Behavioral Dependence

No signs of
psychological   ←——————————————————→   Psychologically
dependence   dependent

Cognitive Impairment

Psychoactive drugs can also have acute (temporary) or chronic (long-term) effects on cognitive functioning, adaptive abilities, and intelligence. Depressant drugs (like alcohol, tranquilizers, and sedatives) can impair memory, attention, reaction time, and learning abilities during the period of intoxication. This is an important reason why driving under the influence is illegal. With long-term use, alcohol and certain other psychoactive drugs can also produce chronic, even irreversible, mental impairment.

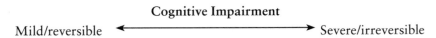

Cognitive Impairment

Mild/reversible   ←——————————————————→   Severe/irreversible

Medical Harm

Many psychoactive drugs also have the potential to damage physical health. Some harm is due to the acute effects of intoxication, such as risk taking, aggression, and overdose. Other forms of medical harm are related to chronic use. There are well-documented links of smoking to heart disease and cancer. Heavy drinking is associated with increased rates of various cancers, heart disease, and damage to the liver and other organ systems. Alcohol/drug use can also damage health indirectly by diminishing normal self-care, displacing nutrition, and compromising the management of chronic conditions such as diabetes.

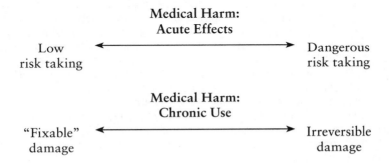

Motivation for Change

Finally, motivation for change is commonly recognized as an important dimension of addiction and recovery. Reluctance to recognize the need for change and take action is a common problem in addiction. Historically it was believed that a person with addiction had to "hit bottom" and experience sufficient suffering before being ready to change, but there are now many tools to help enhance motivation for change (see Chapter 10).

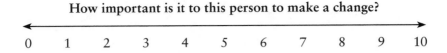

Studying addiction is in a way like the fabled blind men encountering an elephant. One touches the trunk and concludes that an elephant is like a firehose. Another touching the elephant's side says that it is like a wall. One who holds the tail finds elephants to be like snakes. Another hugs a leg and reports that an elephant is much like a tree. An elephant is none of these and all of these. A complete understanding requires combining different perspectives; any one part reveals only a little about other aspects or about the whole elephant.

BOX 2.1. Applying Your Knowledge: Thinking about the Different Dimensions of Addiction

In the previous section, we described seven different dimensions of addiction. Consider the following case example and think about where this individual would fall on the seven dimensions of addiction:

Steven is a 28-year-old male who comes in to your clinic because he tested positive for cocaine on a random drug test at work and is required by his employer to get drug counseling. He reported using cocaine twice in the past 12 months, both times while at parties with old college buddies. He reported that he snorted one line on both occasions and woke up the next morning without any side effects of withdrawal. He is a marathon runner and is training for a triathalon, with a "clean bill of health" from his primary care physician. When asked about some of the not so good things about using cocaine, he reported concern about possibly losing his job as a result of this positive drug test and some fears about what cocaine use might do to his body, specifically how it might impact his marathon time. Steven told you, "I'm done with using cocaine. I won't ever be using it again. This event made me realize that I need to grow up and start acting my age. I'm not some dumb college kid any more, and I want to be successful in my career and continue to improve my marathon times in order to qualify to run in the Boston marathon. I know cocaine isn't going to help me do either of those things."

Where would you say Steven is on each of the seven dimensions, given what you know so far? What else would you want to know?

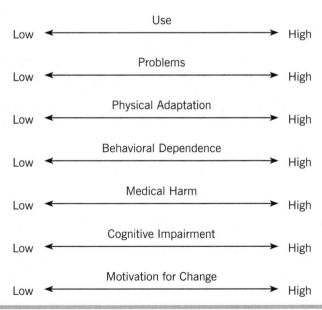

Use
Low ◄─────────────────────► High

Problems
Low ◄─────────────────────► High

Physical Adaptation
Low ◄─────────────────────► High

Behavioral Dependence
Low ◄─────────────────────► High

Medical Harm
Low ◄─────────────────────► High

Cognitive Impairment
Low ◄─────────────────────► High

Motivation for Change
Low ◄─────────────────────► High

HISTORY OF THE DSM

Technically speaking, there was no alcoholism prior to 1849. That is when the Swedish physician Magnus Huss coined the term "alcoholism" to describe adverse consequences of excessive drinking (Sournia, 1990). There was drunkenness, inebriety, and intemperance, but no alcoholism. Since then, society has struggled to define what constitutes addiction and to puzzle over its causes.

The history of diagnoses in the DSM illustrates the evolving concept of addiction. Each DSM has offered criteria for deciding whether specific diagnoses fit a particular person's case. The diagnostic decision is binary—present or absent—even though reality may be more of a continuum. To make a yes/no diagnostic decision, then, often means drawing a somewhat arbitrary cutoff point along a continuum of severity. In the DSM this is typically done according to the number of symptoms present.

In the early 1950s, the first edition of the DSM grouped both *alcoholism* and *drug addiction* with sociopathic personality disturbances, indicating that people with addiction suffered from "deep seated personality disturbance" (DSM-I; American Psychiatric Association, 1952, p. 34). The sociopathic personality category also included sexual deviations and antisocial behavior, suggesting that individuals with addiction were a threat to societal order. Unlike the detailed lists of criteria that are used to classify disorders today, the first edition contained only a brief paragraph that focused almost entirely on the presumed etiology of the disorder. According to the DSM-I, addiction was likely a symptom of an underlying brain or personality disorder and was a clear departure from culturally acceptable behavior. The signs and symptoms displayed by someone with an addiction to drugs or alcohol were not clearly described.

In the second edition (DSM-II; American Psychiatric Association, 1968), several new terms were proposed as types of alcoholism, including *episodic excessive drinking, habitual excessive drinking*, and *alcohol addiction*. This reflected conceptions from a classic book by E. M. Jellinek (1960), *The Disease Concept of Alcoholism*, that used "alcoholism" as a broad and generic term for alcohol-related disorders (as Magnus Huss had done), and hypothesized various subtypes. Similarly, *drug dependence* was expanded in DSM-II to include subcategories by specific drug class. Physiological signs of dependence, such as withdrawal and tolerance, were described as signs and symptoms of these conditions. As in DSM-I, however, these disorders remained as subcategories of "personality disorders and certain other nonpsychotic mental disorders." The placement of these conditions implied once again that addiction represented a disorder of the personality that caused the individual to use alcohol or other drugs excessively.

During the 1970s, clinical research indicated a need to further differentiate substance use disorders. The *Feighner criteria* were developed in an effort to diagnose alcoholism on research-based decision rules (Feighner et al., 1972). This trend toward differential diagnosis was reflected in the third edition of the DSM (DSM-III; American Psychiatric Association, 1980).

DSM-III was the first to identify substance abuse and dependence as separate pathological conditions. This differentiation was based, in part, on findings from longitudinal research indicating that many people with a history of alcohol problems never progressed to dependence (Cahalan, 1970; cf. Hasin, Grant, & Endicott, 1990), suggesting the possibility of two separate disorders. As of DSM-III, "alcoholism" was no longer used as a formal diagnosis. Another significant change in DSM-III was the creation of a separate category for substance use disorders, removing the prior implication that they represented underlying personality disorders.

DSM-III more generally avoided tying disorders to specific etiologies. With regard to addiction, DSM-III suggested that social and cultural factors were important contributors to the onset and continuation of abuse and dependence. This suggestion further underlined the shift away from thinking of addiction as personal pathology, toward something more akin to a public health model that considered environmental factors. *Substance abuse* was defined as problematic use with social or occupational impairment, but with the absence of significant tolerance and/or withdrawal. The DSM-III definition of *substance dependence* emphasized the physiological symptoms of tolerance (needing to take much higher doses of the substance to obtain the same effect) and withdrawal (having a distinct pattern of physiological changes after stopping or reducing use), and required the presence of one or both of these criteria in order to make a dependence diagnosis. In both disorders, impairment in social and occupational function was a prominent aspect of the definitions, creating a significant overlap between the criteria for substance abuse and dependence. In essence, "abuse" was the presence of drug-related problems in the absence of a history of significant physiological adaptation.

Meanwhile, a changing conception of substance dependence was already emerging, a shift away from strictly physiological symptoms toward a broader behavioral syndrome. This shift was strongly influenced by the work of Griffith Edwards (1986; Edwards & Gross, 1976) who conceptualized alcohol dependence as a cluster of interrelated behavioral, psychological, and physiological elements, all varying in severity. Common elements of the dependence syndrome included a narrowing of the drinking repertoire (increasingly patterned and predictable), drink-seeking behavior, tolerance, withdrawal, drinking to relieve or avoid withdrawal symptoms, subjective awareness of the compulsion to drink, and a return to drinking after a period of abstinence. Also contributing to a shift toward emphasis

---

BOX 2.2. Is There an Addictive Personality?

In the mid-20th century it was believed that people with substance use disorders had a particular predisposing personality, with high levels of immature defense mechanisms such as denial. Treatment programs were designed to confront and "break down" these pathological defenses since they were seen as a primary cause of addiction. Yet decades of research have revealed few commonalities in the personality of people with addiction problems. People with substance use disorders vary widely on other dimensions, and when their defenses have been measured specifically they appear no different from other people (Donovan, Hague, & O'Leary, 1975). In other words, many different kinds of people succumb to addiction. There are some developmental factors related to risk of subsequent addiction—difficult temperament, childhood conflicts with the law and authorities, and impaired self-control—but no characteristic abnormal personality.

So if people do not walk through the door of addiction treatment programs all with the same personality, what behaviors caused counselors to perceive their clients as in *denial*? Often it came down to disagreement with the counselor over a diagnosis or label, and the client showing (from the counselor's perspective) insufficient distress, acceptance of help, compliance with particular treatment prescriptions, and change—factors that tend to get clients labeled as "unmotivated." Treatment providers tended to perceive clients as "motivated" when they agreed with the provider, accepted the provider's diagnosis or label, expressed a desire for help, showed appropriate distress, voiced a need for the provider's assistance, complied with treatment prescriptions, and succeeded in changing. Clients' resistance and defensiveness, which often were attributed to their difficult personalities, are highly responsive to counseling style (see Chapter 16). A suspicious, authoritarian, confrontational style substantially increases resistance and defensiveness, not only in people with addictions but in most human beings. This creates a self-fulfilling prophecy, with clients who are initially ambivalent digging in their heels and becoming adamant about *not* changing. In contrast, a respectful, listening, and compassionate therapeutic style (see Chapter 4) tends to reduce resistance and promote change.

---

on behavioral aspects of dependence was classic work by Brady and Lucas (1984) showing that laboratory animals can be taught to self-administer psychoactive drugs. Once animals learned to self-administer an addictive substance, most would expend enormous amounts of time and effort to obtain additional doses. This drug-seeking behavior also proved difficult to extinguish, particular when the administered substance was one with high abuse liability in humans (such as stimulants or opiates).

In 1987, DSM-III was revised (DSM-III-R; American Psychiatric Association, 1987) in a way that gave the behavioral aspects of substance use disorders equal weight to the physiological components. The DSM-III-R category of *psychoactive substance abuse* was defined as a pattern of use that continues despite knowledge of adverse consequences or by drug use in situations in which it is physically dangerous. As before, the "abuse" diagnosis was a residual category for people who had never met criteria for dependence.

DSM-IV (American Psychiatric Association, 1994) largely continued the definitions of DSM-III, now defining over 100 different substance-related disorders for 12 different classes of drugs (see Chapter 3). In addition to abuse and dependence, there were diagnoses for drug-related intoxication, withdrawal, delirium, dementia, amnestic disorder, psychotic disorders, mood disorders, anxiety disorders, sexual dysfunction, and sleep disorders. Unlike its predecessors, DSM-IV clearly separated the criteria for dependence from those of abuse. Dependence in DSM-IV was a syndrome involving compulsive use, with or without tolerance and withdrawal. Abuse was defined as problematic use without compulsive use, tolerance, or withdrawal. A transitional text revision (DSM, 4th ed., text rev.; American Psychiatric Association, 2000) defined substance abuse as meeting any one of four criteria revolving around recurrent problems related to the substance, and dependence as meeting three or more of seven physiological or behavioral criteria. This created a problem of "diagnostic orphans" who, for example, evidence none of the criteria for abuse and only one or two symptoms in the dependence category.

The fifth edition of the DSM, planned for release in 2013, revisits this terminology yet again. Under consideration is a transition from the abuse/dependence terminology and back to a general term of "addiction" with categories of severity (e.g., mild, moderate, and severe), similar to the approach we have taken in this book. Factor analyses found that the abuse and dependence criteria actually loaded on a single factor and are interrelated with each other (Martin, Chung, & Langenbucher, 2008; Mewton, Slade, McBride, Grove, & Teesson, 2011). This transition marks further recognition that addiction occurs along a continuum of severity, and that "abuse" is not separate from or necessarily antecedent to dependence.

Moving away from the separate categories of *dependence* and *abuse* is something that we support. The terms "abuse" and "abusers" have always been moralistic and pejorative in tone. (A colleague once quipped that "alcohol abuse" is mixing a single-malt scotch with root beer.) And while the term "dependence" has served to broaden thinking, it has also been confusing because of its changing meanings. Many providers, particularly those in medical settings, still equate dependence with physiological adaptation, as was the case in DSM-III. (Of course the same can be said of "addiction" as a generic.) Another reason we favor abolishing these separate categories is that the change in nomenclature more accurately represents the continuum of severity, and eliminates the problem of diagnostic orphans who don't meet prior categories yet still have significant problems related to substance use.

WHERE IS THE LINE FOR ADDICTION?

Diagnosis historically has focused on a binary, black-or-white decision: Does the person "have" a particular condition or not? Sometimes it's vital to know that. Presence or absence matters with regard to a brain tumor or the human immunodeficiency virus (HIV). Many other conditions, however, involve shades of gray, a gradual continuum of severity, and addiction is one of those. How much is too much? When has a person who drinks or uses other drugs crossed "over the line" to addiction? As illustrated by the evolving DSM, the answers change over time.

The idea that there is a black-or-white line has itself been a source of problems in personal and social response to alcohol/ drug use. At the time of DSM-II, the prevailing belief was that alcoholism was a binary, present-or-absent condition, like pregnancy. One could not be "a little" alcoholic—either you were or you weren't. In this view, alcoholics were unable to handle alcohol, whereas normal people could drink with impunity. It thus became a source of significant argument whether a particular person was or wasn't alcoholic. In the common situation where a professional (or relative) diagnosed someone as being over the line, a person who disavowed the diagnosis was said to be "in denial" (Carr, 2011). Because alcoholism was then believed to be a personality disorder, and denial a characteristic defense mechanism of the disorder, this often was seen as confirming the diagnosis. A complementary belief was that only alcoholics had problems with alcohol, a view that discouraged social controls on alcohol or caution in its use by those presumed to be nonalcoholics. Within this perspective, the main approach to prevention would be to identify and educate those unfortunates who have the condition.

> The idea that there is a black-or-white line has itself been a source of problems in personal and social response to alcohol/drug use.

The recognition of addiction as a continuum has led to a different approach. Certainly people with severe dependence deserve humane and effective care. It is also clear that alcohol is a hazardous substance that warrants special social controls (Babor, 2010). A majority of those who are harmed or endangered by alcohol use are not dependent drinkers (Institute of Medicine, 1990). Arguing about whether a person is on one side or the other of a diagnostic line misses the point. We find that it is common for clients to balk at a diagnostic label or the idea of "having a problem." Yet if we ask them to tell us about ways in which alcohol or other drugs have caused problems or hassles for them, there is usually a list, sometimes a long one. The more important issue is to understand how substance use is affecting people's lives, and what they need or want to do about it.

A clear current reflection of this broader conception is the recommendation of "safe drinking limits" by the World Health Organization, the

U.S. National Institute on Alcohol Abuse and Alcoholism (NIAAA), and other bodies. Working from epidemiological data, such guidelines inform people about levels of consumption that are linked to increased risk of illness and injury. Regardless of diagnosis, there are levels of alcohol use that are simply risky in terms of short- and long-term health consequences. In a "Rethinking Drinking" website, the NIAAA defined at-risk drinking as consuming more than four drinks on any day or 14 drinks per week for men, or more than three drinks on any day or seven drinks per week for women (*rethinkingdrinking.niaaa.nih.gov* as of May 2011).

This change in thinking toward a continuum of severity is also occurring in general medicine with regard to chronic conditions such as diabetes, heart disease, and asthma. The arbitrary cutoff points for "normal" versus "elevated" blood pressure, glucose, or cholesterol have been decreasing over the years, with earlier intervention indicated. In the past, diabetes was not treated until the patient became symptomatic. This has shifted toward identifying those who are prediabetic so that physicians can intervene prior to organ damage. For patients with identified risk factors, such as being overweight or having a family history of diabetes, the routine procedure is to regularly assess fasting glucose or HbA1c levels and encourage lifestyle changes to prevent the development of diabetes.

The idea of intervening prior to someone developing more severe consequences also parallels trends in mental health. For example, there are good reasons to prevent a *first* occurrence of depression. Once a person experiences one episode of major depression, there is an increased likelihood of having another, suggesting the idea of biological *kindling*: the first episode makes that person more vulnerable to future episodes. This finding has increased efforts to intervene early (Muñoz, Le, Clarke, Barrera, & Torres, 2009). For those at high genetic risk of developing depression, there are effective strategies to prevent the first episode. There are also treatment guidelines based on the number of depressive episodes a person has experienced. For example, if someone has three or more episodes, prophylactic maintenance on antidepressant medications is often recommended.

> It is common to use different treatment strategies depending on the level of severity.

It is common, therefore, to use different treatment strategies depending on the level of severity. Treatment for hypertension, diabetes, depression, and many other medical and psychological conditions varies depending on where the individual is on a continuum. The parallels to addiction are straightforward. Yet addiction has often been treated as though it could be cured through acute care. If addiction at least resembles a chronic illness, then one should not expect the problem to be resolved by an episode of treatment, and ongoing care is as important as it would be with asthma or diabetes.

Historically people seldom received addiction treatment before substantial problems and dependence had developed. In the 21st century, there is a trend toward recognizing, treating, and preventing both alcohol and other drug problems at an earlier stage, through screening and intervention within more general health and social service settings (Miller & Weisner, 2002). The efficacy of even relatively brief opportunistic counseling is well documented (Bernstein et al., 2007; Monti et al., 1999; Spirito, 2004), even though these individuals were not actively seeking addiction treatment and may not even have been thinking about making a change in their drinking or drug use. Prevention is discussed in more detail in Chapter 23, and brief intervention is discussed in more detail in Chapter 9.

Another important reason for addressing addiction within primary health care, mental health, and social service settings is the high rate of co-occurrence with other health and social problems (see Chapter 18). Whether or not they know it, professionals in such settings most likely are regularly treating people with addiction problems. In children and adolescents, alcohol/drug use is a common element in clusters of problem behaviors (Jessor & Jessor, 1977). In adults, addiction seldom occurs in isolation. In people with serious mental illnesses, addiction is the most frequently coexisting disorder, occurring at three times the general population rate (Substance Abuse and Mental Health Services Administration, 2009).

Before moving on to consider causes of addiction, we add one more practical recommendation. Don't waste time and effort arguing with people about whether they warrant a diagnostic label. Great emphasis has sometimes been placed on making clients "accept" or "admit" an identity such as "alcoholic" or "addict." There is no good evidence that this is a prerequisite to change. Plenty of people recover without ever accepting a diagnosis or receiving treatment. Clinicians also know that there are many who readily accept a diagnostic label and yet continue to struggle. Don't get stuck trying to impose a label. Within the original 12-step philosophy, one never imposes the label "alcoholic" on someone else; it is for each individual to decide whether this identification fits and is helpful (Alcoholics Anonymous [AA] World Services, 2001). The writings of Bill W., cofounder of AA, reflect great patience to work with people wherever they are at present (Miller & Kurtz, 1994).

> Don't waste time and effort arguing with people about whether they warrant a diagnostic label.

ETIOLOGIES OF ADDICTION

The *etiology* of a condition is its cause or origin. We turn now to consider the etiologies of addiction, those factors that influence its onset, severity, and course. Identifying and understanding these factors is different from diagnosing addiction. Beginning with the third edition in 1980, the DSM has separated diagnosis from etiology.

So what causes addiction? Is it a shortcoming of character or will? Can anyone become addicted? Can the blame be placed on the drugs themselves, as addictive substances? Is the fault in our genes or personality, with some people more prone to addiction, in the same manner that they are predisposed to diabetes or depression? Should we look to the social environment for causes? To some extent, the answer to all of these questions is "Yes." There is a certain amount of truth to each.

Personal Responsibility Models

In most societies, problems with alcohol and other drugs have been regarded to some extent as a failure of self-control, a violation of moral, ethical, or religious standards. Most religions have prohibitions regarding the use of certain psychoactive substances. In Jewish and Christian Scriptures, for example, alcohol is not proscribed, but drinking in a way that risks or causes harm is described as sinful. The remedies suggested by this model include legislation, education, repentance, punishment, and social sanctions. This perspective is still very much evident in social responses to and sometimes even in treatment of addictions. Underlying these models in general is the assumption that alcohol/drug use is a voluntary, chosen behavior, and that the person could have done otherwise. This is exemplified in social views and practices with regard to driving under the influence. Few would accept a defense that someone just couldn't help but use drugs or drink before driving. Intoxication is rarely a defense or mitigating factor in crime. Substance use is still regarded as a choice for which one is responsible.

Some models place particular emphasis on spiritual factors. Prominent among these is the 12-step approach begun in 1935 from the experience of its cofounders Bill W. and Dr. Bob when, "in the kinship of common suffering, one alcoholic had been talking to another" (Kurtz, 1979, p. 8). The 12-step programs, which do not endorse any particular model of etiology, nevertheless place considerable emphasis on character flaws as a contributor to addiction. The importance of spirituality is even more central in the 12-step program for recovery. In this perspective, people are powerless to resolve addiction on their own, and the help of a higher power is essential. AA and other 12-step programs (see Chapter 14) provide recommendations for a program of spiritual awakening and personal recovery. This spiritual awakening is understood as the means to move from destructive independence to proper dependence on God and others (Kurtz, 1991). A spiritual path to recovery was also emphasized in Moral Rearmament, another international program that, like AA, had its roots in Rev. Frank Buchman's Oxford Groups in the 1930s (Lean, 1985).

Agent Models

Agent models place primary emphasis on the strong effects of the agent (the drug) itself. In this view, anyone who is exposed to the drug is at risk because of its addictive and destructive properties. The U.S. temperance movement, which originally promoted caution and moderation (temperance) in the use of alcohol, became a prohibition movement, placing primary blame on the drug itself. In 1919, the 18th Amendment to the U.S. Constitution was ratified, making it illegal to manufacture, sell, transport, or import "intoxicating liquor," only to be repealed by the 21st Amendment in 1933. To be sure, the hazardous qualities of alcohol and tobacco are well documented, and if they were to be introduced as new drugs today, knowing what we know, they would be unlikely to be legalized. An agent model was implicit in the "war on drugs" of the late 20th century. The primary remedy it implies is to rid society of the drug itself.

Dispositional Models

Dispositional models, in contrast, place the primary cause of addiction within the person. They share this emphasis with moral models, but typically construe the cause as constitutional and beyond the individual's willful control. Among these is a disease model that regards people with addiction as constitutionally different from others and incapable of controlling their own use. In this view, the person is not responsible for having the condition. Disease models did much to argue for humane treatment rather than punishment of addiction. Of relevance to dispositional models, various genetic risk factors have been documented that increase the likelihood of developing addiction to particular substances. Other dispositional models have emphasized stable and perhaps irreversible changes that occur in the brain with chronic use and that compromise self-control. While a dispositional model may absolve people of blame for their condition, the responsibility for recovery necessarily remains with the individual, who is typically counseled to adopt permanent abstinence as the only sure way to prevent further progression and harm.

Social Learning Models

Other models emphasize the role of experience in shaping addiction. The use of alcohol and other psychoactive drugs is clearly responsive to both classical (stimulus–response) and operant conditioning (contingent reinforcement and punishment). Even highly dependent individuals modify their choices and use of substances in response to changes in the social environment. Drinking and drug use practices are also clearly influenced by modeling (learning by observing others), particularly from family and peers. As the psychology of learning embraced human thought processes in the late 20th century, the role of cognition in addiction was also examined. An important factor highlighted by this research is drug *expectancies*, beliefs and expectations about the likely positive or negative effects of drug use (Brown, Christiansen, & Goldman, 1987; Goldman, Del Boca, & Darkes, 1999). Interventions from a social learning perspective focus on changing the individual's relationship to the social environment: changing patterns of reinforcement for drug use and nonuse (Chapter 11), social support, family interactions, high-risk situations, expectancies, and cognitive-behavioral coping skills (Chapter 12).

Sociocultural Models

A still broader viewpoint emphasizes the influence of societal and cultural factors. The ease of availability and the price of alcohol, tobacco, and other drugs clearly affect the level of use in a community. Social environments with high levels of use (such as drinking in the military or in college fraternities) tend to increase consumption levels in new and continuing members. Advertising and media programming also influence expectancies and perceived norms. Interventions within this perspective typically focus on alcohol/drug policy. Examples include the licensing and regulation of sales outlets, training of alcohol servers to prevent intoxication and impaired driving, and taxation to increase the price of legal substances.

A Public Health Perspective

In seeking to prevent, treat, and contain threats to health, the most common approach is a broad one that takes into account all of the above influences. Usually called a *public health* perspective, it groups causal factors into three categories: those involving the *agent* (in this case, the drug itself), the *host* (personal characteristics of an individual), and the *environment*. In containing a flu epidemic, for example, one would consider the particular virus family involved (agent), personal factors that increase or decrease an individual's risk of infection (host), and environmental factors that promote or diminish spread of the disease. The history of addiction treatment has often been characterized by passionate debates about which of these factors is most important, which model is "correct." A public health perspective takes all important factors into account and considers their interactions with each other.

> A public health perspective takes all important factors into account and considers their interactions with each other.

The agent dimension was discussed above, focusing on characteristics of the drugs themselves. Substances have addictive properties, including rapidity of onset, tolerance, and interaction with neurotransmitter systems.

The faster a drug reaches the brain, the more reinforcing its use tends to be. Once in the brain, psychoactive drugs mimic or influence neurotransmitters (see Chapter 3). Many, for example, increase the release of dopamine, which is one of the primary neurotransmitters in the experience of pleasure. Substance-induced dopamine transmission is three to five times greater than that of natural reinforcers, like food or sex. It is sensible, then, that drugs may be preferred over natural rewards because of this rapid and intense pleasure. It is possible to classify drugs according to their potential to produce addiction. Toxic side effects of drugs like alcohol and tobacco are also well documented. The effects of drugs also pose particular risks in certain situations (e.g., when driving, during pregnancy). Thus the drugs themselves deserve attention in social policy.

Much is also known about host factors in addiction, where attention is focused on characteristics of individuals that place them at risk. Propensity for addiction is related to gender, family history of addiction, age, and temperament (Substance Abuse and Mental Health Services Administration, 2009). Tarter's construct of neurobehavioral disinhibition comprises a cluster of emotional tendencies, behavioral symptoms, and problems in cognitive function that indicate that a child has not adequately developed psychological self-regulation (Tarter et al., 2003). The construct includes many symptoms that characterize attention-deficit/hyperactivity disorder (ADHD), conduct disorder, and oppositional defiant disorder. Escalating psychosocial problems in youth, particularly conduct problems, have long been identified as a predictor for later alcohol/drug problems (Jones, 1968; Sartor, Lynskey, Heath, Jacob, & True, 2007). Temperament is, of course, itself partially inherited. It is estimated that genetic risk factors explain about 50% of the vulnerabilities leading to heavy drinking (Schuckit, 2009) but the picture is less clear for genetic predispositions to other drug addiction (Buckland, 2008).

The environmental dimension includes factors outside of the individual. The environment includes the broader community, such as the legal environment (alcoholic beverage control laws, laws regarding driving under the influence, minimum purchase age laws, zoning), the economic environment (pricing, tax rate, promotions), and the normative environment (social attitudes and beliefs regarding substances). The environment also includes the physical aspects of the person's environment, such as the setting or context in which drinking and other drug-using behavior occurs. Another environmental influence is a person's associates, including their family, friends, coworkers, and other peers, who in turn carry ethnic, religious, and educational influences. Environmental or cultural stress levels may also influence substance use. Certain religious group affiliations may increase or decrease risk for alcohol/drug use and addiction (Gorsuch, 1995).

These agent, host, and environment factors also interact with each other. A child who inherits a difficult temperament and risk for poor self-regulation may be protected by intensive parenting (Diaz & Fruhauf, 1991). An individual who lives and works in a hard-drinking environment may be protected by religious affiliation. People differ in the inherited extent to which their brains "light up" in response to particular drugs. Explanations that focus on a single cause or model are clearly too simplistic. Effective treatment and prevention efforts consider the range of factors involved and address those most likely to yield benefit for the particular person or community.

KEY POINTS

🔖 Addiction occurs along a continuum of severity, or rather along at least seven continuous dimensions of use, problems, physical adaptation, behavioral dependence, cognitive impairment, medical harm, and motivation for change.

🔖 Knowing where an individual falls on one of these dimensions tells little about the rest of the clinical picture.

🔖 Diagnosis is about classification according to decision rules, which have changed markedly over time.

🔖 Explanatory models of addiction have also evolved over time, often emphasizing one causal factor to the exclusion of others.

🔖 A public health view of addiction embraces host, agent, and environmental factors and their interactions, providing a more comprehensive perspective for guiding treatment and prevention.

REFLECTION QUESTIONS

💬 Of the various etiological models described in this chapter, which one(s) have you most strongly embraced in your own views of addiction? Which one(s) most closely match your own current perspective?

💬 In your own mind, when does a behavior cross the line and become an addiction?

💬 To what extent do you think people are responsible for developing their own addiction(s)?

CHAPTER 3

How Do Drugs Work?

In Chapter 1 we explained why addiction treatment is a matter not only for specialists in this area, but also for health and social service professionals in general. The training and experience of behavioral health professionals in particular provides excellent background for helping people overcome alcohol/drug problems.

Yet even in the 21st century, the training of such professionals still seldom provides sufficient background and encouragement to treat addictions. Although generalist professional training may provide 80% of the competence needed to help people with substance use disorders, the remaining 20% of information and skills are important. Lacking this preparation, clinicians may overlook addiction problems or refer them elsewhere for treatment. One of our main goals in writing this book is to fill in that remaining 20%.

One important core competence, of course, is at least a basic working knowledge of psychoactive drugs and their effects. That is the primary focus of this chapter. Let us say at the outset, however, that nonmedical practitioners need not have memorized all of the chemical and street names or understand in detail the psychopharmacology of each and every drug. Medical colleagues are available for consultation on such issues, and much of what you don't know about street savvy, your clients can teach you. Compared to clinicians, clients often have much more firsthand knowledge about the drugs they use, although of course street information can also be dangerously inaccurate. Drug users' practical knowledge might be thought of as a daunting disadvantage for the health professional, but it also means that clients are a constant source of learning about lives and cultures that may at first be quite alien to those who have survived the rigors of postgraduate training. We, the authors of this book, have learned much about addictions from our clients. Of course we also constantly examine such learning, as well as our own hunches and beliefs, in the light of the best science available.

ROUTES OF ADMINISTRATION

A good starting point, before considering major classes of drugs, is to understand the various and sometimes surprising routes by which people self-administer psychoactive drugs. They fall into four major categories, all of which begin with "in": (1) ingestion, (2) inhalation, (3) intranasal, and (4) injection. These do not encompass all possible routes of administration that have been devised (such as placement under the eyelid, insertion into the rectum or vagina, or absorption through the skin as by "patches"), but they do encompass about 99.9% of drug misuse.

Ingestion

By far the most common way to self-administer a psychoactive drug is by mouth: to eat it, drink it, chew it, swallow it, or let it dissolve under the lips or tongue. Drinking is the exclusive route for the most common problem drug: ethyl alcohol. Prescription and other drugs in pill form are swallowed. Hairspray can be sprayed into a jug of water, shaken, and allowed to settle—a preparation known as *ocean* because of its frothy appearance— that is then drunk. Teas are brewed from various substances including khat and valerian root. The original active ingredient in Coca-Cola was cocaine, from which it derived its name.

Other drugs are chewed, absorbed through the gums, or placed under the tongue in solid or liquid form. Coca leaves, khat root, tobacco, and nicotine gum can be chewed, and their active ingredients absorbed through saliva and the rich supply of blood vessels in the mouth. Some drugs can be introduced through foods that are eaten and then absorbed through the stomach, such as marijuana in brownies, alcohol-injected fruit, or rum-saturated cake.

Psychoactive drugs ingested by mouth pass into the gastrointestinal system, where they are absorbed into the bloodstream through the lining of the stomach and large intestine. Drugs in liquid form (such as alcohol) tend to be absorbed more rapidly. Absorption is usually slowed by the presence of food in the stomach, which is why drinking on an empty stomach produces faster intoxication. It can take from one to several hours to absorb most of a drug dosage taken by mouth.

Inhalation

The second most common way to administer psychoactive drugs is to inhale them as smoke or vapor, absorbing them primarily through the lungs. The lungs have a rich blood supply, and drugs that are inhaled can be in the bloodstream within seconds. This is, of course, the usual route of administration for tobacco and marijuana. Cocaine in its usual hydrochloride salt form is destroyed by burning, but it can be reduced by various methods to a concentrated base form (such as "crack") that is smokable to deliver very high doses. Other misused drugs are termed *inhalants* because they are self-administered by breathing them in through the nose or mouth as a gas (such as nitrous oxide) or a vapor (such as "sniffing" glue or "huffing" gasoline).

Intranasal

A third common route of administration is by snorting a drug into the nose, which also has an extremely rich supply of blood vessels in the mucous membranes. Snuff is a preparation of tobacco that can be drawn up into the nose in this manner. Snorting is a common method for self-administering "lines" of cocaine hydrochloride. Heroin is also sometimes taken intranasally.

Injection

Finally, drugs of abuse can be introduced into the body by shooting them via syringe into a vein (intravenous), a muscle (intramuscular), or beneath the skin (subcutaneous). Intravenous injection is the most common route of administration for heroin and certain other opiates. It is also a popular method for taking methamphetamine ("crank"), which may be combined with heroin. Intravenous injection is, of course, the most rapid method for getting a drug into the bloodstream, producing the fastest and most intense effects. It is also the most dangerous. When used regularly for injection, veins begin to collapse. As veins in the arms become unusable, injection drug users may make use of blood vessels in the hands, feet, legs, and neck. Bacterial infections and abscesses can occur if sterile procedures are not used. The sharing of syringes by drug users is a major cause of the spread of blood-borne infections such as HIV and the various forms of hepatitis. Containing the spread of such diseases is a principal purpose of *needle exchange programs* where users can obtain new sterile syringes and safely dispose of used needles free of charge. Injection is also the most common route of fatal overdoses of illicit drugs, precisely because the drug effects are so immediate, intense, and often difficult to reverse.

DRUG DISTRIBUTION AND ELIMINATION

After a drug has been introduced, it moves through the body in more or less predictable ways (*pharmacokinetics*) until finally it is eliminated. Drugs first travel from the point of entry into the bloodstream, as by absorption through membranes, unless it has already been placed directly into the circulatory system by intravenous injection. Once a drug enters the

Once a drug enters the bloodstream it is circulated throughout the body within about a minute.

bloodstream it is circulated throughout the body within about a minute. To reach its principal site of action in the central nervous system, however, a psychoactive drug must further cross from the bloodstream through the *blood–brain barrier* and into the brain, where it interacts with nerve cells (*neurons*) to produce its effects.

Most psychoactive drugs do not circulate in the bloodstream for long. They are gradually eliminated through the body's filtering systems. They are broken down or *metabolized* by the liver, excreted through the kidneys in urine, even expelled in air from the lungs, in sweat through the skin, or in breast milk. Drug testing makes use of this by analyzing expelled air (as in alcohol breath tests) or urine for the presence of psychoactive drugs or their metabolites.

The speed with which a given drug is eliminated from the body is usually expressed in terms of its *half-life*, which is the length of time required for the body to reduce the drug level by half. Within one half-life, the level of a drug would be reduced to 50% of its starting level. It takes two half-life periods to eliminate 75%, and after three half-life periods the amount of drug in the body would be down to about 12% of its original level. Drugs vary dramatically in their half-life. Ethyl alcohol, for example, is cleared from the body far faster than is methyl alcohol. Methadone has a longer half-life than heroin, making it a better substitution drug* because its effects are distributed across 1–2 days instead of an hour or two (for heroin). Speed of elimination can also be influenced by factors including age, gender, health of the liver, interactions with other drugs, and hereditary traits.

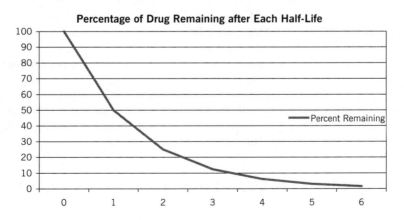

Percentage of Drug Remaining after Each Half-Life

---

*Substitution medications are used to replace illicit drugs that the person has been using. They may be used both for detoxification (see Chapter 6) and as longer term maintenance medications (see Chapter 15).

DRUG EFFECTS

Once they reach the brain, psychoactive drugs interact with particular neural systems to produce their characteristic effects. The brain's communication system relies upon tiny electrical currents transmitted through chains of neurons. Each neuron fires in response to particular chemicals known as *neurotransmitters*. When one of these chemicals comes into contact with a nerve cell to which it is related (by virtue of the cell having receptors for it), the molecule fits like a key into a lock. By fitting into the receptor, it can increase or decrease the cell's ability to transmit electrical signals to other nerve cells farther along in the chain.

A neuron consists of the cell body, *dendrites* that receive chemical messages from previous neurons in the chain, and a tail-like fiber called an *axon* that communicates with subsequent neurons in the chain. Many axons have a *myelin sheath* that speeds up the transmission of information. When a neuron fires, it releases one or more special neurotransmitters from its axon into a *synapse*, the fluid space between nerve cells. The released chemical comes into contact with the dendrites of other neurons and may cause them to fire. The neurotransmitter is then normally reabsorbed from the synapse by the neurons from which it was released, a process known as *reuptake*.

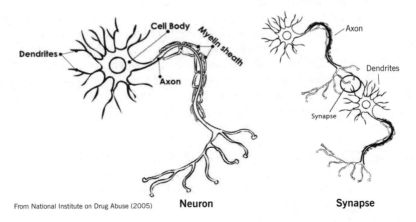

From National Institute on Drug Abuse (2005) **Neuron**   **Synapse**

The human body was not designed to respond to most drugs that are misused. Some psychoactive drugs work because they closely resemble molecules that occur naturally within the body. For example, the central nervous system includes a remarkable capacity to reduce pain through the release of natural neurotransmitters known as *endorphins*. Opioid drugs such as heroin closely resemble these natural molecules. They stimulate the endorphin (opiate) receptors, artificially activating the body's system for relieving suffering and inducing a pervasive sense of well-being. A drug that can thus mimic the effects of a natural neurotransmitter is called an *agonist* for that system. Most drugs of abuse are agonists, activating or amplifying transmitter systems in the brain, usually in a way that is much more intense than normal experience.

One problem with artificial activation, however, is the phenomenon of *drug tolerance*, discussed in Chapter 2. Heroin-dependent people often report that the most intensely pleasant rush of their lives happened during their first exposure to heroin, and that they have spent the rest of their lives chasing that same high. For a variety of reasons, psychoactive drugs tend to lose their potency with repeated use, so that in order to experience the same high the person must use ever larger doses. The system becomes saturated, and natural neurotransmitter activity is reduced in response to artificial activation. Eventually the person uses the drug just to feel normal.

Just as some drugs serve as agonists, others serve as *antagonists* for specific neurotransmitters. An antagonist molecule binds to the receptor and blocks it, reducing activation by either the natural neurotransmitter or by its artificial agonists. Some drugs can serve both agonist and antagonist functions; they are *partial agonists* stimulating activity in a specific neurotransmitter system, while also blocking further stimulation by other agonists. We discuss agonists, partial agonists, and antagonists further when we consider therapeutic medications that are used to treat drug dependence (Chapter 15).

Resembling a natural neurotransmitter is not the only way in which drugs can influence the central nervous system. Some drugs exert effects not by mimicking neurotransmitter molecules, but by acting on neurons in other ways. Alcohol is a prime example. Although some of alcohol's many effects do seem to involve activation of receptor systems, alcohol also impacts the entire brain by altering nerve cell membranes in ways that are only partially understood at present. Other drugs exert their effects by blocking reuptake, causing a neurotransmitter to remain longer than normal in the synaptic space and thus continuing to act on postsynaptic neurons.

MAJOR DRUG CLASSES AND THEIR ACUTE EFFECTS

This section outlines major classes of drugs that are used illicitly and how they affect the central nervous system. For each drug class we describe the common sought-after effects of intoxication ("the peak") and the rebound period that follows use ("the valley"). These descriptions are necessarily brief. Several classic resources are available that describe in more detail the pharmacokinetics, pharmacodynamics, and specific effects of psychoactive drugs (Hart, Ksir, & Ray, 2008; Julian, Advokat, & Comaty, 2007; Preston & Johnson, 2009; Stahl, 2009).

Some common street names for major drug classes are listed in Box 3.1. There are hundreds of such street names, which vary among geographic areas, with new slang names appearing regularly. Box 3.2 on page 37 summarizes the neurotransmitter systems particularly affected by the various classes of drugs discussed below.

BOX 3.1. Some Street Names for Drugs

Alcohol	Booze, hooch, juice, sauce
Amphetamine	Speed, crystal, ice, crank, chalk, crystal, glass, meth, uppers, bennies
Barbiturates	Barbs, downers, reds, ludes, goofballs
Benzodiazepines	Benzos
Cannabis	Pot, dope, grass, weed, herb, hemp, rope, Mary Jane, hash, ganja, tea
Cocaine	Coke, C, crack, snow, crystal, rocks, toot, cola, nose candy, heaven, white
Heroin	Horse, shit, smack, junk, H, skag, fix, China white, whack, brown
LSD	Acid, 25, tabs, sugar, blotter, microdots, paper mushrooms
Mescaline, peyote	Buttons, mesc, mess, cactus
Phencyclidine	Angel dust, PCP, elephant, hog
Psilocybin	Mushroom, shroom, sacred mushrooms, magic mushrooms

Stimulants

Stimulants can be ingested, taken intranasally, or injected intravenously. By reducing them to a *base* form, stimulants can also be inhaled in smoke. As a class of drugs, stimulants exert their psychological effects by increasing activity in three key neurotransmitter systems: dopamine, norepinephrine, and serotonin. Cocaine does so by blocking the reuptake of these chemicals from synapses. Amphetamines resemble the neurotransmitter epinephrine (adrenalin), and exert their stimulant effect primarily by the dumping of increased amounts of dopamine and norepinephrine into neural synapses. Stimulants activate the brain's positive reinforcement system, which normally rewards activities that promote survival and well-being. In essence they directly and intensely trigger the brain system that says "Do that again!" It is no mystery, therefore, why these drugs have such a high capacity for habitual use and dependence.

The Peak

Stimulants have been called "power drugs" because they induce euphoria and a grandiose sense of personal power and achievement. They can be used to remain awake and alert, promote persistence, and suppress fatigue and hunger—effects that historically made these drugs useful to soldiers and to others like students and truck drivers wanting to stay awake and alert. In general they speed up functioning: the person thinks faster, talks faster, moves faster. With higher or repeated doses, the user may develop paranoia or other delusions.

The Valley

As with many drugs of abuse, the stimulant high is followed by a low, a "crash." The rebound from stimulant use is substantial, and not surprisingly involves the opposite of the drug's acute effects. During the postdrug valley the user may experience anxiety, depression, fatigue and drowsiness, increased appetite, and persisting paranoia.

Two other widely used stimulants are nicotine (primarily in tobacco) and caffeine (in coffee, tea, soft drinks, and chocolate). Like other stimulants, both nicotine and caffeine activate reward channels in the brain, and increase alertness. Caffeine blockades receptors for the inhibitory neurotransmitter *adenosine*, thereby increasing acetylcholine and dopamine activity. Nicotine directly stimulates one subtype of acetylcholine receptors, releasing adrenalin into the bloodstream and increasing heart rate and blood pressure. Like other stimulants, nicotine also suppresses appetite. Withdrawal symptoms from caffeine are generally mild, characterized by headache and some disruption of concentration, whereas nicotine quickly produces dependence as tenacious as that for cocaine or opiates. Nicotine withdrawal involves a substantial and often prolonged rebound, potentially including depression, anxiousness, agitation, insomnia, increased appetite, and emotional volatility.

Sedatives

Sedative drugs have as their general effect a suppression (and in higher doses, shutting down) of the central nervous system. They all enhance the activity of GABA (gamma-Aminobutyric acid), a class of inhibitory neurotransmitters that broadly decrease neural activity. Relatedly, they tend to suppress the NMDA (N-methyl-D-aspartate) subtype of glutamate, which is an activating neurotransmitter. In sum, they enhance neurochemicals that close down the central nervous system and interfere with neurochemicals that activate it. This is true of alcohol, sedative–hypnotic drugs like barbiturates, and tranquilizers such as benzodiazepines.

The Peak

Sedatives are downers and shutdowners. In lower doses they tend to reduce feelings of anxiety and induce mild euphoria. These drugs also interfere with memory and can be quite effective in producing partial or total amnesia ("blackout") during a period of intoxication. They progressively slow down nervous system functioning, and are therefore quite dangerous when combined with driving, operating machinery, or engaging in other potentially risky activities that require clear attention and coordination. The sedative "high" is physiologically more like a low and includes dream-like intoxication, damping of distress and memory, loss of inhibitions, and a sense of well-being or at least unconcern. In short, they make the world (especially an unpleasant world) go away.

The Valley

The rebound (hangover) from sedative intoxication involves agitation and unpleasant arousal. The higher the level of sedative intoxication, the greater the rebound. Sedative hangover can include irritability, anxiety and restlessness, insomnia and nightmares, racing heart, nausea, headache, and sweating. Such symptoms tend to be quickly alleviated by redosing with a sedative ("a bit of the hair of the dog that bit you"), which in turn can encourage cyclic and escalating use. Drug withdrawal with severe alcohol or other sedative dependence can be life-threatening (see Chapter 6 on detoxification).

Similar sedative effects result from inhaling solvents (gasoline, nail polish remover) and other volatile substances such as glue and aerosols. The intoxicating effects closely resemble those for alcohol, but most inhalants are far more toxic.

BOX 3.2. Neurotransmitters Particularly Affected by Psychoactive Drugs

Drug Classes	Receptor Systems Activated	Receptor Systems Suppressed
Alcohol	GABA, endorphin	NMDA glutamate, acetylcholine
Barbiturates	GABA	NMDA glutamate
Benzodiazepines	GABA	
Stimulants	Dopamine, norepinephrine, serotonin	
Caffeine	Dopamine, acetylcholine	Adenosine
Nicotine	Acetylcholine	
Opioid analgesics	Endorphin	
Marijuana	Cannabinoid	Glutamate
Psychedelics	Serotonin, dopamine	Acetylcholine (PCP suppresses NMDA)
Steroids	Steroid (testosterone)	

Opiates

The body has a built-in system for *analgesia*, the relief of pain. At the center of it are naturally produced neurotransmitters known as *endorphins* that decrease pain and enhance the sense of well-being. *Opioid analgesics* (or "opiates") mimic endorphins and thereby artificially stimulate the body's analgesic system.

The Peak

Opiates flood the person with a euphoric sense of well-being, combined with drowsiness and relief of pain. Breathing is slowed and in higher doses is suppressed completely—the usual cause of opiate overdose deaths.

The Valley

Unlike withdrawal from sedatives, the discomfort involved in rebound from opiate use is not life-threatening, though it can be much feared by users. It has been likened to a very bad case of the flu: sweating, insomnia, aches and pains, agitation, anxiousness and restlessness, a general feeling of being sick—and, of course, a hunger for more of the drug.

Psychedelics

Psychedelic drugs differ in a number of important ways from other drugs of abuse. One of these is that primates and lower mammals will self-administer nearly all psychoactive drugs that humans misuse, but will not use psychedelic drugs (with the exception of PCP) when given free access to them. Furthermore, they produce no significant withdrawal syndrome, so that even with prolonged exposure, animals show no inclination to continue the use of psychedelics. Thus, whereas most drugs of abuse produce neural effects that appear to be inherently reinforcing for mammals, the effects of psychedelics are found reinforcing only and uniquely by humans.

The Peak

The experience of loss of control is central to psychedelic experience. Other misused drugs produce effects that are fairly predictable, so that a user knows what to expect and can replicate the experience of prior use (though tolerance often diminishes such effects). One who uses a psychedelic drug, however, does not know what to expect in subjective experience, as illustrated by the "bad trip" experience associated with higher doses. Within a dream-like state, the person experiences sensory and perceptual distortions and hallucinations, often accompanied by disorientation and amnesia. Psychedelic drugs have long been used to evoke or intensify spiritual experiences (Casteneda, 1985; Griffiths, Richards, Johnson, McCann, & Jesse, 2008).

The Valley

There is virtually no withdrawal associated with the use of psychedelics. The person's mental functioning gradually returns to normal within a few hours, without apparent rebound (although it is unclear what would constitute a rebound). *Flashbacks* to distressing subjective experiences sometimes occur in the weeks or months following psychedelic drug use.

Cannabis

Because of some overlapping effects, marijuana has sometimes been classified with the psychedelics, but its effects are quite different. Tetrahydrocannabinol (THC), the active ingredient in cannabis, stimulates particular cannabinoid receptors that are ordinarily activated by the neurotransmitter *anandamide*. Cannabinoids suppress glutamate and thereby exert a general sedating effect like alcohol, slowing reflexes and movement, decreasing attention and concentration, impairing memory and learning, lengthening reaction time, and lowering core body temperature. Unlike alcohol, however, THC appears to decrease aggression.

The Peak

The overlap with psychedelic effects is found in a dream-like state involving time distortion and sensory-perceptual alterations, albeit of a more predictable variety. Cognitive processes tend to be loosened up by THC, leading to less controlled and more unusual mental associations. Intoxication usually induces a sense of euphoria and well-being, although higher doses can amplify negative emotions.

The Valley

Cessation of regular marijuana use has been associated with various forms of discomfort including insomnia, anxiousness, restlessness, irritability, and nausea, representing a rebound from the sedative effects of THC.

Steroids

Testosterone is a naturally occurring hormone that functions as a neurotransmitter in both men and women (as do many other hormones). When testosterone and related synthetic compounds are taken, they override the

---

BOX 3.3 The Eyes Have It

Some drugs of abuse are well known for effects that can be seen by looking into the user's eyes. *Dilated (wide-open) pupils* occur with the use of stimulants and psychedelics. *Constricted (pinpoint) pupils* accompany opiate use. *Bloodshot eyes,* with red streaks in the whites of both eyes, are common soon after marijuana use.

---

body's normal process to self-regulate the circulating level of testosterone. The predictable result of regular use is a substantial increase in masculine characteristics, muscle mass, and aggression.

The Peak

There is little or no acute high from the use of steroids. Typically they are taken over a span of time to increase muscle mass, enhance athletic performance and aggressiveness, and increase masculine appearance. The payoff is primarily in terms of self-perception and, in the case of female and male athletes, enhanced performance. The effects are quite noticeable and have become increasingly attractive to adolescent boys as well as adults.

The Valley

When steroid use is stopped, unwanted changes usually follow. Besides the gradual loss of muscle mass, people often experience restlessness and depression, decreased self-esteem, insomnia, and decreased appetites including sexual desire.

DRUG INTERACTIONS

> Drug misuse is seldom limited to one drug.

Drug misuse is seldom limited to one drug. Most alcohol-dependent people also smoke tobacco. Those who use marijuana have a much greater likelihood, relative to the general population, of also using alcohol, tobacco, cocaine, heroin, and other drugs.

The effects described above become far more complicated when drugs are combined.

Drugs within the same class, for example, often show *cross-tolerance.* People who are dependent on and have a high tolerance to alcohol also have heightened tolerance to other sedatives including barbiturates, benzodiazepines, and general anesthetics. Alcohol-dependent people undergoing surgery may therefore require a significantly higher dose of general anesthetic to induce or maintain unconsciousness and amnesia.

At the same time, drugs within the same class when combined tend to *potentiate* each other's effects. For a person already sedated by benzodiazepines, a dose of alcohol will have a much larger effect than it would if taken alone. Furthermore the potentiation is not merely additive. The total amount of sedation is more than the combined effect of alcohol alone plus benzodiazepines alone. Here is a case where two plus two can equal six. The reason for this is that sedatives also inhibit each other's metabolism: in the presence of benzodiazepines or barbiturates, the body breaks down alcohol more slowly, and vice versa. Thus each drug remains in the body longer than it would have had it been taken alone. This is one reason why the combination of sedatives with each other or with opiates carries a high risk of lethal overdose.

Similarly, the pharmacological effects of two different drugs can combine in dangerous and unpredictable ways. Even in relatively low doses, either marijuana or alcohol alone significantly impairs the mental and physical functions required to operate a motor vehicle safely. Use of both drugs together multiplies the impairment of driving ability and of judgment regarding one's ability to drive safely.

LONG-TERM EFFECTS

Contrary to lore about denial, by the time people have developed alcohol or other drug dependence they are usually well aware of the dangers and harm related to their drug use. Most smokers, for example, clearly know that they are

> By the time people have developed alcohol or other drug dependence they are usually well aware of the dangers and harm related to their drug use.

at increased risk for cancers and heart disease because of their tobacco use. Though they may staunchly reject a label such as "alcoholic" or "problem drinker," most heavy drinkers can readily list ways in which alcohol has put them at risk or created harm and problems. It is no secret that misusing drugs is a gamble, risking long-term harm for short-term pleasure.

Certain risks pertain to specific drugs. For example, sudden stroke or heart attack in a young person without a history of heart disease is particularly associated with the use of stimulants, and to a lesser extent with alcohol intoxication. During pregnancy, sedatives (such as alcohol and inhalants) can inflict particularly devastating effects on the unborn child.

Many of the adverse long-term effects of substance abuse, however, are similar across diverse drugs. In this final section we describe several groups of common long-term effects, pointing out as applicable where certain drugs pose particular risks.

Dependence

One of the obvious risks of long-term drug abuse is the development of dependence on the drug. One dimension of dependence is physical addiction, in which withdrawal (abstinence) from the drug produces unpleasant symptoms that are relieved by renewed use of the same or a similar drug. As described in Chapter 2, however, dependence involves much more than physical withdrawal symptoms, and in fact drug dependence can occur without such physical addiction. Within this larger perspective, becoming dependent involves having one's life increasingly centered around acquiring, using, and recovering from effects of the drug. Psychoactive drugs vary widely in their potential to produce dependence. For some drugs with very high potential, there are few users who are not dependent. Others have very low potential to produce a drug-dependence syndrome (see Box 3.4).

Acute Events

Some long-term consequences can result from even short-term use. Much of the injury, tragedy, and mortality associated with alcohol and other drugs results from acute events related to drug acquisition, use, and intoxication. Many psychoactive drugs significantly impair human judgment about what is safe, reasonable, or acceptable to do. Consequently during intoxication, people are more likely to take risks and violate social norms as well as their own values. Intoxication not only affects appraisal of dangerousness, but also tends to impair mental and physical functions that are important to safety (such as reaction time and coordination). The result can be a tragedy that lasts for (or ends) a lifetime. Up to half of all deaths by falls, fire, drowning, and other "accidents"; by violence; and of pedestrians and driv-

---

BOX 3.4. Potential to Produce Drug Dependence

Drugs differ in how likely they are to produce dependence. The following ratings are based on the proportion of users who are drug-dependent.

Potential to Produce Drug Dependence	Drug
Very high	Amphetamine, cocaine, nicotine, heroin, and other opiates
High	Caffeine, PCP
Moderate	Alcohol, marijuana, benzodiazepines
Low	Psychedelics, steroids
Very low	Antidepressant, antimanic, and antipsychotic medications

ers involve victims or participants under the influence of alcohol or other drugs.

Drug intoxication also increases the likelihood of committing acts with long-term or irrevocable consequences. In Western nations, a majority of people in prison are there for crimes committed under the influence of or otherwise related to drug use (particularly alcohol). Stimulants, alcohol, steroids, and psychedelics all significantly increase aggression, particularly in males. Alcohol influences males to overperceive hostile intent in the actions of others and to respond more aggressively (Ogle & Miller, 2004). A substantial proportion of people who commit suicide were under the influence of or dependent on drugs (particularly alcohol) at the time.

Toxicity

Beyond these acute events, many drugs of abuse also exert toxic effects on body organs including the brain, liver, lungs, heart, and gastrointestinal system. Heavy use of alcohol or tobacco is associated with greatly increased risk of a variety of cancers. For people who are both drinkers and smokers, cancer risk is not additive but multiplicative. This includes cancers of the lung, breast, mouth, larynx, esophagus, stomach, intestines, and rectum. Alcohol and inhalants are particularly toxic to the central nervous system, and long-term abuse of these drugs is associated with increasing impairment of memory, learning, and cognition.

Of all misused drugs, those that suppress the central nervous system have the highest potential for lethal overdose. These include (1) alcohol, barbiturates, benzodiazepines, and other sedatives; (2) heroin and other opiates; and (3) most inhalants.

There is increased risk and exacerbation of heart disease associated with some drugs of abuse. The nicotine and carbon monoxide in tobacco smoke increase blood pressure and arterial disease, in turn increasing the risk of coronary disease and heart attack. While moderate use of alcohol has been linked to decreased risk of coronary disease, heavier drinking clearly increases risk for hypertension and congestive heart disease.

Adverse Consequences

Health Consequences

Damage to health also occurs because of poor self-care associated with alcohol/drug problems and dependence. Nutrition may suffer from the use of drugs that suppress appetite and induce anorexia (e.g., stimulants), or from the replacement of dietary calories by ethyl alcohol. Major and enduring dental problems are common among people who have been drug-dependent because of a variety of factors including poor oral hygiene and infrequent dental care. The combination of poor hygiene, injuries, infections, and immune suppression can yield a plethora of skin diseases and lesions.

Interpersonal Consequences

Family, friendship, and intimate relationships often suffer in relation to addictions, which are associated with high rates of divorce, alienation, and loss of child custody. Ties are often broken with people who would encourage sobriety, and replaced by relationships with peers who practice and support drug use.

Intrapersonal Consequences

Substance abuse and dependence also take their toll on personal happiness. Negative emotions increasingly dominate drug-free hours: depression, anxiety, loneliness, anger, and resentment. Stimulant use is linked to other psychiatric problems, particularly drug-induced paranoia and psychosis.

Social Consequences

The progression of drug dependence also typically involves deterioration in social functioning. As life becomes ever more centered on drug use, prior interests, activities, and responsibilities fall away. Impaired work performance, absenteeism, and job loss are common. Illicit drug use, of course, also carries the risk of criminal sanctions and associated long-term social consequences. Financial problems and the decay of relationships contribute to social instability, sometimes leading to cycles of unemployment and homelessness.

Fetal Effects

> Virtually all of the commonly misused drugs cross the placental barrier.

Virtually all of the commonly misused drugs cross the placental barrier; thus when the pregnant mother uses, so does the unborn child whose body does not have adult capacities to metabolize drugs. Exposure to certain drugs can interfere with normal development and injure the fetus, producing long-term effects on the child's health and behavior. Significant damage can be done during early development, even before the mother realizes that she is pregnant. Nevertheless, stopping drug use at any point in pregnancy is associated with better outcomes.

The use of some drugs can interrupt pregnancy, leading to spontaneous abortion, premature delivery, and stillbirth. These risks are increased by the use of tobacco, stimulants, and alcohol during pregnancy. Drug-using mothers may also take less care of themselves in other ways (e.g., nutrition, rest, exercise, and prenatal care) that influence fetal health.

Retardation of fetal growth is another effect of some drug use during pregnancy. Physically smaller babies (e.g., low birth weight, smaller head circumference) may be born to mothers who used tobacco, stimulants, or alcohol during pregnancy. Tobacco use interferes with the delivery of oxygen to the fetus, which can impair development and later intellectual functioning. Amphetamine, cocaine, and other stimulants similarly reduce blood supply to the unborn child. Depending on the particular point in pregnancy, reduced blood flow can disrupt normal development of the brain, heart, or other organs. Babies who have been exposed to regular doses of dependence-producing drugs show withdrawal syndrome in the hours and days after birth. Nicotine and other stimulant use during pregnancy has been linked to increased risk for ADHD when the child reaches school age.

The most devastating effects on unborn children, however, are those associated with maternal use of alcohol or other sedative drugs. A clear fetal alcohol syndrome (FAS) has been described, involving mental and growth retardation, birth defects of the face and limbs, and behavioral problems including ADHD. Alcohol is by far the largest preventable cause of mental retardation. Short of full FAS, a variety of alcohol-related birth defects have been described, mostly lower level individual components of the syndrome. No safe level of drinking during pregnancy has been established, and women who are seeking to or have already become pregnant are best counseled to abstain from alcohol completely.

The Web of Addiction and Related Problems

All of this underlines that the treatment of addiction should be closely integrated with a broader spectrum of health and social services. Most people with alcohol/drug problems also have a daunting array of other life, health, social, and psychological problems. Often the resolution of

> The treatment of addiction should be closely integrated with a broader spectrum of health and social services.

these other problems is a higher priority for them than addressing their substance use, and not without reason. A mother who is homeless is likely to be more urgently concerned with safety, shelter, and feeding her children than with abstaining from drugs. A man suffering from depression, panic attacks, and PTSD may not perceive alcohol abstinence as a high priority. To be sure, getting free from alcohol and other drug use often leads to improvement on other dimensions, but it is no longer adequate to treat addiction in isolation from other concerns. As discussed in Chapter 1, people with alcohol/drug problems are mostly likely to seek help for other, related problems. Often they are seen dozens or even hundreds of times in health care, social service, legal, correctional, welfare, and hospital systems before they seek specialist treatment for addictions, if ever they do. They have not one problem, but many.

KEY POINTS

- Drugs can be taken into the body in various ways, but principally by ingestion, inhalation, intranasal, or injection routes of administration.

- A drug is distributed throughout the body via the bloodstream, affecting neurotransmitter systems in the brain until it is ultimately eliminated from the body.

- Acute intoxication (peak) effects vary by drug class, as do withdrawal (valley) effects, which often are mirror opposites of the drug's initial effects.

- Different drugs can interact in the body in various ways such as cross-tolerance and potentiation.

- Longer term effects vary according to the drug that is being used and can include dependence, toxicity (also to an unborn child), and adverse consequences resulting from acute or chronic use.

REFLECTION QUESTIONS

What implicit messages about drug use are conveyed through advertising of prescription and over-the-counter medications?

What interventions do you think are appropriate to prevent permanent damage to an unborn child from maternal alcohol/drug use?

To what extent can drug problems be explained by the biological effects of drugs? What proportion of responsibility for drug dependence might you assign to the drugs themselves? Does your estimate of this proportion vary depending on the drug (e.g., alcohol, tobacco, marijuana, cocaine, heroin)?

PART II

A Context for Addiction Treatment

Before exploring specific evidence-based methods in Part III, we discuss five more general aspects of addiction treatment. First we address the important subject of counseling style, one's professional manner in working with people affected by substance use disorders. There is strong evidence that relationship, the manner in which one delivers services, substantially influences treatment outcomes. Any attempt to provide evidence-based services should therefore attend to these important determinants of outcome. In Chapter 4 we present a broad client-centered approach that has been shown to promote change. In Chapter 5 we take up practical matters of screening and evaluation, offering recommendations for cost-effective assessment methods. An important minority of people with substance use disorders require special care for a period of detoxification to carry them safely through withdrawal from the drugs they use. Chapter 6 addresses how to evaluate the need for detoxification and the process of stabilization that precedes rehabilitation. It is now widely accepted that "one size does not fit all" in addiction treatment, but how does one go about determining what services people need? In Chapter 7 we describe a four-phase model of treatment and the process of matching treatments to individuals. Finally, if addictions truly are chronic disorders, then it makes sense to treat them as such (McLellan, Lewis, O'Brien, & Kleber, 2000). One does not expect to resolve diabetes, heart disease, or asthma with an acute treatment episode. As with other chronic disorders, the management of addiction is a long-term process. Chapter 8 provides a chronic disease management perspective and discusses the important role of ongoing case management.

CHAPTER 4

A Client-Centered Foundation

The central theme of this chapter is that effective addiction treatment is not just a matter of *what* you do, but is also strongly influenced by *who* you are and *how* you work with your clients. One of the better predictors of clients' likelihood of successful treatment outcome is the particular style of the counselor who works with them. How you relate to your clients is, in turn, strongly influenced by how you think about them and the problems they face. Research documenting the impact of counselor style on treatment outcome has actually been around for a long time, but as often happens, it was slow to influence practice (Rogers, 1995). We place this chapter early in the book, because counseling style has at least as much impact on client outcomes as the particular treatment methods you use (Imel, Wampold, & Miller, 2008; Project MATCH Research Group, 1998d).

THERAPEUTIC EMPATHY

One striking finding in research on the treatment of substance use disorders is that clients' outcomes differ dramatically depending on the counselor to whom they are assigned (Najavits, Crits-Christoph, & Dierberger, 2000; Najavits & Weiss, 1994). Even when ostensibly delivering the very same manual-guided treatment, therapists differ in their effectiveness (Project MATCH Research Group, 1998d). What accounts for such differences among counselors?

One of the strongest predictors of a counselor's effectiveness in treating sub-

> One of the strongest predictors of a counselor's effectiveness in treating substance use disorders is empathy.

stance use disorders is empathy. In one study, among nine therapists all delivering the same behavior therapy, clients' drinking outcomes were strongly predicted by the extent to which the counselor practiced empathic, reflective listening during treatment. Clients of the most empathic counselor showed a 100% improvement rate, whereas those of the least empathic counselor showed a 25% improvement rate (Miller, Taylor, & West, 1980). Even 2 years later, clients' drinking outcomes were strongly related to how empathic their counselor had been during treatment (Miller & Baca, 1983). Another early study demonstrated a strong relationship between client relapse rates and the counselor's skillfulness in client-centered counseling. The more empathic and client-centered the counselor's style, the lower the relapse rate of his or her clients after counseling (Valle, 1981).

What is this quality of empathy? Some associate the term with the ability to *identify* with one's clients by virtue of having had similar experiences. In fact, personal recovery status neither increases nor decreases one's success in treating substance use disorders, even when delivering a 12-step-based treatment (Project MATCH Research Group, 1998d). What *does* make a difference is therapeutic empathy, which is not the same thing as being able to understand a client based on your own personal experience. If anything, being *early* in one's own recovery could get in the way of effective counseling by fostering identification and countertransference (Manohar, 1973).

Carl Rogers (1959) identified *accurate empathy* as one of the three critical conditions that a counselor must provide to promote growth and change in clients. (The other two were interpersonal warmth, or *unconditional positive regard*, and personal honesty, or *genuineness*.) These "conditions" can be linked to particular counselor skills and practices. What Rogers meant by "empathy" was the ability to listen to your clients, and accurately reflect back to them the essence and meaning of what they have said. Such reflection, which was termed *active listening* by Rogers's student Thomas Gordon (1970), serves at least three purposes. First, it allows you to ensure that you are correctly understanding what your client means. Second, it communicates respect, understanding, and acceptance. Third, and most important in Rogers's theory, it helps clients to clarify their own internal processes—thoughts, feelings, associations—and to experience them in a nonjudgmental atmosphere. It fosters the opposite of the avoidant coping style referred to by the psychoanalytic term *denial*. Clients are encouraged to explore their real experiencing, whatever it is, and to do so in the company of someone who continues to regard them with unconditional loving acceptance.

Learning accurate empathy is no quick and easy task. Those who are good at reflective listening make it look simple and natural, but it is actually a skill that is honed over years of practice. Happily, as we will discuss below, your clients can teach you how to do it.

Beneath empathy is an attitude of total interest in and focus on understanding how your client perceives things, on seeing the world through his or her eyes. The empathic listener suspends, at least for the time being, all of her or his own material—advice, questions, suggestions, stories, brilliant insight—and focuses entirely on the person's own experience. It is a challenging, sacrificial, and much underrated way of being with people (Rogers, 1980).

Why focus so fully on what your client thinks, feels, values, and believes, when you could be conveying your own wisdom? Herein is another of Carl Rogers's assumptions about human nature that we share. He believed that within each person is a seed waiting to blossom. In each client there is wisdom, a desire to be well and whole, a natural tendency to move in a positive direction given the proper conditions, just as a seed grows to its potential if given air, water, soil, and sunshine. The counselor's job, Rogers believed, is not so much to plant the seed as to provide the right conditions for its growth. Like a midwife, you help with the birthing process but don't provide the baby. Rogers trusted his clients' own experiencing, wisdom, and resourcefulness. If you don't share that belief, then it might well seem a waste of time to be listening to what your clients have to say.

The counseling style that we are describing here is one that communicates not "I have what you need," but rather, "*You* have what you need, and together we will find it." That's not to say that you never give advice, make suggestions, teach new skills, or share personal experiences. There is a time and a way to offer your professional expertise. Here we depart a bit from Rogers, in that we combine the client-centered foundation described in this chapter with other effective and more directive treatment methods described in subsequent chapters.

One reason why we devote an entire chapter to this counseling style is that it works. Being empathic is itself an evidence-based practice (Bohart & Greenberg, 1997; Norcross, 2002; Zuroff, Kelly, Leybman, Blatt, & Wampold, 2010). As described above, counselors who have honed their skill in empathic, reflective listening are simply more effective in treating people with substance use disorders. This counseling style meshes well with other treatment methods, including cognitive-behavioral and 12-step approaches (Longabaugh, Zweben, LoCastro, & Miller, 2005; Miller, 2004). In fact, the related client-centered method of *motivational interviewing* (Chapter 10) appears to amplify the effectiveness of treatment approaches with which it is combined (Hettema, Steele, & Miller, 2005). Empathy is also a quality that clients want in their therapist, above and beyond the type of treatment they receive (Swift & Callahan, 2010; Swift, Callahan, & Volliver, 2011).

There is also evidence that a low level of empathy in addiction treatment can be toxic, that clients whose counselors show low levels of skill in accurate empathy have particularly poor outcomes relative to clients with high-empathy counselors (Valle, 1981), and even relative to no treatment (Miller et al., 1980). In Valle's (1981) study, clients whose counselors showed low levels of the critical skills described by Carl Rogers were two to four times more likely to be drinking at each follow-up interval, relative to high-skill counselors' clients. Studies have illustrated that certain counselors are outliers in terms of their clients having outstandingly poor outcomes (Luborsky, McLellan, Woody, O'Brien, & Auerbach, 1985; McLellan, Woody, Luborsky, & Goehl, 1988; Project MATCH Research Group, 1998d). Screening for empathic skill in hiring addiction treatment personnel is not only possible (Miller, Moyers, et al., 2005), but well justified as an evidence-based practice to improve client outcomes. First, do no harm!

> Screening for empathic skill in hiring addiction treatment personnel is not only possible, but well justified as an evidence-based practice to improve client outcomes.

In sum, empathy is not something that you *have* so much as something that you *do*. It is a learnable skill. Most counselors already think of themselves as "good listeners," but accurate empathy is a particular kind of listening that does not come naturally to most. Once you learn it, however, you have a remarkable gift to give not only to your clients, but to others around you.

REFLECTIVE LISTENING

It sounds easy enough. Just repeat back what the client says. It is the substance of parodies of Carl Rogers and of counselor characters in situation comedies.

Skillful reflective listening actually does far more than repeat what a client says. Simple repetition just tends to go around in circles. Try it for a while and you'll probably feel like you are getting nowhere. Instead, skillful reflective listening moves ahead, if only just a little. It considers what the person has *not* quite spoken, but may mean. Instead of merely repeating what the client has just said, complex reflections offer what *might* be the next, as yet unspoken, sentence of the person's paragraph.

How do you know what a client *hasn't* said? There are many ways. Sometimes you pick it up from the person's nonverbal cues. Sometimes you're trying out a hypothesis about what the client might mean by a word or phrase that you heard. Perhaps you are voicing what, based on your own clinical experience, the person may be feeling in relation to what was said, or perhaps you remember something your client said two sessions ago and you make a connection. Not all reflections make brilliant leaps to the unspoken. Sometimes you do mostly repeat what the client said, or just substitute a synonym, particularly when you're not clear what is meant. If the person keeps on talking, keeps exploring, tells you something more, then you know you did it right.

In fact, that's how you learn this skill. What you are really doing when you offer a reflection is making a guess. Based on your experience and what you heard, you're stating to the best of your ability what you think the person may have meant. It is a hypothesis, and you are testing it. When you state your hypothesis in the form of a good reflection, the client will either confirm or revise it. If you hit it on the head, the person is likely in some form to say "Yes ... " and will continue to elaborate. If you missed it, the person will probably in some form say "No ... " and will continue to elaborate. Thus there is no penalty for missing. Either way you learn more about the client's experiencing, and so does the client. When your client continues to elaborate, that's your signal that you reflected well.

Sometimes, though, a person does not respond with a yes or no followed by elaboration. Sometimes what you see instead is a kind of resistance—a backing off, closing down, taking back, or arguing. That's usually a sign that your reflection was not accurate, or perhaps that you jumped too far ahead of your client. Analysts call it a "premature interpretation." It might also have something to do with your tone of voice. (The simple reflective statement "So you don't see any problems with your drinking" is quite different from a sarcastic "So YOU don't see ANY problems with your drinking!") When you reflect well, the person accepts (even if correcting) what you said, and moves ahead. Once you know what to look for, you will continue for the rest of your counseling career to receive accurate feedback from your clients that helps you improve your skillfulness in reflective listening. That also, by the way, is how you get to be more accurate in your empathy. After listening reflectively to people for years and receiving immediate feedback about whether you got it right or not, you simply get better at knowing what people mean. You're more likely to guess it right, and sometimes your clients regard you as a kind of wizard. "How did you know that?" It's not magic. It's practice with constant feedback.

Reflective listening is not an easy skill to learn. Be patient with yourself at first. This is a complex and demanding skill, but one very worth the time it requires. It is also something at which you can become increasingly adept through all the years of your life.

So what is a good reflection? First of all, it is a *statement* and not a question. The natural tendency is to ask your client if this is what he or she means. After all, you're not sure. Your reflection is just a hypothesis. You might be wrong. Wouldn't it be better to *ask* your client if you are right? Here is one place where the natural instinct is misleading. Even though your intention in asking a question (rather than making a statement) is respectful, the actual *effect* of questioning is often to cause the person to step back. Questions demand something of the person. Statements do not. Consider the difference between these two counselor responses:

"You're angry with me?"
"You're angry with me."

Say them out loud. The first one is subtly different from the second. If your clinical antennae are like ours, the first one is more likely to cause the person to back away from the feeling, to deny it or qualify it. A simple statement, on the other hand, gives permission to continue exploring and experiencing. Until you're accustomed to this, it can feel unnatural. The worry is that you are "putting words in the person's mouth," dictating what he or she means. Very rarely do people perceive good reflective listening in this way. They just keep going.

So a good reflection is a statement. It doesn't need any fancy words at the front. Stereotypic counselor responses such as, "What I hear you saying is that you ... " are unnecessary window dressing, and can be annoying after a few times. The only thing you need in most cases in order to begin a good reflection is the word "You." Consider this snippet from an initial session with a 33-year-old woman:

CLIENT: I'm not really sure why I'm even here, actually. There is so much going on in my life right now, I don't know if this is what I should be doing.

THERAPIST: You're feeling confused right now, and pretty overwhelmed.

CLIENT: Well, I'm just about to be kicked out of my apartment, and my ex says he's not going to pay child support any more. I already owe my lawyer a lot of money and I can't run up any more lawyer fees.

THERAPIST: You're feeling at the end of your rope. So you wonder if you should even be here.

CLIENT: I just don't know what to do, and I know drinking is part of the problem, but is that what I should be focusing on right now?

THERAPIST: Seems like there might be more important things for you to worry about.

CLIENT: Like my kids. How am I going to feed them?

THERAPIST: You care a lot about your kids.

CLIENT: They're all I have! I just want them to grow up and be happy.

THERAPIST: And that, in part, is why you're here.

CLIENT: I guess so. I don't want them to have a drunk for a mother.

All of the therapist responses above are reflective listening statements. None of them is a straight parroting of what the client said. Also, all of them are statements rather than questions. Consider the potentially different impact if the counselor had instead asked:

"Are you feeling overwhelmed?"

or

"So you think there are more important things to talk about than your drinking?"

or

"Do you care about your kids?"

or

"So is that why you're here?"

The difference may not seem very large, but the tone is changed if you turn it from a statement into a question just by inflecting your voice upward rather than down at the end, or adding question words like "Do you ... " It puts the person on the defensive, if only just a little, even though you didn't have that intention. Good reflections are typically statements rather than questions.

When you're listening with accurate empathy, there are also a lot of things that you're not doing. You're not giving advice, offering solutions, or asking questions. Neither are you warning, educating, persuading, or sympathizing. You're not agreeing or disagreeing, analyzing or diagnosing. Your whole attention is focused on understanding and following the person's own perspectives, and that's work enough in itself.

Of course reflection is not everything that you do, even at the outset of counseling. While it is an interesting and challenging exercise to try 100% reflective listening for even 10 minutes, counseling normally involves a dance back and forth between reflection and other types of communication. We emphasize accurate empathy first, both because it appears to be a key to effective counseling and because other responses (like asking questions) are so much easier that it's tempting to overuse them when it might be better to listen.

OARS: FUNDAMENTAL COUNSELING SKILLS

Reflection is one of four fundamental skills that form a client-centered foundation and safety net in counseling. When you're just getting started, or whenever you're lost and aren't sure what to do next, you can always fall back to these fundamental four and be reasonably sure that you are helping and not harming your client. These four skills are summarized by the acronym OARS: Open questions, Affirmation, Reflection, and Summaries.

> ## BOX 4.1. Personal Reflection: Learning to Listen
>
> The main emphasis in my own graduate training was on a fairly directive behavioral style, but along the way we were also exposed to the humanistic client-centered approach of Carl Rogers and the particular skill of accurate empathy. I found it very challenging and clumsy at first, but something about it just felt right to me. I also found that clients responded very well even to my stumbling early efforts to listen to them in this way. When subsequently on internship, I found myself working on a ward for the treatment of people with alcohol dependence, I fell back on these listening skills, mostly because I knew almost *nothing* about addictions. I let the clients be the experts on their own lives and problems and educate me. It turned out to be a helpful and enjoyable approach for both of us. I quickly developed both a real respect and appreciation for these people and their struggles and a curiosity that led me to the primary focus of my professional career. I have always enjoyed talking with people with addiction problems. The ability to listen in this way has also greatly enriched my personal as well as my professional life.
>
> What really surprised me, though, was how important empathy turned out to be in my subsequent treatment outcome research. I taught my own students both behavioral and client-centered treatment methods, as I had been trained, and it turned out that this ability to listen empathically was a very strong predictor of successful outcomes, even within a highly structured behavioral approach. That finding ultimately led me to the development of motivational interviewing, and to focus on the quality of counselor–client relationships.
>
> —W. R. M.

O: Open Questions

The first of these is asking open questions, with an emphasis on the O (open) rather than the Q (questions). Many counselors, we find, ask far too many questions, a majority of which are closed questions, ones that have a short answer. Open questions, in contrast, are not easily answered with a yes or no or with short-answer information. They leave the clients some room to move, to think, to explore. They invite reflection.

A reasonably good rule of thumb is *never ask three questions in a row.* After an open question you should usually be listening and reflecting. Asking a question is not listening; rather, it creates an opportunity for you to listen. Another simple rule of thumb is to offer about two reflections for each question that you ask: a two-to-one ratio. Give it a try! Listen to a tape of an ordinary counseling session and count up the number of questions that you asked and the number of times you offered a reflective listening statement. We find that it's not uncommon for counselors to ask 10 or more questions per reflection.

BOX 4.2. Closed and Open Questions

CLOSED QUESTIONS

"How old are you?"
"Do you live with your parents?"
"When did you last use marijuana?"
"Do you want to quit drinking?"
"How many drinks did you have yesterday?"
"Have you ever had a blackout?"
"Isn't it time to do something different?"
"Do you think you're an alcoholic?"
"What do you want to do about cocaine—keep using, cut down, or quit?"
"Whose idea was it to call us?"
"How long has it been since you went for a few days without drinking?"
"Do you belong to a church?"

OPEN QUESTIONS

"What brings you here today?"
"Tell me about your family."
"What do you like about marijuana?"
"And what's the other side … in what ways has drinking not been so good to you?"
"How does alcohol affect you?"
"So what are you thinking about your drinking at this point?"
"What do you want to do about cocaine?"
"How have you been feeling this week?"
"How did you happen to call us?"
"Tell me about the last time you felt really good without drugs or beer."
"How, if at all, is religion or spirituality important in your life?"

There are times, to be sure, when you need to ask more questions. Many treatment programs require a structured intake interview, such as the Addiction Severity Index (see Chapter 5), that involve asking a preset series of questions. Here we offer two suggestions. First, try not to start off your counseling with a slew of questions. Asking a number of questions in a row, particularly closed questions, tends to create a mind-set of passivity in the client. If possible, just sit down and listen to your client for a while, even just for 15 minutes, before you start questioning. Ask an open question like "What brings you here today?" and then listen and reflect.

Second, put a frame around the questions so that your client does not confuse them with the normal course of treatment. "In a little while I have a whole series of specific questions that I will need to ask you [the frame], but before I do, I just want to hear in your own words what brings you here today [open question and opportunity for you to reflect]."

A final working rule of thumb that we recommend is to ask more open than closed questions. Of the questions that you do ask, try to make more than half of them be open questions that give you an opportunity to listen to something more than a short answer, and to reflect.

So when it comes to using questions in counseling:

- Try listening before you ask a lot of questions.
- Avoid asking three questions in a row.
- Shoot for more than half of your questions to be open questions.
- Offer about two reflections for each question you ask.

A: Affirm

The second of the four OARS skills is to *affirm* your client. This sounds easy enough. Look for opportunities to comment positively. Thank your client for being on time or for coming in at all, even if late. Find things that you can genuinely appreciate, admire, respect. Reframe client experiences as laudable strengths.

> CLIENT: I've been on the street for 3 years, and I've had to do some bad stuff to get drugs. I've been beaten, busted, OD'd, hungry, cold—you name it.
>
> COUNSELOR: You've been through an awful lot. You're a real survivor. I don't know if I could handle what you've been through.

Look for successes, even small ones, in the client's past or present and affirm them. Here's the familiar choice of half-full or half-empty. After years of having between 8 and 12 drinks every night, and some initial success in cutting back, a client wanted to make it through a whole week without drinking at all. On Monday she came back to the clinic looking dejected and defeated. She had had six alcohol-free days, but on the weekend she had 2 drinks on Saturday. You could shame her: "I thought you said that you weren't going to drink this week! What happened?" Why not instead congratulate her on her first six days of sobriety in years, be impressed that she somehow managed to go from about 70 drinks a week down to 2, and ask her how she did it?

Where did the crazy idea that if you can just make people feel bad enough then they will change come from? Most clients, we find, have already been rather thoroughly shamed, humiliated, and blamed

Where did the crazy idea that if you can just make people feel bad enough then they will change come from?

in their lives before coming to see us, and more of the same is unlikely to help. One of the many insights of Carl Rogers was that when people feel unacceptable they are immobilized, unable to change. It is, paradoxically, when people experience acceptance that they are freed to change.

R: Reflect

This one we have already discussed. Reflective listening is perhaps the most important of the four OARS skills.

S: Summarize

Beyond immediate reflections, it is helpful to pull together in short summaries what your clients say. This shows and requires, of course, that you have been listening carefully, which is an important communication in itself. Summaries also allow you to emphasize and integrate what a client has offered. At least three kinds of summaries can be helpful.

First, there are *collecting* summaries. These happen in the midst of a counseling session, and pull together a variety of related things the person has said. If, for example, you have asked about ways in which drug use has had negative effects in the person's life, you begin collecting those mentally, and in addition to reflecting them as you go, you also periodically give them back to the client like a small bouquet. Then you continue the process by asking, "What else?"

> "So far you've told me that you don't like how you feel in the morning when you get up, and you know that your work has suffered some from being hungover. Your daughter has also been worried about you, and has told you she thinks that you drink too much—which kind of annoys you. You've also noticed that sometimes you don't remember things that happened. What else?"

Second, there are *linking* summaries, which make a connection between something that the person has just said and material that was offered earlier, perhaps in a prior session. Again you are communicating that you remember and regard as important what your client tells you. Beyond this, the point of a linking summary is to suggest a connection, to test a hypothesis that two things you've learned might be related.

"I wonder if this feeling of panic that you're talking about is somewhat like how you felt when your husband suddenly announced that he wanted a divorce. Both of them seem to involve a feeling of being out of control, which really upsets you."

There is obvious similarity here to analytic interpretations, where the therapist does not want to be too far ahead of the person's current awareness. The primary purpose of a linking summary is to increase understanding (both your own and the client's) of what the client is experiencing.

Finally, there are *transitional summaries*. These tend to be a bit longer, and are used to end a session or to shift from one task or topic to another within a session. They draw together what has gone before, and point toward something new.

"OK—here's what I understand about your situation from what you've told me today, and let me know if I've missed something important. You came here primarily because your probation officer sent you, and you understand now that you could get treatment somewhere else if you're not happy here. What got you in trouble was the misfortune of having cocaine in your car when you were pulled over, and it also turned up in the drug test they gave you. It seems to you that it's really nobody's business what you do, and that you were just unlucky, but now you have this probation officer watching over you. There have been some times when you used quite a bit more than you meant to, and felt scared and paranoid. And you've spent a lot of money on cocaine, which has created some financial problems for you. You don't like having to be here, but as you've said, you might as well make the best of it. Did I miss anything?"

With these four fundamental OARS skills, you can often make substantial progress. This client-centered style can be quite helpful in itself. It's a good way to begin a counseling session, and as we've said, you can always fall back on the OARS when you're not sure what to do. Confident skillfulness in this way of being with people is an excellent foundation for further counseling interventions.

STAYING FOCUSED

A simple but important principle in effective treatment is to be professional and focused in your counseling. That may sound self-evident, but a surprising amount of time in addiction treatment can be devoted to informal "chat" that is unrelated to clients' treatment needs (Martino, Ball, Nich, Frankforter, & Carroll, 2009). In one study with Hispanic clients, the amount of such off-topic chat was *inversely* related to client motivation for change and retention in addiction treatment (Bamatter et al., 2010). This is consistent with the more general finding in psychotherapy research that better outcomes are associated with the therapist's adherence to an organized, coherent theoretical approach (Beutler, Machado, & Neufeldt, 1994).

TAKING AN ACTIVE INTEREST IN YOUR CLIENT

It is important for clients to be actively involved in their own recovery. That is one reason for a client-centered foundation in counseling, rather than leaving clients in a passive role. A good predictor of successful behavior change is the extent to which a person is actively doing things, taking steps toward making that change.

At the same time, active involvement in counseling is a two-way street. It should be clear to clients that you are actively engaged and interested in working with them. Don't hesitate to take steps that can facilitate change. Consider the example of making a referral. Is it best just to give your client the phone number, leaving the responsibility to him or her to make the call, or might it be better to place the call while the person is still in your office? Some favor the former, thinking that it is vital for clients to take personal responsibility (which it is). Consider, however, that clients are about three times more likely to actually complete the referral if you place the call together while they are still in your office (Kogan, 1957). Perhaps they should get there first, and then work on personal responsibility! Similarly, it has been known for a long time that people are about twice as likely to return after an initial visit or after a missed appointment if you send them a short handwritten note of encouragement (not a form letter) or give them a simple telephone call to say that you look forward to working with them (Gottheil, Sterling, & Weinstein, 1997a; Koumans & Muller, 1967; Koumans, Muller, & Miller, 1967; Nirenberg, Sobell, & Sobell, 1980; Panepinto & Higgins, 1969). Such simple messages of caring and active interest require little time, but can make a big difference.

Menschenbild

The client-centered counseling style described in this chapter has been shown to improve client outcomes in the treatment of addictions, and it can meld well with other counseling methods. It is unclear exactly why this particular therapeutic style works so well, but we suspect that it has something to do with the underlying assumptions about people. Each therapeutic approach, at least when put into practice, includes an implicit picture of human nature. A useful noun for this is the German *Menschenbild*—

literally, one's picture of people. A similar noun, *Weltanschauung*, may be more familiar to psychotherapists, referring to one's broad assumptions about the nature of the world and reality. *Menschenbild* is more specific: it's how we think about people.

Within the context of counseling, your *Menschenbild* can make a great difference. One important dimension has to do with belief in people's potential to change. In a classic study, researchers conducted psychological testing with clients in three alcoholism treatment programs, and in appreciation for the staff's cooperation they identified those clients who had particularly high alcoholism recovery potential according to the tests. Sure enough, the staff did find that those clients were more motivated, attended sessions on time, and worked harder in treatment. Indeed, a year after discharge, these clients were more likely to be abstinent and employed, and had had fewer slips and longer spans of sobriety. The secret of the study was that these "high potential" clients had actually been chosen at random, and were in no way different from others in the same treatment programs, *except* that their counselors believed that they would do well (Leake &

| Believing in clients' potential or lack thereof is a self-fulfilling prophecy. |

King, 1977). Believing in clients' potential (or lack thereof) is a self-fulfilling prophecy. In a still older study, researchers listened to doctors' tone of voice when interviewed about people with alcoholism, having filtered out the content so that raters could not understand what was being said, only how it was being said. Voice tone strongly predicted whether patients would complete a referral: the more anger and irritation in the doctor's voice, the less likely it was that the person would seek treatment (Milmoe, Rosenthal, Blane, Chafetz, & Wolf, 1967).

The client-centered approach that we advocate focuses primarily on the person's own strengths, motivations, and potential for change. An opposite perspective focuses on *deficits*, that which clients are assumed to lack. As discussed earlier, a deficit model communicates to the client "I have what you need, and I'll give it to you," whereas a client-centered approach implies that "*You* have what you need, and together we'll find it." It communicates *potential*: hope, empowerment, and responsibility.

Another important dimension of *Menschenbild* has to do with the counselor's degree of support for client autonomy (Deci & Ryan, 2008). At one extreme pole of this dimension is the assumption that people (in this case, people with addictions) are fundamentally flawed and must have external controls. They cannot be given choice, allowed to think for themselves, or trusted to make good decisions. They simply lack the necessary insight, honesty, maturity, skills, character, or self-control. This view, of course, suggests the need for a no-nonsense, authoritarian approach. At the opposite pole is the *Menschenbild* of Carl Rogers and the human potential movement: that people have within them an inherent tendency and potential to grow in a positive direction, given the proper therapeutic conditions. Each person has a natural and positive self that can be realized or suppressed. Somewhere in between these extremes is a *tabula rasa* view that people have no inherent nature at all, but are shaped by their environment. Depending on this view of human nature, a counselor might be more trustful or less inclined to honor the client's autonomy and choice.

There is a sense, however, in which client autonomy is simply a reality. Short of extreme restriction of freedom (as in imprisonment), people do in fact determine their own goals and make their own decisions. To tell someone "You can't drink" does not acknowledge the truth. In one early and somewhat naïve study, problem drinkers were randomly assigned to either an abstinence or a moderation goal (Graber & Miller, 1988). People in both groups felt equally free to reject the goal that had been set for them. A belief that "You can't let clients choose" implies an impossible level of counselor power. The ability to choose cannot be taken away. Frankl (1969) observed that even under the extreme privations of a concentration camp, people still made life-shaping choices about how they would think and be. Suicide crisis counselors know that people in distress do ultimately retain autonomous choice, and yet there is much that can be done to help them. We find it helpful to acknowledge, honor, and work within the client's autonomy.

Finally, we commend thinking of your client as your partner, as a collaborator or co-counselor (Gordon & Edwards, 1997). No one knows more about clients than they do themselves, and it is vital to draw on their own expertise and wisdom. After all, recovery is a long-term process, and the hours we share with clients represent but a tiny part of their lives. A collaborative partnership allows you to move together toward change.

BUT I DON'T HAVE *TIME* FOR LISTENING!

Many professionals don't have the luxury of 50-minute hours for counseling, and feel the pressure of heavy caseloads with short visits. The temptation is to fall back on a director role and just tell people what to do.

> Think of your client as your partner.

Yet empathic listening is a valuable skill that can be practiced for just a couple of minutes if that's all you have, and even brief spans of good listening can make a difference (see Chapter 9). Empathic listening also turns out to be a good tool even for collecting information and making sure you're not missing something important. Just a few minutes of good listening can help the people you serve feel cared for and understood. If you have a lot to do—information to collect and convey, multiple problems to address, dual roles to fulfill—it may be all the more important to listen well in the time you have. There is a paradox here: slow is fast and fast is slow. If you act like you only have a few minutes, it seems to take a long time to get a task done.

If you act (and feel) like you have all day, it may only take a few minutes (Roberts, 2001). Don't be afraid that if you open the door to listening you'll never be able to close it again. Sometimes people keep talking and repeating themselves precisely because they're not sure you are hearing them.

KEY POINTS

- Treatment providers vary widely in effectiveness. A significant determinant of clients' outcomes is the counselor with whom they work.

- It matters not only what treatment you provide, but also how you provide it. Counseling relationship matters.

- Accurate empathy—the learnable skill of reflective listening—has a particularly positive impact on addiction treatment outcomes, and its absence can be detrimental.

- Think of your clients as partners in the change process. They are experts on themselves, and get to make their own choices about whether and how they will change.

- Counselor perceptions of clients can become self-fulfilling prophecies. To some extent in counseling, what you expect is what you get.

REFLECTION QUESTIONS

- Given your life experience thus far, how optimistic or pessimistic do you feel about the likelihood that people will recover from addiction?

- Listen to a recording of your own counseling and count the OARS.

- After treating people with addictions, do you feel more like you've been dancing or wrestling with them?

CHAPTER 5

Screening, Evaluation, and Diagnosis

M any treatment professionals and agencies place a premium on assessment, on gathering information. This also fits with helping professionals' natural interest in people and the privilege of entering into the inner world of strangers. Yet, from a practical perspective, assessment is useful only to the extent that it informs practice. There are also some risks in spending too much time on assessment in early contacts. Asking questions implies an expert role: once I have enough information, then I will have the answer for you. It places the client in a passive role, awaiting expert judgment. When the goal is behavior change, it is important for clients to be very actively involved in their own treatment. Answering a lot of questions is not very engaging, and it can be off-putting. What good is gathering a lot of information if the person doesn't come back?

In this chapter we consider the uses of screening and evaluation in addiction treatment. We don't think of evaluation as a prelude to but rather as an ongoing part of treatment. What do I *need* to know now in order to proceed with helping this person? Gathering information can be fascinating and naturally appeals to one's curiosity about and interest in people, but how will this information be useful? Treatment begins from the very first contact, and evaluation (at least ideally) is done in the service of identifying and achieving treatment goals.

The functions of screening and evaluation also depend in part on the context. People with substance use disorders and their family members turn up in many different settings including emergency rooms, primary care and mental health clinics, correctional systems, and social service agencies (Rose & Zweben, 2003; Rose, Zweben, & Stoffel, 1999). Some examples might include a pregnant woman who is seen in a mental health clinic for intimate partner violence, a professional man coming to an employee assistance program for poor job performance, a 24-year-old single woman treated in an emergency room after a motor vehicle accident, and a 75-year-old depressed man seen in a social service agency. In these settings, staff may be unfamiliar with symptoms of addiction that are masked as injuries, family problems, or mental health problems. They may be unfamiliar with screening protocols for detecting alcohol or drug problems. Consequently, despite the high incidence of addictive disorders in health and social service settings, drug and alcohol problems are often missed (Miller & Weisner, 2002). Without adequate knowledge and screening, health and social service workers are likely to recognize only the more debilitated individuals. This means that many people who might benefit from addiction treatment do not receive it (Dawson, Grant, Stinson, & Chou, 2006).

Throughout this book, we emphasize the importance of recognizing and addressing the full range of substance use problems (see Chapter 23). In this chapter we take up three interrelated tasks, screening, evaluation, and diagnosis, and how they inform treatment and change planning.

Screening ➜ Evaluation ➜ Diagnosis ➜ Change Plan

SCREENING FOR SUBSTANCE USE DISORDERS

> Screening is sometimes confused with diagnosis and evaluation.

Screening is sometimes confused with diagnosis (confirming the presence of a disorder) and evaluation (doing a more thorough evaluation in order to understand a problem). By definition, screening procedures are meant to be overinclusive, to detect the *possible* presence of a problem and the need for further evaluation.

There are two kinds of possible mistakes that can occur in screening. One is a false positive and the other is a false negative. Think of a drug screen. A false positive occurs if the screen says that a drug is present (e.g., in breath or urine) when in fact it is not. A false negative happens if the test says that a drug is not present when in fact it is. The relative frequency of these mistakes is determined by where one sets the test's "cutoff point": the threshold at which the test says "yes" versus "no" (Cherpitel, 1995). A false negative indicates no need for further evaluation, which means that a potentially important condition is missed. A false positive results in unnecessary additional evaluation to confirm the absence of a condition. In the case of drug screens, a positive finding typically results in a different (usually more expensive) test to confirm or disconfirm the presence of the drug. Ideally a screen would give no false negatives or false positives, but in reality this is rarely achievable. In order to have a lower false negative rate, it is necessary to accept a larger number of false positives. A test's *sensitivity* is its ability to accurately detect true positives and not make false negative errors. A test's *specificity* is its accuracy in not making false positive errors. The cutoff point of a screening test is meant to offer the right balance between sensitivity and specificity.

Consider a situation in which many people are seen for health or social services, and the goal is to identify which people also have addiction problems that may complicate outcomes and that need to be addressed. The service is already busy, so ideally a screening procedure would be fairly simple and not require much time. It should also be fairly sensitive in case finding (to avoid missing people with addiction problems) but also reasonably specific (so as not to suggest unnecessary additional evaluation). Add to this the complexity that addiction problems occur all along a continuum of severity plus a desire to detect problems early rather than waiting for them to be severe and entrenched, and screening can become quite a complex task (Cooney, Zweben, & Fleming, 1995).

People seeking help in specialist addiction treatment settings are more likely to be aware of and open about their substance use problems. This is in part because they have usually already experienced significant consequences of addictive behaviors (e.g., loss of job, family conflict, and incarceration) as well as pressure from family and friends to seek help. In a way, just walking through the door of an addiction treatment setting is a positive screen indicating a need for further evaluation.

In contrast, individuals seen in general health and social service settings may not have yet experienced severe consequences or pressures resulting from their substance use. Consequently they often do not think of themselves as having "a problem," let alone a need for addiction treatment. They come for help with other concerns such as medical or emotional problems, and may or may not have made the connection between their concerns and their substance use (Cooney et al., 1995). Such hesitancy may also be related to the stigma attached to addiction treatment. Thus people seeking health and social services are sometimes surprised, even defensive, about being screened for substance use disorders. In particular settings (such as child welfare services, employee assistance, and criminal justice) there may be particular obstacles to honesty about substance use, such as a fear of losing parental custody (Zweben, Rose, Stout, & Zywiak, 2003).

A few guidelines can be helpful in presenting and discussing screening questions or instruments, particularly when used outside specialist addiction services:

- Give clear instructions as needed to complete the screening task.
- Provide appropriate and accurate assurances about privacy and confidentiality.
- Explain (as appropriate) that this is a routine procedure used with all clients.

- Listen to and reflect any concerns that are raised (see Chapter 4) —for example, "You're wondering why we're asking about your alcohol/drug use when you came into the emergency room to be treated for your injury."
- Answer the person's questions honestly.

Screening Tools

A variety of screening tools are available, many of them in the public domain and thus free of charge. Considerations in selecting an appropriate screener include the instrument's demonstrated sensitivity and specificity, its feasibility in your setting (e.g., length, cost), and the particular populations with whom it is to be used (e.g., language and reading level).

Clinical Questions

Perhaps the most common screening approach is to ask one or more carefully worded questions during the course of conversation and evaluation. Substance-focused items can be intermixed with questions about other health or social issues to reduce defensiveness.

A simple alcohol screen, recommended by NIAAA (National Institute on Alcohol Abuse and Alcoholism, 2005), is a single question about heavy drinking:

- For men: "How many times in the past year have you had five or more drinks in a day?"
- For women: "How many times in the past year have you had four or more drinks in a day?"

(If you're not familiar with a standard drink unit, see Box 23.2 in Chapter 23.) In one study, this single question identified 86% of individuals who had an alcohol use disorder (Williams & Vinson, 2001). Similarly, a simple single question yielded good results (100% sensitivity, 74% specificity) in screening for substance use disorders in primary care: "How many times in the past year have you used an illegal drug or used a prescription medication for nonmedical reasons?" (Smith, Schmidt, Allensworth-Davies, & Suitz, 2010).

Other screening questions probe for problematic patterns and effects. An early four-question screener for alcohol problems was the CAGE (Ewing, 1984). The usual cutoff point indicating a need for further evaluation is two "Yes" answers. It is sensible to precede these questions by asking "Do you sometimes drink beer, wine, or other alcohol beverages?" because the "have you ever" format of these questions can produce false positives for people who have quit drinking.

Various modifications of the CAGE have been developed and tested. A modification based on the 4-item Rapid Alcohol Problems Screen (RAPS4) further improved on the sensitivity of the CAGE (Cherpitel, 2006). The CAGE-AID (Brown & Rounds, 1995) changed the wording of questions to address alcohol and other drugs simultaneously. Other modifications of the CAGE have been developed specifically for use with pregnant women (Russell, Martier, & Sokol, 1994) and older adults (Fleming, 2002).

Questionnaires

Many screening instruments are longer than a few questions, and can be administered either in written form or as an interview. One of the earliest of these was the Michigan Alcoholism Screening Test (MAST; Selzer, 1971). Although the MAST has a reasonably good track record in screening, its age shows in its construction. It contains a mixture of content, and the time referent differs across items, varying from present tense ("Do you feel ... ") to lifetime ("Have you ever ... "), which is one reason that it can have a high false positive rate for current alcohol disorders (Connors, Donovan, & DiClemente, 2001; Luckie, White, Miller, Icenogle, & Lasoski, 1995). A Drug Abuse Screening Test (DAST) was developed by Skinner (1982), which shares the strengths and limitations of the MAST.

The Alcohol Use Disorders Identification Test (AUDIT) is a state-of-the-art screening instrument developed by the World Health Organization (Babor & Grant, 1989; Babor, Higgins-Biddle, Saunders, & Monteiro, 2001). It has been validated cross-culturally, in various nations and languages. Its 10 items deal with amount and frequency of drinking, alcohol dependence symptoms, personal problems, and social problems. Scores of 0–7 are indicative of low problem severity, while those of 26–40 are suggestive of high problem severity. Unlike the MAST, it has a consistent time reference for items (i.e., the last 12 months), and its specificity remains strong with individuals having psychiatric disorders (Hulse & Tait, 2003). The AUDIT has also been adapted as a screening tool for detecting both alcohol and drug problems called the AUDIT-ID (*Includes other Drugs*; Campbell, Hoffman, Madson, & Melchert, 2003). There is a parallel Drug Use Disorders Identification Test (DUDIT) focused on illicit drugs (Berman, Bergman, Palmstierna, & Schlyter, 2005; Durbeej et al., 2010).

The National Institute on Drug Abuse (2010) encourages screening and brief intervention in general medical settings and produced an instrument that can be used for this purpose, the Modified Alcohol, Smoking and Substance Involvement Screening Test (NM-ASSIST) based on a World Health Organization instrument (WHO ASSIST Working Group, 2002). A longer interview, it first queries lifetime and then recent use in 12 drug classes, then the presence or absence of various diagnostic signs of alcohol/drug problems.

Biological Markers

In some cases it might be helpful to include biological measures such as lab tests along with self-reports to obtain accurate screening data, particularly where honesty of self-report is in question. Such might be the case for people whose employment or legal status is at risk due to drinking or drug use. One advantage of biological measures is that, unlike self-report measures, they cannot be influenced by motivational or cognitive factors (Babor & Higgins-Biddle, 2000). Biological measures may also increase the accuracy of self-report by serving as a "bogus pipeline," that is, individuals are more likely to provide accurate drinking or drug use data if they believe that the information will be corroborated by other measures such as laboratory tests. Two markers of recent heavy drinking are gamma glutamyl transpeptidase (GGTP) and carbohydrate deficient transferin (CDT). Hair analysis is also a useful means for verifying self-report, even for heavy drinking (Morini & Polettini, 2009). Such tests are not a replacement for self-report, however. By themselves, laboratory tests have low sensitivity (high false negatives), identifying only 10–30% of problem drinkers (Anton, Lieber, Tabakoff, & CDTect Study Group, 2002; Babor & Higgins-Biddle, 2000). Further, GGTP and CDT levels are significantly affected by age, gender, and smoking status, and GGTP is heavily influenced by liver disease and medication use. Similar problems have been found in assessing drug use. Urine screens for cocaine, opiates, and amphetamines have only a 2–3 day window for detection, and more than a week window for heavy marijuana use (Anton, Litten, & Allen, 1995). The urine screen is strongly influenced by the individual's metabolism, use of legally prescribed drugs, how the drug was taken (injection or orally), and its potency (Connors, Donovan, et al., 2001). False negatives are common. For all these reasons, it is recommended that lab tests serve mainly as adjunctive aids in screening for harmful substance use; that they only be used in combination with standardized screening devices, clinical interviews, and collateral reports; and that they be employed mainly when self-reports are considered to be suspect (Anton et al., 2002; Babor & Higgins-Biddle, 2000).

Subtle Tests

> Subtle screening scales don't work any better than simpler, more direct, free scales.

In response to concerns about honesty, many attempts have been made since the 1950s to develop subtle or indirect screening instruments that detect possible substance use disorders despite respondents' denial and fabrication. Such indirect scales have typically included items that bear no obvious relationship to alcohol/drug problems, but are purported to have high sensitivity and specificity even in the face of intentional dishonesty. A short summary of decades of research on indirect scales is that they don't work any better than simpler, more direct, and free public domain scales that ask about alcohol/drug use, such as those described above (Feldstein & Miller, 2007; Miller, 1976).

EVALUATING ADDICTION PROBLEMS

Screening casts a wide net to identify a broad range of people with substance use problems. Diagnosis, as discussed below, identifies a subset of these people who fall above a certain level of severity. Neither screening nor diagnosis, however, provides much information about what is actually happening in a particular person's life and substance use, why problems are emerging, and what treatment options would be most appropriate to try. These tasks—to understand the nature and causes of the individual's particular situation and to consider possible routes to change—lie at the heart of evaluation. A more comprehensive evaluation of this kind generates working hypotheses about what is most likely to help, and what concerns may need priority attention. This in turn yields information to formulate change goals and treatment plans (see Chapter 7).

Conducting a Multidimensional Evaluation

Addictions, like diamonds, have multiple facets. Knowing about one dimension may tell you surprisingly little about the others. For example, the amount and pattern of substance use is only modestly correlated with the extent of negative health and social consequences or the person's level of substance dependence. There are also important contextual factors to consider. What events or conditions are most likely to interfere with establishing and maintaining sobriety? How does the person's substance use relate to and affect his or her employment, family, social networks, emotional states, and stressors? What resources does the person have in terms of coping skills, personal strengths, and social support? What motivates this person; what does he or she care about?

Obviously such a thorough evaluation can take some time, and we do not encourage thinking of evaluation as a prerequisite to treatment. Being asked questions is of very limited value from a client's perspective (after all, the client already knows all this), and we think it is important to provide something useful and heartening quite soon in consultation. Early dropout is common in addiction treatment, and it is important to provide

> Think of treatment as beginning with the very first contact.

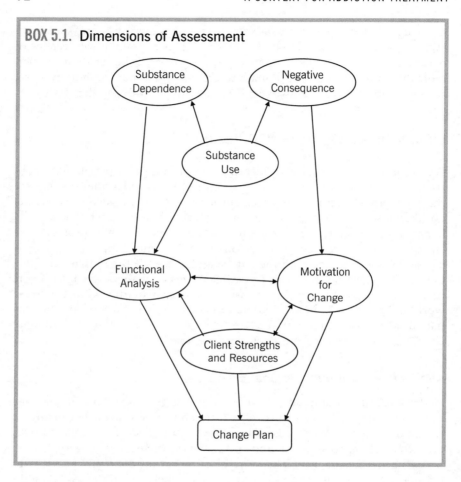

BOX 5.1. Dimensions of Assessment

something useful in the very first contact, just in case the person never returns. Doing so, of course, makes it more likely that a client *will* return. We encourage you to think of treatment as beginning with the very first contact ("intake"), and to consider evaluation and treatment as interweaving rather than sequential processes. What do you really *have* to know during the first session? Evaluation can be completed in pieces, and indeed as treatment proceeds it becomes clearer what you need to know next.

With that said, we discuss four broad domains for evaluation that encompass seven dimensions of addiction discussed in Chapter 2, areas in which to gather information over time during the process of treatment: (1) nature and severity of substance use and problems, (2) motivation for change, (3) client strengths and resources, and (4) functional analysis.

Nature and Severity of Substance Use and Problems

SUBSTANCE USE

One obvious domain to assess in addiction treatment is substance use. What drug(s) has the person been using during the past few months? How were the drugs taken (orally, intravenously, etc.), how much how often, and what is the pattern (e.g., steady maintenance, periodic binge use). This can quickly devolve into a very long series of closed questions, which is not an optimal way to establish rapport and engage the client (see Chapter 4). A simple start is to ask clients to tell you about what they have been using, how, and how often (an open question), and then listen.

If more detail is truly needed, there are some structured interview formats to make sure you cover all the possibilities. These include the above-mentioned ASSIST instrument (WHO ASSIST Working Group, 2002) and the Form-90 interviews (Miller, 1996a; Tonigan, Miller, & Brown, 1994; Westerberg, Tonigan, & Miller, 1998), both available free of charge in the public domain. They survey patterns of use for a dozen drug categories. The Form 90 uses a modified time line follow-back method (Sobell & Sobell, 1992, 1996), reconstructing drug use across a 90-day calendar.

NEGATIVE CONSEQUENCES

One indication of the severity of addiction is the extent to which substance use has caused adverse consequences in the person's life and family. The Drinker Inventory of Consequences (DrInC; Forcehimes, Tonigan, Miller, Kenna, & Baer, 2007; Miller, Tonigan, & Longabaugh, 1995) was designed as a relatively pure measure of alcohol-related problems. It is in the public domain, easily administered in paper-and-pencil form, and covers five problems areas: physical, social responsibility, intrapersonal, impulse control, and interpersonal. Scores derived on the measure can be placed along a continuum of severity. The parallel Inventory of Drug Use Consequences (InDUC; Tonigan & Miller, 2002) assesses negative consequences of alcohol/drug use more generally. These instruments can be motivationally useful as well, because they connect drinking and drug use with current problems and hassles that the client might want to change (Maisto & McKay, 1995).

The Addiction Severity Index (ASI; McLellan, Kushner, Metzger, & Peters, 1992; McLellan et al., 1990) is a psychometrically sound, multidimensional public domain interview examining severity of problems in five different areas that may be affected by alcohol or drug abuse: medical, employment, legal, family relations, and psychiatric. Clients' perceptions of problem severity along with interviewers' perceptions of severity are rated for each of the five areas. Interviewers typically require special training in the ASI to obtain valid information. A commercial computer-administered version of the ASI is also available (Butler et al., 2001). Along with motivational feedback, the ASI can be useful to develop a treatment plan specifically targeting problem areas that abstinence alone may not resolve. Clients who receive additional services to address these troublesome areas fare better than those who do not (McLellan et al., 1997, 1999).

SUBSTANCE DEPENDENCE

Another indication of severity is the extent to which clients have developed behavioral or/or physiological dependence on their preferred drugs. The potential for withdrawal syndrome and need for supervised detoxification is one important issue for clients who use dependence-producing drugs (see Chapter 6). The broader behavioral spectrum of substance dependence outlined in the DSM-IV (American Psychiatric Association, 1994) has been well validated and is reliably measurable (e.g., Skinner & Horn, 1984; Stockwell, Sitarthan, McGrath, & Lang, 1994).

Motivation for Change

A second important domain is the client's current motivation for change in substance use. Motivation is one of the more consistent predictors of how clients will perform in addiction treatment. Higher levels of motivation have been found to be associated with better adherence rates and more favorable outcomes in several addiction treatment trials (Burke, Arkowitz, & Dunn, 2002; Donovan & Rosengren, 1999; Litt, Kadden, Cooney, & Kabela, 2003; Zweben & Zuckoff, 2002). Again this dimension can become apparent within a clinical interview, which can include a structured question such as: "On a 0–10 scale, how important would you say it is for you to make a change in your _____ use?"

Public domain questionnaires assessing motivation are also available for clients to complete in or between sessions. Some of these are open-ended, and can be applied to any particular behavior change. The original "stages of change" measure is the University of Rhode Island Change Assessment (URICA; Abellanas & McLellan, 1993; DiClemente & Hughes, 1990). The URICA has good reliability and predictive validity with alcohol clients (Carbonari & DiClemente, 2000; DiClemente, Doyle, & Donovan, 2009; Prochaska & DiClemente, 1992). Items refer to problems generically but can be focused specifically toward substance use. Various subscales were developed by clustering items reflecting the four stages of change (i.e., precontemplation, contemplation, action, and maintenance). Individuals are categorized as being in a particular stage of change based on receiving a higher score on a specific subscale. Research has supported the clustering of items in accordance with the four subscales in an addiction population (Connors, Donovan, et al., 2001; Donovan, 1995). For clinicians limited by

BOX 5.2. Personal Reflection: How Useful Is Assessment?

I must admit that I am rather ambivalent about assessment. I have personally devoted countless hours to developing and evaluating clinical assessment scales for the addiction treatment field. I know well how challenging it is to measure things reliably, even substance use itself. And there is something satisfying about having clear objective numbers that allow us to compare a unique individual with broader norms or to measure a degree of change. When I go for a health checkup, my vital signs and lab tests are checked against norms and my past values to see if any of my aging functions are going astray. Somehow that feels more solid than my doctor just looking me over and pronouncing me healthy or not. Reliable measures are also among the tools of clinical science, without which most of the research on which this book is based would not have been possible.

But I also share Carl Rogers's healthy skepticism about the value of all this measuring of human beings. When we have asked a lot of questions and taken some measures, we can feel like we have *done* something, although our clients may not share that confidence. Questions can get in the way of listening, of understanding, of really engaging with our clients. In a treatment program that I directed, the intake process had consisted of about 4 hours of questions before a person ever got to see a counselor. I asked how much we really needed to know in order to get paid for a first session, and it turned out to be about 20 minutes' worth of information. So I had our most senior counselors, rather than clerks, be the first people a new client would see, and I told them to start with this statement: "After a while I'm going to ask you some questions that we need to ask everyone, but right now I just want to know why you're here, what's happening in your life, and what you hope we might be able to do for you." They spent 30 minutes hearing the client's story, using good reflective listening skills, and when the half hour came and it was time to ask our standard questions, they found that they already knew the answers to most of them. Our retention rate went way up; we didn't have so many people drop out during those first visits; and the clients often wanted very much to stay with the counselor who did their intake. They had engaged from the very first session because someone listened to them. Relatively simple systemic changes like this can significantly decrease no-shows and dropouts, reduce waiting lists, and enhance engagement in treatment (Rukowski et al., 2010).

—W. R. M.

time constraints, a shorter 12-item form of the URICA is available (Connors, Donovan, et al., 2001; downloadable from *www.umbc.edu/psyc/habits/content/ttm_measures/index.html*).

A more recent 12-item instrument, the Change Questionnaire, was based on the natural language of motivation for change (Miller & Johnson, 2008). A factor analysis yielded three items (on a 0–10 disagree–agree scale) that accounted for 81% of variance, and that can be incorporated in a clinical interview:

Importance: "It is important for me to _____."
Ability: "I could _____."
Commitment: "I am trying to _____."

Other public domain instruments specifically measure motivation for change in substance use. These include the 12-item Readiness to Change Questionnaire (Rollnick, Heather, Gold, & Hall, 1992) and the 19-item Stages of Change Readiness and Treatment Eagerness Scale (SOCRATES; Miller & Tonigan, 1996).

Another important aspect of motivation is the client's reasons for continuing drug use, which essentially work against change (Brown, Goldman, Inn, & Anderson, 1980; Goldman et al., 1999). In a clinical interview you can simply ask a client, "What do you like about using _____? What does it do for you?" (Miller & Pechacek, 1987). There are also psychometrically sound questionnaires to measure expectancies, particularly regarding alcohol use. The original of these is the Alcohol Expectancy Questionnaire (AEQ; Brown et al., 1987). It contains 90 items designed to assess several dimensions of alcohol-related expectancies. The AEQ has been employed with both help-seeking and non-help-seeking diverse populations and has good psychometric properties (Donovan, 1995). Several adaptations of the scale have added negative as well as positive expectancies (Connors & Maisto, 1988; Fromme, Stroot, & Kaplan, 1993; George et al., 1995; Jones, Corbin, & Fromme, 2001; Rohsenow, 1983).

Client Strengths and Resources

The context of addiction treatment easily lends itself to assessing people's deficits and shortcomings, but there are good reasons also to assess and affirm clients' strengths as well as the social supports that favor change (Corcoran, 2004; Lawrence & Sovik-Johnston, 2010; Rapp, 2002). Exploring these is vital. Most people who recover from addictions do so on their own, without ever seeking treatment. Whatever time you spend with a client is but a small sliver of that person's life. Mobilizing clients' own strengths and social supports is important not only in rehabilitation, but in maintenance as well. Exploring strengths can also bolster clients' self-efficacy, which is a predictor of successful change, and build a working therapeutic alliance.

PERSONAL STRENGTHS

As with all of the topics in this chapter, you can explore clients' strengths as part of normal conversation in clinical sessions. What does this client have going for him or her that can be an asset in changing? What successful changes has this person made in the past? What social support and resources are there to accompany this client on the road to sobriety? What are the values that guide this person's life? What does she or he most want, hope for, envision as a future?

If a little structure helps here, consider using the "Characteristics of Successful Changers" (see Box 5.3), one of many resources from the public domain Combined Behavioral Intervention (Miller, 2004). It is an arbitrary list of 100 positive traits that people may have. Showing this list to a client, ask, "Which of these words best describe you? Which ones are most true of you?" When the client chooses particular adjectives, you can explore "In what way does this describe you?" "Give me an example of when you have been _____," and so on. Listen, reflect, and affirm (Chapter 4).

BOX 5.3. Some Characteristics of Successful Changers

Accepting	Committed	Flexible	Persevering	Stubborn
Active	Competent	Focused	Persistent	Thankful
Adaptable	Concerned	Forgiving	Positive	Thorough
Adventuresome	Confident	Forward-looking	Powerful	Thoughtful
Affectionate	Considerate	Free	Prayerful	Tough
Affirmative	Courageous	Happy	Quick	Trusting
Alert	Creative	Healthy	Reasonable	Trustworthy
Alive	Decisive	Hopeful	Receptive	Truthful
Ambitious	Dedicated	Imaginative	Relaxed	Understanding
Anchored	Determined	Ingenious	Reliable	Unique
Assertive	Diehard	Intelligent	Resourceful	Unstoppable
Assured	Diligent	Knowledgeable	Responsible	Vigorous
Attentive	Doer	Loving	Sensible	Visionary
Bold	Eager	Mature	Skillful	Whole
Brave	Earnest	Open	Solid	Willing
Bright	Effective	Optimistic	Spiritual	Winning
Capable	Energetic	Orderly	Stable	Wise
Careful	Experienced	Organized	Steady	Worthy
Cheerful	Faithful	Patient	Straight	Zealous
Clever	Fearless	Perceptive	Strong	Zestful

From Miller (2004). This material is in the public domain and may be reproduced without further permission. Purchasers may download a larger version of this material from *www.guilford.com/p/miller11*.

Another motivational asset is self-efficacy, a client's belief that he or she is capable of making a particular change (Bandura, 1997). One common way to strengthen this sense of self-efficacy is to explore changes that clients have made successfully in the past. What was the change? How did they do it? What obstacles did they encounter and how did they overcome those? You can tie these into characteristic strengths identified in the "successful changers" method described above. The Abstinence Self-Efficacy scale (DiClemente, Carbonari, Montgomery, & Hughes, 1994), originally focused on alcohol use, describes a variety of situations in which a client may feel able (or less able) to abstain, based on factors originally identified by Marlatt (1996; Marlatt & Donovan, 2005). From this scale you can identify potential situations in which a client feels more confident of being able to refrain from use, and explore how he or she would cope with such situations. Other scales directly assess coping skills and styles (Litman, 1986) that predict maintenance of sobriety (Miller, Westerberg, Harris, & Tonigan, 1996). The Coping Resources Inventory (CRI; Moos, 1993) is a useful measure in evaluating how persons handle stress. It takes about 10 minutes to complete and assesses cognitive, emotional, social, spiritual, and physical components of stress reduction.

SOCIAL SUPPORT

Another potentially important resource is a client's social support system. Including a supportive significant other in treatment tends to improve treatment outcome (see Chapter 13). Who is there in the client's social networks—family, friends, coworkers, support from religious communities and mutual help groups (Zweben, Rose, Stout, & Zywiak, 2003)? The extent to which these people actively support the client's sobriety (vs. favoring continued use) predicts stability of sobriety (Longabaugh, Wirtz, Zweben, & Stout, 2001; Longabaugh, Wirtz, Zweben, & Stout, 1998). The support system can play a valuable role in enhancing treatment engagement and adherence, buttressing motivation and, more important, offering alternatives to a lifestyle of drinking or drug use such as in the AA/NA fellowship (Tonigan, 2001; Tonigan, Connors, & Miller, 2003; Zweben et al., 2003).

The Important People and Activities (IPA) interview (Longabaugh, Beattie, Noel, Stout, & Malloy, 1993) was constructed specifically to measure network support for drinking (in contrast to general social support). Clients are asked to identify people in their social network and rate them on the following: (1) their importance to the client, (2) their response to the client's drinking, and (3) their own drinking behavior. A summary index of network support for abstinence is obtained, and has been found to predict better outcomes at both the 1-year and 3-year follow-ups (Babor

& Del Boca, 2003; Longabaugh, Wirtz, et al., 2001). A shortened form that focuses only on supportive people (and not activities) is also available (COMBINE Study Research Group, 2003).

Functional Analysis of Substance Use

People use alcohol and other drugs for good reasons. It is not for naught that substance use persists despite adverse consequences. A functional analysis seeks to understand what roles or functions substance use is playing in the person's life (Meyers & Smith, 1995; Miller & Pechacek, 1987). It focuses both on *antecedents* (triggers or stimuli that increase the likelihood of use) and *consequences* of substance use (which may reinforce it). These can be explored in a structured interview (Miller & Pechacek, 1987; see Chapter 11), by having clients keep self-monitoring records of use (Miller & Muñoz, 2005), or via self-report questionnaires.

Several questionnaires have been used to identify situations that pose particular risk of return to substance use. The Inventory of Drinking Situations (IDS; Annis, Graham, & Davis, 1987) and the Inventory of Drug Taking Situations (IDTS; Annis & Graham, 1991) cover eight types of potential high-risk situations, again based on the work of Alan Marlatt (1996): unpleasant emotions, pleasant emotions, physical discomfort, testing personal control, urges and temptations, conflict with others, social pressure, and pleasant times. Clients are asked to rate the frequency of drinking or drug use in these situations. A client profile is created identifying areas that pose the greatest and least risk for relapse. Simpler scales (12 or 20 items) that are available free of charge are the Situation Temptation Scales that have three subscales: negative affect, social/positive use, and cravings/habitual use. The underlying assumption with these scales is that there is a causal link between prior use and the likelihood of a recurrence of drinking or drug use in these situations (Donovan, 1999). Individualized risk profiles can inform treatment plans to identify and address high-risk situations (Kadden et al., 1992; Monti, Abrams, Kadden, & Cooney, 1989; Monti et al., 2002; see Chapter 12), particularly when risk level varies across situations (Annis & Graham, 1991).

The Situational Confidence Questionnaire (SCQ; Annis & Graham, 1988) is a companion instrument querying clients' perceptions of their ability to deal with high-risk situations without resorting to substance use (i.e., level of self-efficacy). The situations parallel those contained in the IDS. A client profile is again generated based on levels of client self-efficacy in potential high-risk situations. As with the IDS, profiles on the SCQ can inform treatment goals and strategies. The underlying strategy here is that increased levels of self-efficacy lead to better outcomes (Solomon & Annis, 1990).

It should be noted that the risk or coping situations identified on the aforementioned instruments may not always be pertinent to a particular client's circumstances. The predetermined risk situations described on these questionnaires may not capture an individual's own "slippery slopes." It is therefore useful to invite clients completing these measures to also choose their own high-risk/coping situations (Connors, Donovan, et al., 2001). "What situations were most problematic for you during the past year? How confident are you now in handling these same events?" This can increase the clinical relevance of the process to individual clients.

Assessing all four areas (nature and severity of substance use and problems, motivation for change, personal strengths and resources, and functional analysis of substance use) can help you understand the interrelationships between these different areas and form working hypotheses about what action steps are needed for the client to accomplish and sustain change. Such assessment information can also be used as feedback for your clients to promote motivation for change, increase awareness of risk situations that pose the obstacles to sobriety, and identify targeted strategies for reaching identified change goals. The development of a change plan is a negotiated process, of course, informed by what clients expect, prefer, need, and are willing to do. Box 5.4 lists instruments we recommended above for screening and for each of the four evaluation areas, along with current website sources. Recognizing practical obstacles (such as heavy caseloads and cost) when conducting evaluations in real-world clinical settings, we have emphasized shorter instruments and those available free of charge.

DIAGNOSING ADDICTION PROBLEMS

The purpose of screening is to determine whether further evaluation is warranted. Evaluation is an ongoing process that begins with the first contact, to provide whatever information is needed as treatment proceeds. Diagnosis has a different purpose from both screening and evaluation (Miller, Westerberg, & Waldron, 2003). In etymology, *diagnosis* literally means to know the difference, to recognize patterns that constitute identifiable diseases or conditions. In current practice, as discussed in Chapter 2, diagnosis involves determining whether a person currently meets predetermined criteria for having a particular condition, which in turn may influence eligibility for treatment. Third-party payers typically require a diagnosis as a precondition for reimbursement. A diagnosis is meant to establish the seriousness of a condition and, ideally, suggest what treatments might be most appropriate. However, because most disorders listed in the DSM are not linked to particular etiology, diagnosis alone does not determine how to proceed with treatment.

BOX 5.4. Some Recommended Instruments for Screening and Multidimensional Evaluation

Purpose	Recommended Instruments (Choose those most appropriate to your setting.)
Screening	• Alcohol Use Disorders Identification Test (AUDIT)* *whqlibdoc.who.int/hq/2001/who_msd_msb_01.6a.pdf* • NM-ASSIST* *www.drugabuse.gov/nidamed/screening/nmassist.pdf* • Drug Use Disorders Identification Test (DUDIT)* *www.penalreform.ro/fileadmin/pri/projects/documente/DUDITManual.pdf* • Michigan Alcoholism Screening Test (MAST)* *www.ncadd-sfv.org/symptoms/mast_test.html* • RAPS4* *alcoholism.about.com/od/tests/a/raps.htm*
Nature and severity of substance use and problems	• Addiction Severity Index (ASI)* *www.tresearch.org/resources/instruments.htm#top* • Alcohol Dependence Scale *chipts.cch.ucla.edu/assessment/IB/List_Scales/ADS-Scale.htm* • Drinker Inventory of Consequences (DrInC)* *casaa.unm.edu/inst.html* • Inventory of Drug Use Consequences (InDUC)* *casaa.unm.edu/inst.html* • Severity of Alcohol Dependence Questionnaire (SADQ)* *www.markjayalcoholdetox.co.uk/wiki/sadq.php*
Clients' personal strengths and resources	• Abstinence Self-Efficacy Scale* *www.umbc.edu/psyc//habits/content/ttm_measures/self-efficacy/index.html* • Important People Interview (IPI)* *casaa.unm.edu/inat/Important%20People%20Initial%20Interview.pdf* • Coping Responses Inventory (CRI) *www4.parinc.com/Products/Product.aspx?ProductID=CRI*
Functional analysis of substance use (and high-risk situations)	• Alcohol Expectancy Questionnaire** • Situational Temptation Scales* *www.umbc.edu/psyc//habits/content/ttm_measures/situation/index.html* • Desired Effects of Drinking* *casaa.unm/inst/Desired%20Effects%20of%20Drinking.pdf*

(cont.)

BOX 5.4. *(cont.)*

Purpose	Recommended Instruments (Choose those most appropriate to your setting.)
Motivation for change	• *University of Rhode Island Change Assessment (URICA)* *www.umbc.edu/psyc//habits/content/ttm_measures/urica/index.html* • Stages of Change Readiness and Treatment Eagerness Scale (SOCRATES)* *casaa.unm.edu/inst.html* • Change Questionnaire* casaa.unm.edu/inst.html • Readiness to Change Questionnaire* *www.ncbi.nlm.nih.gov/pubmed/1591525*

*Instruments available free of charge.
**Request in writing to Sandra Brown, PhD, 9500 Gilman Drive (0109), San Diego, CA 92093-0109.

Making a Diagnosis

Two similar classification systems are most commonly used for diagnosing substance use disorders (Hasin, Hartzenbuehler, Keyes, & Ogburn, 2006). One is the DSM of the American Psychiatric Association. International diagnostic practices tend to follow the ICD of the World Health Organization. Both of these systems are updated periodically, and the DSM-5 and ICD-11 are anticipated for release within 5 years.

As described in Chapter 2, diagnostic conceptions and criteria have changed markedly over time. In DSM-IV, substance abuse and substance dependence were separate diagnoses. In DSM-5, this distinction is expected to be removed in favor of a single diagnosis of a substance use disorder, further specifying level of severity (based on the number of criteria met), presence or absence of physiological dependence, and levels of remission. As with screening measures, a somewhat arbitrary severity cutoff point is specified for individuals to meet criteria for diagnosis.

The most common approach to diagnosis is through a clinical interview comparing an individual's current symptoms with the specified criteria (Hersen & Turner, 2003). Where greater precision and reliability are required, structured interview procedures have been developed, the most common of which are the Structured Clinical Interview for DSM (SCID; First, Spitzer, Gibbon, & Williams, 1997) and the Diagnostic Interview Schedule (DIS; Aktan, Calkins, Ribisl, Kroliczak, & Kasim, 1997; Grant et al., 2003). Specialized training is required for reliable use of these structured diagnostic interviews. A computer-administered version of the DIS is also available (Robins et al., 2000; *epi.wustl.edu/dis/Dishome.htm*).

KEY POINTS

🖈 Screening for addictions is appropriate when working with a diverse client population, to identify those for whom additional evaluation is warranted.

🖈 Screening instruments do not establish a diagnosis. Diagnosis determines whether an individual meets certain preestablished criteria for a disorder.

🖈 Evaluation is a process that occurs over time, not merely a prelude to treatment.

🖈 Four broad domains for evaluation are (1) the nature and severity of substance use and problems, (2) motivation for change, (3) client strengths and resources, and (4) a functional analysis of substance use.

🖈 There is a wide array of instruments with documented reliability and validity, many of which are available free of charge in the public domain. It is unwise to develop homemade assessment instruments when evidence-based options are available.

REFLECTION QUESTIONS

💬 If you work in a setting where a wide variety of people seek services, how might routine screening for alcohol/drug problems be implemented?

💬 What assessment measures do you currently use in your own practice, and why? What do you know about their reliability and validity?

💬 What information do you really need in order to begin treatment?

CHAPTER 6

Detoxification and Health Care Needs

The process of physiological dependence involves the body adjusting to drug use so that it can function more normally when the drug is present. Discontinuation of the drug triggers a complementary adjustment process known as a "withdrawal" or "abstinence syndrome." In Chapter 2 we discussed this rebound effect that is opposite to the effects of the intoxication. For example, heroin use produces euphoria and decreases anxiety, and the withdrawal from heroin typically produces the opposite symptoms of *dys*phoria and *increased* anxiety.

Detoxification is the process of removing toxins from the body, readjusting normal function to the absence of the drug. Intoxicated people may be seen in an emergency department or medical clinic seeking palliative care. Detoxification is also offered to stabilize patients in preparation for addiction treatment (see Chapter 7).

Depending on your employment setting, working with individuals who are going through detoxification may be something you do a lot or a little. However, even if you aren't working in a medical setting or a detoxification setting, it is still a good idea to know what drug withdrawal is and what it looks like. For instance, while working with a client who is seeing you for outpatient treatment, the client might tell you that he or she returned to using a substance a few times a day and is now afraid of stopping because of fear of what the withdrawal will be like. Clients might also ask you what withdrawal from a particular substance will feel like, in order to know what to expect. For these reasons, it is a good idea to have a working knowledge of what someone should expect during the detoxification process and to be able to assess the potential seriousness of the withdrawal. The particular interventions used in the detoxification process are determined by the type(s) and amount of drug the person has been using, the person's history of withdrawal, and his or her other current psychosocial and medical needs. The goal of detoxification is to manage symptoms and minimize physical risk or harm during the withdrawal process. Detoxification does not constitute addiction treatment in itself; rather it is a preparation for rehabilitation and maintenance (see Chapter 7). There are three main tasks in the detoxification process: evaluation, stabilization, and transition into treatment (N. S. Miller & Kipnis, 2006).

> Detoxification does not constitute addiction treatment in itself; rather it is a preparation for rehabilitation and maintenance.

EVALUATION

A first step in detoxification is to evaluate what drugs are in the person's body and screen for possible medical and psychiatric conditions that could complicate withdrawal. In addition to the person's self-report, lab tests of blood or urine tests may be used to identify drugs that are present. It is helpful to establish good rapport as quickly as possible in order to foster honesty and cooperation.

Several important decisions are made during the evaluation process. One is the appropriate level of care. The vast majority of detoxification efforts can be done safely in outpatient care (Abbott, Quinn, & Knox, 1995). However, other factors such as homelessness, suicidality, or medical complications may increase the need for residential care and medical supervision. Another decision is whether to use medications to help patients through the withdrawal process. This is determined in part by the person's presenting symptoms, history of past withdrawal, and the substance(s) the person has been using. For example, there are particular medical safety issues involved in withdrawal from alcohol and sedative–hypnotic drugs, depending on severity of dependence.

Some practical guidelines have been developed by the American Society of Addiction Medicine (ASAM, 2001) for deciding an appropriate level of care during detoxification. Individuals are evaluated on six dimensions: (1) acute intoxication or withdrawal potential; (2) biomedical conditions and complications; (3) emotional, behavioral, or cognitive conditions and complications; (4) readiness to change; (5) relapse, continued use, or continued problem potential; and (6) recovery/living environment. The ASAM criteria include five different contexts for detoxification:

Level I-D: Ambulatory detoxification without extended onsite monitoring

Level II-D: Ambulatory detoxification with extended onsite monitoring

---

BOX 6.1. Personal Reflection: Necessity Breeds Discovery

In the early 1980s, the Reagan administration developed the "block grants" program that transferred funding of addiction treatment programs from the federal to the state level. This seemed a good idea, in that individual states would be more likely to understand local needs, and of course there was excitement to have this new stream of funding under state control. What was not so immediately evident, however, was that the total amount of funding provided was being cut in half. The result was a sudden shortage of funding for public programs.

The University of New Mexico at the time was operating two large public treatment programs for substance use disorders. One was a residential 28-day detoxification and rehabilitation center that treated a few hundred people per year. The other was an outpatient treatment facility that served a few thousand people annually. The two programs had similar budgets, and funding was reduced by half. Which one would we close? The answer seemed fairly clear, particularly in that research was already showing similar overall outcomes from inpatient and outpatient treatment (Miller & Hester, 1986).

We were concerned, though, because we had been accustomed to handling detoxification through the inpatient unit, and there were now no beds for this purpose except for emergency hospital beds. How would we handle severe alcohol withdrawal and complex detoxification from multiple drug use? Could more severely dependent clients really be treated on an outpatient basis? For all but the affluent, we had no choice but to find out. What we found was the same thing being discovered across the country: that detoxification (in our case, with good medical supervision) was safe and effective on an outpatient day treatment basis for 99% of our patients, and we had no untoward outcomes (cf. Day & Strang, 2011). In fact, we tended to hospitalize only those patients who required inpatient treatment for some *other* reason in addition to detoxification (such as suicidality or severe medical illness). People who would otherwise be sitting in an inpatient detox bed instead came to the clinic each day for observation and medication as needed, until they were safely through the withdrawal process. This also eased their transition into treatment at the same clinic. We changed because we had to, and in the process discovered that we could serve more people at lower cost without compromising quality of care.

—W. R. M.

Level II.2-D: Clinically managed residential detoxification
Level III.7-D: Medically monitored inpatient detoxification
Level IV-D: Medically managed intensive inpatient detoxification

Some practical questions to help guide this decision include:

What is the person's history regarding the amount and duration of substance use?

How long ago was the last use of each substance?

When was the last time the person went for a few days without using? What happened?

Does the person have a history of delirium tremens or withdrawal seizures?

Is the person taking anything else that might affect his or her withdrawal symptoms?

BOX 6.2. Using the ASAM Criteria

Josephine is a 17-year-old female brought into the emergency department (ED) after her mother called the police. Earlier in the evening, Josephine had gotten into an argument with her father and attempted to throw a knife at him. There was some indication that she was under the influence of substances at the time, and her parents feel like she has been making many bad decisions lately, including hanging out with a "dangerous" crowd and staying out past her curfew. Josephine hasn't been in addiction treatment in the past and told the psychiatric team that she had used alcohol, cocaine, and marijuana several times per week over the past few weeks, including using alcohol and cocaine a few hours prior to her ED visit, but does not show signs of physical withdrawal. She said that she was able to go 3 days without using when she attended a family reunion out of town. Both of Josephine's parents are present in the ED, but Josephine is refusing to speak with them and says that she never wants to return home again.

Josephine is evaluated on the following six clinical dimensions:

1. **Acute intoxication or withdrawal potential:** Though she was intoxicated at home prior to the knife-throwing incident and uses frequently, she is no longer acutely intoxicated and has not been using substances in large enough quantities to suggest complicated withdrawal.
2. **Biomedical conditions and complications:** She is physically healthy and has no current medical complaints.
3. **Emotional, behavioral, or cognitive conditions and complications:** Problems with family discord and anger.
4. **Readiness to change:** Josephine is willing to talk to a clinician. She is angry with her parents for not trusting her. She agrees to treatment, but doesn't want to be at home at least for the next few nights.
5. **Relapse, continued use, or continued problem potential:** High probability that if she returns home tonight, there will be fighting and possibly violence again.
6. **Recovery/living environment:** Josephine's parents are also frustrated with her. They want her in the hospital to reduce the fighting.

Based on the ASAM levels, what context for detoxification do you think would be the best fit for Josephine? Why?

Is there any medical or psychiatric comorbidity (hallucinations, traumatic brain injury)?

Is there any risk of harm to self or others?

Is there any risk of violence at home?

Can the person understand and carry out routine medical instructions?

Does the person have reliable transportation?

Does the person have a supportive person to assist with detoxification?

Screening for Likelihood of Complicated Withdrawal

There are several instruments that can be used to screen for the probability of complicated withdrawal. If you are not a medical prescriber, your main role in this part of evaluation may be to refer people for appropriate medical consultation. Nevertheless, it is important to know some basic information about the withdrawal process, what to expect, and the potential seriousness of withdrawal and complications. Monitoring for signs of withdrawal, such as changes in mental status, hallucinations, seizures, fever, and abdominal pain (Kosten & O'Connor, 2003), can also be part of a multidisciplinary approach to patient care. Such signs and symptoms require immediate medical attention.

Alcohol

There is an advantage to using a validated instrument such as the Clinical Institute Withdrawal Assessment for Alcohol Scale, Revised (CIWA-Ar; Sullivan, Sykora, Schneiderman, Naranjo, & Sellers, 1989) It takes just a few minutes to administer and helps to make the decision about the person's level of need for medical supervision. The CIWA-Ar (Box 6.3) is a public domain instrument that measures 10 subjective signs and symptoms of alcohol withdrawal: nausea, tremor, autonomic hyperactivity, anxiety, agitation, tactile, visual disturbances, auditory disturbances, headache, and disorientation. The CIWA-Ar should be repeated at regular intervals (every 1–2 hours initially) to monitor the client's progress and changes in withdrawal symptoms. People who score less than 10 usually do not need medication for withdrawal.

Cocaine

The Cocaine Selective Severity Assessment (CSSA; Kampman et al., 1998) is an 18-item scale that reliably measures cocaine withdrawal signs and symptoms (see Box 6.4). High scores on the CSSA are correlated with poor outcome (Kampman et al., 1998). The scale is designed to be adminis-

BOX 6.3. Clinical Institute Withdrawal Assessment for Alcohol Scale, Revised (CIWA-Ar)

Patient: _____ **Date:** _____ **Time:** _____

Pulse or heart rate, taken for one minute: _____ **Blood pressure:** _____

NAUSEA AND VOMITING—Ask "Do you feel sick to your stomach? Have you vomited?" Observation.

0 no nausea and no vomiting
1 mild nausea with no vomiting
2
3
4 intermittent nausea with dry heaves
5
6
7 constant nausea, frequent dry heaves, and vomiting

TACTILE DISTURBANCES—Ask "Have you any itching, pins-and-needles sensations, any burning, any numbness, or do you feel bugs crawling on or under your skin?" Observation.

0 none
1 very mild itching, pins and needles, burning or numbness
2 mild itching, pins and needles, burning or numbness
3 moderate itching, pins and needles, burning or numbness
4 moderately severe hallucinations
5 severe hallucinations
6 extremely severe hallucinations
7 continuous hallucinations

TREMOR—Arms extended and fingers spread apart. Observation.

0 no tremor
1 not visible, but can be felt fingertip to fingertip
2
3
4 moderate, with patient's arms extended
5
6
7 severe, even with arms not extended

AUDITORY DISTURBANCES—Ask "Are you more aware of sounds around you? Are they harsh? Do they frighten you? Are you hearing anything that is disturbing to you? Are you hearing things you know are not there?" Observation.

0 not present
1 very mild harshness or ability to frighten
2 mild harshness or ability to frighten
3 moderate harshness or ability to frighten
4 moderately severe hallucinations
5 severe hallucinations
6 extremely severe hallucinations
7 continuous hallucinations

PAROXYSMAL SWEATS— Observation.

0 no sweat visible
1 barely perceptible sweating, palms moist

(cont.)

From Sullivan, Sykora, Schneiderman, Naranjo, and Sellers (1989). This scale is in the public domain and may be reproduced without further permission.

BOX 6.3. *(cont.)*

2
3
4 beads of sweat obvious on forehead
5
6
7 drenching sweats

VISUAL DISTURBANCES—Ask "Does the light appear to be too bright? Is its color different? Does it hurt your eyes? Are you seeing anything that is disturbing to you? Are you seeing things you know are not there?" Observation.

0 not present
1 very mild sensitivity
2 mild sensitivity
3 moderate sensitivity
4 moderately severe hallucinations
5 severe hallucinations
6 extremely severe hallucinations
7 continuous hallucinations

ANXIETY—Ask "Do you feel nervous?" Observation.

0 no anxiety, at ease
1 mildly anxious
2
3
4 moderately anxious, or guarded, so anxiety is inferred
5
6
7 equivalent to acute panic states as seen in severe delirium or acute schizophrenic reactions

HEADACHE, FULLNESS IN HEAD—Ask "Does your head feel different? Does it feel like there is a band around your head?" Do not rate for dizziness or lightheadedness. Otherwise, rate severity.

0 not present
1 very mild
2 mild
3 moderate
4 moderately severe
5 severe
6 very severe
7 extremely severe

AGITATION—Observation.

0 normal activity
1 somewhat more than normal activity
2
3
4 moderately fidgety and restless
5
6
7 paces back and forth during most of the interview, or constantly thrashes about

ORIENTATION AND CLOUDING OF SENSORIUM—Ask "What day is this? Where are you? Who am I?"

0 oriented and can do serial additions
1 cannot do serial additions or is uncertain about date
2 disoriented for date by no more than 2 calendar days
3 disoriented for date by more than 2 calendar days
4 disoriented for place/or person

Total **CIWA-Ar** Score
Maximum Possible Score 67

This assessment for monitoring withdrawal symptoms requires approximately 5 minutes to administer. The maximum score is 67. Patients scoring less than 10 do not usually need additional medication for withdrawal.

tered at each detoxification visit and measures withdrawal over the past 24 hours.

Opioids

Two rating scales that are reliable indicators of the severity of the opioid withdrawal syndrome are the Subjective Opiate Withdrawal Scale and the Objective Opiate Withdrawal Scale (Handelsman, Cochrane, Aronson, & Ness, 1987). The Subjective Opiate Withdrawal Scale (SOWS) is a 16-item questionnaire assessing common motoric, autonomic, gastrointestinal, musculoskeletal, and psychic symptoms of opioid withdrawal. Clients can rate their own symptom severity on a scale of 0 to 4. The sum of the scores on each item is the total SOWS score, which can range from 0 to 64. Higher scores indicate more severe withdrawal. The items are shown in Box 6.5, page 95.

To screen with the Objective Opiate Withdrawal Scale (OOWS; Box 6.5), you would observe a client for about 10 minutes and indicate if any of the 13 signs of withdrawal are present. The OOWS consists of observable signs that reflect common motoric and autonomic manifestations of withdrawal. Scores range from 0 to 13, with higher scores indicating more severe withdrawal. A difference between the SOWS and the OOWS is that the former relies on client self-report, whereas the latter is based on your own observation of withdrawal signs (Handelsman et al., 1987).

Two Models of Detoxification

There are two broad models for detoxification: a medical model and a social model. Medical model programs are directed by a physician and staffed by health care personnel. They may be hospital-based inpatient programs, residential programs, or ambulatory facilities in the community. Social model or "drug-free" detox programs provide nonmedical services to manage withdrawal without medication, drawing on off-site health care facilities if medical services are needed. There are also mixed-model social programs that offer some on-site or on-call medical supervision. The types of psychosocial services offered by social model programs vary widely.

Transitioning from Evaluation to Stabilization

When evaluation is complete, the client's detoxification plan is in place. A determination has been made regarding detoxification model (social or medical) and setting (inpatient or outpatient). Since routes into detoxification often pass through the legal system, emergency department, or primary care, it's possible that some of the evaluation work has been completed by a referring agency. The next step is to begin implementing the plan and to

BOX 6.4. Cocaine Selective Severity Assessment (CSSA)

Symptom   **SCORE**

1. HYPERPHAGIA: [   ]
  0 = normal appetite
3–4 = eats a lot more than usual
  7 = eats more than twice usual amount of food

2. HYPOPHAGIA: [   ]
  0 = normal appetite
3–4 = eats less than normal amount
  7 = no appetite at all

3. CARBOHYDRATE CRAVING: [   ]
  0 = no craving
3–4 = strong craving for sweets half the time
  7 = strong craving for sweets all the time

4. COCAINE CRAVING: (Please rate intensity) 0–7   [   ]

Please rate the highest intensity of the desire for cocaine you have felt in
the last 24 hours:

0	1	2	3	4	5	6	7
No desire at all							Unable to resist

5. CRAVING FREQUENCY: (Please have subject rate intensity) 0–7   [   ]

Please identify on the line below how often you have felt the urge to use
cocaine in the last 24 hours:

0	1	2	3	4	5	6	7
Never							All the time

6. BRADYCARDIA   [   ]

	0	1	2	3	4	5	6	7
Apical Pulse	> 64	64–63	62–61	60–59	58–57	56–55	54–53	< 53

7. SLEEP 1:   [   ]
  0 = normal amount of sleep
3–4 = half of normal amount
  7 = no sleep at all

(cont.)

From Kampman et al. (1998). This scale is in the public domain and may be reproduced without further permission.

BOX 6.4. *(cont.)*

8. SLEEP II: [   ]
   0 = normal amount of sleep
3–4 = could sleep or do sleep half the day
   7 = sleep or could sleep all the time

9. ANXIETY: [   ]
   0 = usually does not feel anxious
3–4 = feels anxious half the time
   7 = feels anxious all the time

10. ENERGY LEVEL: [   ]
   0 = feels alert and has usual amount of energy
3–4 = feels tired half the time
   7 = feels tired all the time

11. ACTIVITY LEVEL: [   ]
   0 = no change in usual activities
3–4 = participates in half of usual activities
   7 = no participation in usual activities

12. TENSION: [   ]
   0 = rarely feels tense
3–4 = feels tense half the time
   7 = feels tense most of the time

13. ATTENTION: [   ]
   0 = able to concentrate on reading, conversation, tasks, and make
       plans without difficulty
3–4 = has difficulty with the above half the time
   7 = has difficulty with the above all the time

14. PARANOID IDEATION   [   ]
   0 = no evidence of paranoid thoughts
3–4 = unable to trust anyone
   7 = feels people are out to get him/her
   8 = feels a specific person/group is plotting against him/her

15. ANHEDONIA   [   ]
   0 = ability to enjoy themselves remains unchanged
3–4 = able to enjoy themselves half the time
   7 = unable to enjoy themselves at all

(cont.)

BOX 6.4. *(cont.)*

16. DEPRESSION   [ ]
  0 = no feelings related to sadness or depression
  3–4 = feels sad or depressed half the time
  7 = feels depressed all of the time

17. SUICIDALITY   [ ]
  0 = does not think about being dead
  3–4 = feels like life is not worth living
  7 = feels like actually ending life

18. IRRITABILITY   [ ]
  0 = feels that most things are not irritating
  3–4 = feels that many things are irritating
  7 = feels that mostly everything is irritating and upsetting

Total Score: _____

assist the person through withdrawal to abstinence. This is also the time for enhancing motivation to continue into the next phase of treatment.

STABILIZATION

During the stabilization phase, the client is assisted safely through acute intoxication and withdrawal. Previously used drugs are cleared from the body, and withdrawal symptoms are managed to minimize risk and discomfort. As indicated above, detoxification is sometimes but not always assisted by medication. An important function of therapeutic medications during stabilization is to help clients achieve an initial period of abstinence. Pharmacological treatment typically involves substituting a longer acting agent for the drug the person is withdrawing from and then gradually tapering the dose. In Chapter 15 we provide more specific information on the types of medications used to help manage withdrawal and to facilitate maintenance of abstinence.

Withdrawal syndromes vary depending on the type(s) of drug being used. In this regard, it is good to know what you might expect during the withdrawal process, information that you may also share with clients (although they may already have considerable knowledge and experience in this regard). Clients feel more comfortable when they know what to expect, and sometimes considerable fear is involved. For example, there is often disproportionate fear surrounding opioid withdrawal. It's important to be

BOX 6.5. Subjective Opiate Withdrawal Scale (SOWS)

Symptom	Not at all	A little	Moderately	Quite a bit	Extremely
1. I feel anxious.	0	1	2	3	4
2. I feel like yawning.	0	1	2	3	4
3. I'm perspiring.	0	1	2	3	4
4. My eyes are tearing.	0	1	2	3	4
5. My nose is running.	0	1	2	3	4
6. I have goose flesh.	0	1	2	3	4
7. I am shaking.	0	1	2	3	4
8. I have hot flashes.	0	1	2	3	4
9. I have cold flashes.	0	1	2	3	4
10. My bones and muscles ache.	0	1	2	3	4
11. I feel restless.	0	1	2	3	4
12. I feel nauseous.	0	1	2	3	4
13. I feel like vomiting.	0	1	2	3	4
14. My muscles twitch.	0	1	2	3	4
15. I have cramps in my stomach.	0	1	2	3	4
16. I feel like shooting up now.	0	1	2	3	4

From Handelsman, Cochrane, Aronson, and Ness (1987). This scale is in the public domain and may be reproduced without further permission.

empathic with these concerns, while also providing realistic assurance and information to assuage fears and reduce ambivalence. Box 6.6 describes the signs and symptoms of intoxication from specific drugs and alcohol as well as the characteristics, duration, onset, length, and complications of withdrawal.

Methods for "ultrarapid" opiate detoxification have received public attention and attracted some interest. These occur in hospital settings under medical supervision, and involve general anesthesia or deep sedation so that the patient is unconscious during the uncomfortable withdrawal from heroin, methadone, or other opioid drugs (Cucchia, Monnat, Spag-

BOX 6.6. Examples of Drug Withdrawal Symptoms

	Cocaine	Alcohol	Heroin	Cannabis (marijuana)
Onset	Depends upon type of cocaine used: for crack will begin within hours of last use	24–48 hours after blood alcohol level drops	Within 24 hours of last use	Some debate about this, may be a few days
Duration	3–4 days	5–7 days	4–7 days	May last up to several weeks
Characteristics	Sleeplessness *or* excessive restless sleep, appetite increase, depression, paranoia, decreased energy	↑ blood pressure, ↑ heart rate, ↑ temperature, nausea/vomiting/diarrhea, seizures, delirium, death	Nausea, vomiting, diarrhea, goose bumps, runny nose, teary eyes, yawning	Irritability, appetite disturbance, sleep disturbance, nausea, concentration problems, nystagmus, diarrhea
Medical/ Psychiatric Issues	Stroke, cardiovascular collapse, myocardial and other organ infarction, paranoia, violence, severe depression, suicide	Virtually every organ system is affected (e.g., cardiomyopathy, liver disease, esophageal and rectal varices); fetal alcohol syndrome and other problems with fetus	During withdrawal individual may become dehydrated	

Based on N. S. Miller and Kipnis (2006).

noli, Ferrero, & Bertschy, 1998). The usual procedure is to transition the patient directly onto naltrexone, which triggers immediate opiate withdrawal (Rabinowitz, Cohen, Tarrasch, & Kotler, 1997), or to buprenorphine for maintenance (Tornay et al., 2003). With hospital supervision this procedure is relatively safe, and early reports suggested that it may increase adherence in maintenance on naltrexone (Albanese et al., 2000). It is far more costly than routine detoxification procedures, however, and it is questionable whether outcomes are any better (Lawental, 2000; Rabinowitz, Cohen, & Atias, 2002; Singh & Basu, 2010).

What about people who enter detoxification using several substances simultaneously? Increasingly polydrug use is the norm rather than the exception. The individual intoxicating effects of the various drugs can interact, amplify, and complicate each other. Similarly, the body's adjustments to simul-taneous withdrawal of several drugs can interact in

> Increasingly polydrug use is the norm.

complex ways. Withdrawal time curves for individual drugs can overlap or prolong each other. Priority is usually given to determining which of the used drugs poses the most serious withdrawal risks (N. S. Miller & Kipnis, 2006). Alcohol and sedative–hypnotics typically get priority of attention because their withdrawal syndromes can be fatal.

Addressing Other Health Care Needs

During the stabilization process it is also important to identify and address acute health and social problems that need imminent attention. Here are some common issues related to physical health.

Nutritional Needs

Malnutrition is a common concern with people entering detoxification. Alcohol is calorie-dense, and tends to displace food intake. People who are using drugs or alcohol may also have irregular eating habits and poor dietary intake. Alcohol and other drugs can also interfere with nutrient uti-lization and storage. For example, opioids tend to decrease calcium absorp-tion (Cardenas & Ross, 1976) and alcohol can cause thiamine deficiencies (Singleton & Martin, 2001). Thus a nutritional evaluation is often war-ranted during stabilization, accompanied by appropriate dietary counsel-ing. When poverty contributes to malnutrition, stabilization includes con-necting people with community food supplementation resources.

Psychiatric Needs

Diagnosing co-occurring disorders is tricky during acute intoxication and withdrawal because substances can often mimic psychiatric disorders (see Chapter 18). Nevertheless, as withdrawal symptoms abate, co-occurring disorders may become more apparent. Professional consensus is increas-ingly to address addiction and co-occurring disorders simultaneously, rather than waiting for one to resolve before treating the other (Mueser & Drake, 2007; Sacks & Ries, 2005). This suggests linking clients with the appropriate treatment services during the stabilization process.

Immediate mental health needs, however, may require more rapid attention. Suicidal ideation is common for clients presenting for detoxifica-tion. When combined with intoxication and withdrawal symptoms that cloud a person's reasoning, it is particularly important to be attentive to suicide risk. Emotional lability is also common, and protocols for staff and client safety should be in place as a way to manage clients who are angry and act aggressively toward others.

Infectious Diseases

Drug use is associated with risk behaviors such as sharing of contaminated needles and unsafe sexual practices that contribute to the transmission of certain infectious diseases. There are elevated rates of tuberculosis (TB), hepatitis B and C, HIV, and sexually transmitted diseases (STDs). Identifying at-risk clients is the first line of defense, and the stabilization period provides an opportunity to assess and address these concerns. There is a misconception that it is only injection drug users who are at risk of infectious diseases. In fact, this risk crosses the substance use disorders (Rehm et al., 2010). In addition to needle sharing, poor nutrition, poor hygiene, unprotected sex, contact with other substance users, incarceration, and institutionalization all increase the risk of infections.

Screening for infections such as STDs, TB, HIV, and hepatitis is an important health care function during stabilization. In addition to curing or managing the infection itself, interventions should seek to reduce the risk of future infections, and to locate and test others who may have been exposed (Semaan, Neumann, Hutchins, D'Anna, & Kamb, 2010). Needle and syringe exchange programs are effective in reducing HIV transmission (Palmateer et al., 2010).

TUBERCULOSIS

TB is a contagious bacterial infection that mainly involves the lungs, but may spread to other organs. The primary stage of the disease usually doesn't have symptoms. The symptoms of the active disease include fatigue, cough, fever, coughing up blood, chest pains, excessive sweating, and unintentional weight loss. All clients entering treatment programs (and those who treat them) should receive a skin test for TB (Mulligan, 1995). HIV-positive people are at particular risk for developing TB following recent exposure because of the immunosuppression associated with HIV infection. Treatment requires taking medications for about 6–9 months, and close adherence to the prescribed regimen is important. Medications for TB may interact with pharmacotherapies used for people with addictions such as methadone and disulfiram, so medical monitoring is obviously important.

HEPATITIS B

The hepatitis B virus (HBV) spreads through blood, semen, vaginal fluids, and other body fluids. Infection can occur when people have blood transfusions, are stuck with a contaminated needle, or have unprotected sex with an infected person. Many people with HBV have few or no symptoms and may not feel sick, even though they are infectious. Again, routine screening for HBV is indicated. A vaccine is available, and all at-risk individuals (including those who regularly treat patients with addiction) should be vaccinated. Symptoms may not appear for up to 6 months after the time of infection. Early symptoms may include appetite loss, low-grade fever, muscle and joint aches, nausea and vomiting, yellow skin and dark urine due to jaundice, and fatigue. Certain medications such as methadone and disulfiram may be contraindicated for people who have ongoing liver disease because of a hepatitis infection.

HEPATITIS C

Among substance users, especially injection drug users, the prevalence of the hepatitis C virus (HCV) is high. HCV most often spreads through direct contact with blood and contaminated needles, but can also be sexually transmitted. As with HBV, many people with HCV do not have symptoms. If the infection has been present for many years, the liver may be permanently scarred, a condition called cirrhosis. Symptoms that can emerge with HCV infection include abdominal pain, fatigue, jaundice, nausea, vomiting, and loss of appetite. Treatment for HCV currently involves 6–12 months of chemotherapy with interferon or related medications, with longer courses yielding better long-term suppression. Again, close adherence to medication regimens is important. Because HCV affects liver functioning, other medications such as methadone and disulfiram may be contraindicated during treatment.

HIV AND AIDS

Infection with HIV is associated with a progressive disease process. HIV is a chronic medical condition that can be treated, but not yet cured. Most cases are transmitted sexually through intimate sexual contact where there is exposure to body fluids such as semen, blood, and vaginal secretions. HIV can also be spread by the use of contaminated needles and syringes. Once someone has contracted HIV, there are effective ways to prevent complications and to delay progression to AIDS. Symptoms related to HIV are usually due to an opportunistic infection in part of the body and include diarrhea, fatigue, fever, headache, mouth sores, rashes, sore throat, and swollen lymph glands.

Under the influence of alcohol and other drugs, people are more likely to engage in risky sexual practices. Effective counseling methods are available to reduce rates of unprotected sex for both men (Calsyn et al., 2009) and women (Tross et al., 2008). These treatment modules include information about HIV transmission, self-risk assessment, discussion of safe sex options, assertive communication and negotiation skills, and exploration of ways to have enjoyable sex without drugs. Therapist guidelines for these evidence-based modules are available for free download at *www.ctndis-seminationlibrary.org*.

OTHER STDS

Screening and treatment for STDs is appropriate given the high correlation of drug use with unprotected and risky sexual behaviors. More than 30 organisms can cause STDs. Four of the most common STDs among people seeking addiction treatment are syphilis, gonorrhea, chlamydia, and genital herpes.

Transmission of *syphilis* infection *may* occur after sharing needles with injection drug users who are infected with syphilis, though in most cases it is sexually transmitted. The bacteria that cause it spread through broken skin or mucous membranes. If left untreated, syphilis progresses through several phases. Initial symptoms of syphilis may include painless sores and swollen lymph nodes. These usually occur within 3 weeks of infection and may go unnoticed. In the second stage, symptoms can include fever, fatigue, rash, aches and pains, and loss of appetite. Tertiary syphilis damages the heart, the brain, and the nervous system. Syphilis is responsive to treatment with antibiotics. People who have syphilis should be encouraged to have testing for HIV infection, since syphilis may increase the risk for infection with and transmission of HIV.

Symptoms of *gonorrhea* usually appear 2–5 days after infection. In women, these symptoms can be very mild and nonspecific, but may include vaginal discharge, burning and pain while urinating, increased urination, painful sexual intercourse, severe pain in the lower abdomen, and fever. In men, symptoms such as burning and pain while urinating, increased urinary frequency or urgency, discharge from the penis, red or swollen opening of the penis, and tender or swollen testicles may take up to a month to appear. About half of women diagnosed with gonorrhea are also infected with chlamydia, another very common sexually transmitted disease that can result in sterility. Immediately treating a gonorrhea infection helps prevent permanent scarring and infertility.

Chlamydia is a bacterial infection transmitted mainly through sexual intercourse with an infected person. Chlamydia has a high prevalence, is easily transmitted, and is associated with gonorrhea. It is very common for both men and women to not experience symptoms of chlamydia. In men, symptoms of chlamydia are similar to those of gonorrhea and may include a burning sensation during urination, discharge from the penis, testicular tenderness or pain, and rectal discharge or pain. Symptoms that may occur in women include a burning sensation during urination, painful sexual intercourse, vaginal discharge, rectal pain or discharge, and symptoms of pelvic inflammatory disease. Screening is strongly encouraged, particularly for high-risk pregnant women, adolescents, and people with multiple sexual partners. Asymptomatic infection can lead to infertility if untreated. Chlamydia can be treated with an antibiotic regimen; clients should be told to refrain from sexual intercourse until treatment is completed.

Genital herpes is a viral infection that can be treated but currently cannot be cured. It is easily transmitted through genital contact. Initial symptoms in the first week after exposure can be mild and vague, such as fatigue, malaise, headache, or fever. A first outbreak usually occurs during the first month after exposure and can include genital pain, blisters, sensitivity and itching, swollen lymph nodes, fever, and fatigue. Outbreaks typically last for about 2 weeks, and often recur for months or years. Even in the general U.S. population, about one in four adults have been infected. The virus can be passed from mother to newborn baby during vaginal delivery, which can be fatal due to the infant's undeveloped immune system.

Routine medical screening for STDs is an important service to link with addiction treatment. As described above, initial symptoms of STDs are often unnoticed or ignored. The presence of one STD increases risk for other STDs including HIV. Screening is particularly important with pregnant women because of risks for transmission to the child. Bacterial STDs are curable and viral STDs are treatable. Counseling for safe sex practices should also be routine with sexually active clients to reduce the spread of infections.

Other Health Care Needs

People presenting for addiction treatment often have other untreated health problems. These may be related to injuries, nutritional and hygiene practices, and the toxic effects of alcohol and other drugs. As part of case management, it is important to ensure and facilitate each client's linkage with a primary care provider. Oral health is also a common problem related to substance use disorders, and one that can impact health more generally. Ask whether clients are receiving routine dental care, and, if not, help them to do so. Such coordination is facilitated when addiction and health care services are located together or nearby.

TRANSITION TO TREATMENT

After stabilization it has been common for people to receive no further treatment. There are several reasons for this. Sometimes clients become discouraged and distressed during stabilization and leave against medical advice. On the other hand, stabilization may give them the relief they wanted, and feeling better they see no immediate need for further treatment. Geographic separation of detoxification and treatment facilities also hinders transition, as do waiting lists and other barriers to receiving treatment services. The result is the familiar "revolving door" phenomenon whereby people turn up repeatedly in detoxification, hospital, social service, and correctional systems. For this reason, transition to treatment is a third important function in detoxification, along with evaluation and stabilization. Detoxification in itself is insufficient treatment, and very unlikely to change substance use.

Timing is an issue. When the withdrawal process is particularly severe, it is wise to wait for mental functions to clear and physical distress to subside. It's somewhat like working in an emergency department: if someone is coding and in imminent danger of death, that is not the moment for a substance use consult! Yet there is also a risk in waiting too long. The acute discomfort of detoxification can make the need for treatment more salient, and people are sometimes discharged prematurely. As soon as feasible, begin discussing and enhancing motivation for the next phase of treatment (see Chapter 7). Doing so and attending to clients' other needs can also decrease the likelihood of their leaving detoxification prematurely.

Enhancing Motivation for Change

In a subsequent chapter we emphasize that motivation for change is not a client trait, but rather something that emerges in interpersonal context. It is not necessary to wait for people to become "ready" for treatment. Motivation for treatment is very influenced by what you do and how you interact with clients (Miller, 1985; Walitzer, Dermen, & Connors, 1999). Chapter 10 in particular addresses strategies for strengthening client motivation, so here we will mention just a few key aspects.

Compassion

> First and foremost, offer a welcoming atmosphere of acceptance, respect, and compassion.

First and foremost, offer a welcoming atmosphere of acceptance, respect, and compassion. Someone entering the service should feel cared for from the outset. A good model of this is found in AA, where people are always welcomed back. A program is there to serve the clients, not vice versa. Admittedly, it's challenging to feel and show compassion for someone who has just thrown up on your shoes, but it's entirely possible even if you're not Mother Teresa. Motivation for change is promoted by therapeutic acceptance, not rejection; by compassion, not judgment. In several studies, just a brief, compassionate, client-centered conversation in the emergency room significantly increased motivation for change in substance use (Bernstein, Bernstein, & Levenson,

1997; Bernstein et al., 2009; Bernstein et al., 2005; Chafetz, 1961; Chafetz et al., 1962; Monti, Colby, & O'Leary, 2001).

Discrepancy

Although you might like to install motivation in a client, what really matters is the client's *own* motivation for change. One way to think about this internal motivation is as a discrepancy between the current reality and goals that are important to the client (Miller & Rollnick, 2002). Help clients to give voice to their own goals and values, and how changing their substance use could help to achieve them (see Chapter 10).

Hope

Clients are not the only people who can become discouraged. It's common for clinical staff to feel disheartened or annoyed to see the same person coming back again and again for detoxification and to wonder, "What makes this time any different from the last?" It is a good question to ask, in part because it suggests that perhaps it is time to try something different from the last time. It's important to treat clients, even "frequent fliers," with compassion and hope. Because the consequences of substance use are often so readily apparent during detoxification, this is a useful window of opportunity to try different strategies to enhance motivation for change (see Chapter 10). Most people do ultimately escape from the cycle of addiction, and one reframe is that each turn around the circle brings the person one step closer to change. Clients may feel very little hope of their own on returning to detox, so you may need to lend them some of yours (Yahne & Miller, 1999).

Case Management

Addressing barriers to treatment such as housing, child care, transportation, and career assistance can help improve engagement in treatment. There are basic needs clients may have during the detoxification process, including food and clothing, financial assistance, and access to a safe living environment. If these needs are not met, it is harder for the person to commit to a longer course of treatment. It is important to begin assertive case management during detoxification to link the person with needed services (see Chapter 8).

Linkages to Treatment

Once clients have progressed past the most severe withdrawal symptoms and are medically stable, it is appropriate to prepare them for the transition to rehabilitation (see Chapter 7). Whether they take this next step is influenced by a number of factors including:

- The client's level of motivation which, as mentioned above, can be increased by specific clinical strategies. People are more likely to initiate and remain in treatment if they believe the services will help them with specific life problems (Fiorentine, Nakashima, & Anglin, 1999). Find out what clients want, need, and prefer from treatment and actively assist them in finding a good fit.

- Direct linkage. Making a specific appointment with a specific service while the person is still in detox can roughly double the chances of completing the referral, compared to just giving the information to clients and asking them to make the contact.

- Convenience. The farther clients have to travel in order to get to outpatient treatment, the less likely it is that they will persist.

- Transportation. Even among those who make an appointment for addiction treatment, a substantial proportion may not show up (Gottheil, Sterling, & Weinstein, 1997b). Scheduling a staff member or significant other to transport and accompany the client to the appointment will increase arrival. It can also be helpful for the client to have such an advocate along in order to persist through any frustrations or administrative hurdles.

- Minimal wait. The longer clients have to wait for treatment services, the less likely it is that they will engage (Carroll, 1997a).

KEY POINTS

🔖 Detoxification and stabilization represent a preparation for rehabilitation and can usually be accomplished without hospitalization.

🔖 Stabilization involves identifying and addressing urgent needs including detoxification, nutritional and other health care problems, infectious diseases, and pressing psychiatric disorders or psychosocial needs.

🔖 It is important in addiction treatment to assess the likelihood of withdrawal, which can range from none to severe.

🔖 Detoxification is offered in both residential and ambulatory settings, and within each there are both medical and social (drug-free) programs.

✤ Detoxification is not rehabilitation. A primary task during stabilization is to facilitate motivation for and transition to additional treatment.

REFLECTION QUESTIONS

How do you help or refer patients who need medical evaluation during the stabilization process? Is such medical consultation available within your setting?

What experience(s) would help you be more comfortable and competent to assess and manage drug withdrawal?

Dropout after detoxification is a common problem. How can you help ensure that patients make the transition into further treatment?

CHAPTER 7

Matching: Individualizing Treatment Plans

We begin this chapter by reemphasizing that addiction treatment, like that of other chronic conditions, is a process that should begin with the very first contact and continue with follow-up management to help people maintain their own changes and health. Too often treatment in this field has been thought of as a discrete event, a particular dose such as 28 days of residential care or 12 weeks of outpatient treatment that is sandwiched in between an intake process and discharge. Although addiction is commonly regarded as a chronic illness, treatment has not yet adjusted accordingly. Within a good health care system, someone who presents with symptoms of heart disease will receive immediate attention, and care does not end with that episode of treatment. To be effective, addiction treatment should follow a similar path. The most common course of recovery involves successive changes over time, often with two steps forward and one step back.

> Although addiction is commonly regarded as a chronic illness, treatment has not yet adjusted accordingly.

Both addiction and recovery occur over time within a person's ongoing life course. Typically, problems and dependence develop gradually, and it is common for their severity to wax and wane over a period of years. Although people tend not to seek treatment (if ever they do) until problems and/or dependence are well developed, self-change efforts often begin earlier and can extend over many years (Venner & Miller, 2001). It takes time to adjust one's life after having a heart attack or receiving a diagnosis of diabetes. Recovery from addiction can similarly be a long and continuing journey.

We believe it is better to think of treatment in particular and recovery in general as processes that extend over time. Smokers often have three or four serious quit attempts before they finally stop. Similarly, people with alcohol/drug problems commonly go through several episodes of treatment before getting free. The "success rate" of any particular treatment event is, therefore, much lower than the rate of eventual recovery from addiction, and specific treatment episodes are only a small part, timewise, of the recovery process. If addiction is truly like a chronic disease, then it is a mistake to ask how many treatment episodes it takes on average to "cure" it. Chronic diseases are not cured by treatment episodes, but are managed over time to support the person's health and quality of life, and medical care is only part of the picture. With such chronic conditions, long-term health has very much to do with motivation for and practice of self-care.

FOUR PHASES OF TREATMENT: A CONTINUUM OF CARE

Within this bigger picture of managing a chronic condition over time, it is helpful to think about phases of care. Where is this person in the process of recovery? What does he or she need help with at present? This is part of matching treatment to the client. The goals and processes of treatment vary depending on where clients are in their journey. There are various stage models of treatment for addiction, and we think in terms of four phases: palliative care, stabilization, rehabilitation, and maintenance (see Box 7.1).

Phase 1: Palliative Care

Phase 1 actually precedes what many people would think of as "treatment" for addiction. Palliative care for people with addictions is what normally happens when they seek health care. They may see no need at all to be treated for alcohol/drug problems; they may not even think of their drinking or drug use as problematic. A provider may encourage the person to seek formal help (Phase 2 or 3), but it is common for such referral attempts to fail. What then? Should providers ignore or give up on their patients' addiction problems? People still deserve to be cared for, and there is concern to protect not only them, but their families and society from harm.

Some general goals in Phase 1 are to keep the person in contact with systems of care; reduce risks of illness, harm, or death; increase motivation for change in substance use; and facilitate access and entry to Phase 2 or 3 services. The person may be willing to consider options short of formal treatment, such as self-help materials (Apodaca & Miller, 2003) or referral

BOX 7.1. Four Phases of Care

Phase of Care	Specific Tasks
Phase 1: Palliative care	• Prevent drug-related death. • Maintain user's contact with care systems. • Enhance self-care to reduce health risks and harm for the user. • Decrease risks and harm to society. • Identify and support family members, as appropriate. • Strengthen motivation for change in substance use. • Facilitate access and entry to Phase 2 or 3 services.
Phase 2: Stabilization	• Detoxify—safely eliminate drugs from the body. • Enhance retention in and completion of Phase 2. • Stabilize—address acute health and welfare needs. • Initiate case management. • Increase motivation for treatment/rehabilitation (Phase 3). • Facilitate access and entry to Phase 3 services.
Phase 3: Rehabilitation	• Establish an empathic therapeutic relationship. • Enhance retention in Phase 3. • Negotiate and clarify goals for change. • Develop a clear and realistic change plan (including treatment plan). • Implement change plan to stabilize initial change in substance use. • Assess client strengths and resources. • Identify and involve family/support network, as feasible. • Initiate sampling of and participation in mutual help groups, as appropriate. • Address the most pressing concomitant problems and disorders. • Increase motivation for continuation of changes and personal growth (Phase 4). • Initiate a maintenance plan to prevent recurrence. • Facilitate access and entry to Phase 4 services.
Phase 4: Maintenance	• Support motivation for maintenance of change. • Negotiate and clarify goals and plan for maintenance of change. • Implement maintenance plan to prevent recurrence. • Continue case management, facilitate access to needed services. • Continue monitoring and treatment contact as appropriate and desired. • Establish and maintain rewarding drug-free activities and relationships. • Facilitate spiritual development. • Maintain mutual help group involvement, as appropriate.

to a mutual help resource such as 12-step groups (Chapter 14). Although most addiction treatment programs are not seeing people during Phase 1, this is an important phase of care. Most people with diagnosable substance use disorders are not receiving Phase 2 or 3 treatment, and many *never* seek such treatment. Though our primary focus in this book is on Phases 2–4, we will reconsider broader palliative care in Chapter 23.

Phase 2: Stabilization

Given the range and severity of addiction's possible effects on people's health, social, and psychological functioning, it is sometimes necessary to stabilize them in preparation for Phase 3 treatment. This can include detoxification and attention to basic health care needs, as discussed in Chapter 6. There may be pressing social problems that require attention, such as a need for housing, food, or child care. A person may also be in acute crisis or suicidal, and need crisis and case management (see Chapter 8). All of these issues may need to be addressed before a person is sufficiently stabilized to begin Phase 3 treatment.

The transition to Phase 3 is also by no means automatic. There is a familiar revolving door phenomenon of people with addictions returning repeatedly for Phase 1 (e.g., emergency room) or Phase 2 (e.g., detoxification) services without changing their substance use. A vital function in Phase 2, then, is to enhance the person's motivation to change his or her substance use and, as appropriate, to seek help in doing so. Methods for strengthening motivation to change will be discussed in Chapter 10.

Phase 3: Rehabilitation

Historically, Phase 3 services are what most addiction treatment programs have provided. For this phase of care we prefer the term *rehabilitation*— literally, to make able again.

Phase 3 has its own unique goals. One of these, of course, involves changing prior substance use, but most people have a much broader range of problems and needs. In fact, changing substance use may be well down the person's list of priorities. The beginning of Phase 3 is the time to develop a problem list, negotiate and clarify goals for change, and agree upon a clear and realistic change plan. Enhancing motivation to achieve the negotiated goals is an important up-front task (see Chapter 10), and early attention to factors that promote retention in treatment is wise. Phase 3 then proceeds into implementation of the initial change plan, all the while building motivation to maintain the gains that are made (Phase 4). All of this relies upon the establishment and maintenance of an empathic working relationship with your client (Chapter 4).

One reason why we are so enthusiastic in encouraging behavioral health professionals to treat addictions is that addictions seldom occur in isolation (Chapter 18). Those who treat people with substance use disorders encounter the entire DSM, as well as a host of employment, family, legal, medical, and social life problems. Counselors who are prepared only to treat addictions face the challenge of what to do about this host of con-comitant problems and disorders: ignore them, put them on hold, assume they are secondary to the addiction, try to treat them without adequate professional preparation, or refer out for other services? Professionals who are also competent to treat a broader panoply of health and psychological problems are, we believe, better prepared to help people with substance use disorders.

Phase 4: Maintenance

The real challenge with addictions is not making the initial change so much as maintaining it. Mark Twain quipped that quitting smoking is easy—he had done it dozens of times. As with chronic medical illnesses, there is a need for ongoing care and monitoring. Treatment is not over when a Phase 3 episode has ended. People with asthma, diabetes, or heart disease nor-mally receive ongoing monitoring and treatment from a primary care pro-vider, with occasional acute care visits (e.g., to an emergency room) to deal with recurrences. Addiction has been, arguably, the only chronic disease for which there is typically only acute and specialist care with no primary care (McLellan at al., 2000). We discuss Phase 4 care in Chapter 19.

STAGES OF CHANGE

Another perspective that we find helpful in thinking about how to individu-alize treatment is the transtheoretical model (Prochaska, 1994; Prochaska & DiClemente, 1984; Prochaska & Norcross, 2009). In particular, the conception of *stages of change* has had substantial influence in addiction treatment. The overall transtheoretical model is much more complex, but we will focus our discussion on the stages because of their relevance to treatment planning.

People differ in their readiness to change. Some smokers, for example, entirely reject the idea of quitting, others are thinking about it, and still oth-ers are trying. The transtheoretical stages of change began with research on smoking, but can be applied to a broad range of behavior change topics.

First of the five stages is called *precontemplation*, during which the person is not even thinking about or considering change. This may be because the person has never regarded the behavior to be a problem and thus sees no need for change. It may also be, as discussed below, that the person has tried and failed and, thus discouraged, is not thinking about trying again. A usual time frame is half a year, so people are said to be in the precontemplation stage if they are not considering making a change within the next 6 months. At this stage, people need help to begin considering the possibility of change.

As the name of the first stage suggests, the second stage is termed *contemplation*, wherein the person *is* thinking about making a change within the next 6 months. The emphasis here is on contemplating or thinking about change; no decision has yet been made. People in the contemplation stage are typically *ambivalent* about change—they want to change (or see reasons to do so), and they don't. People here need help in resolving their ambivalence in the direction of change. Chapter 10 addresses ways to work with people in precontemplation or contemplation.

Then something happens that tips the balance, and the person is, at least for the time being, in the *preparation* stage. He or she is planning to change, but has not yet decided when and how to do it. People here need help in developing a change plan. The remainder of this chapter is about how to help people at this stage.

Having decided on a course of change, the fourth stage is *action*, which involves implementing the change plan. In this stage, the person is actively trying to change. This corresponds to Phase 3 treatment in the continuum of care described earlier, and is the task most familiar for many programs and providers: that of helping people carry out change. Most of this book is focused on strategies appropriate for people in the action stage.

Finally, as discussed above, the next challenge is *maintenance*, which is the name given to the fifth and final stage of change. The task here is to hold onto and continue gains made through action (see Chapter 19). This is sometimes called "aftercare," but ongoing care is an important part of treatment and not an afterthought.

The transtheoretical stages have sometimes been shown with a sixth stage called *relapse*, involving a recurrence of substance use. In addition to our reservations about the term "relapse" itself (see Chapter 19), this is essentially just a recycling through the stages. The person who resumes drug use may spend a period of time not even considering change (precontemplation), then thinking about change (contemplation), planning for (preparation) and implementing change (action), and back to maintenance. It is also not uncommon for a person to step from a recurrence (a "slip") right back into maintenance. The clinician's task is to help the person not get stuck in early stages, but to resume change plan action and maintenance as soon as possible.

People can and do move back and forth between these stages, in either direction around the circle shown in Box 7.2. Sometimes even within a single counseling visit a person may seem to shift among stages. We also emphasize not only that people move around, but also that the stages are just hypo-

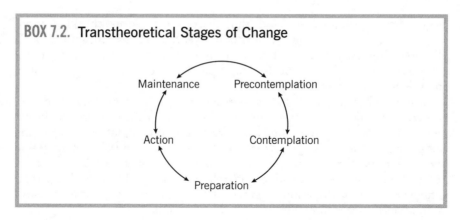

BOX 7.2. Transtheoretical Stages of Change

thetical concepts that simplify much more complex underlying processes of motivation. We do find them helpful in thinking about what a particular person may need at present. We don't favor using these to stick labels on people ("You're a precontemplator"), or assuming that because you have decided on a person's stage you know exactly what he or she needs.

NEGOTIATING AND DEVELOPING A CHANGE PLAN

An early task in Phase 3 treatment (and for people at a preparation stage) is to develop a change plan to which the person can agree and commit. A change plan is broader than a treatment plan, though related. Helping people to develop a change plan is a useful step in treatment. A good change plan lists the client's specific goals for change, and for each the particular steps or strategies to move toward that goal. Not all of these will involve additional treatment, and sometimes none of them do. Getting professional help is one possible strategy to pursue a change goal. A treatment plan therefore represents a subset of the change plan: those parts of the change plan for which additional treatment is anticipated.

Setting Goals

A first step in developing a change plan is to clarify the client's goals. What changes would your client welcome? This is a process of negotiation. Although your aspiration for someone might be that they would stop all drug use immediately and permanently, what change is the person interested in and willing to pursue? The "miracle question" from solution-focused therapy (DeShazer et al., 2007) is one way to get at this: "If a miracle happened, if you woke up tomorrow and all of the problems that you have described were magically gone, how would you know? How would things be different?"

Often there is a need to move from broad or vague desires to more specific goals. A good change goal is one you can get your "ARMS" around (Miller & Mee-Lee, 2010b):

- A—It is *Achievable*. It's fine for a goal to be challenging, but it should be realistic, something that is actually possible for the person to accomplish.
- R—It should be *Rewarding*. A good goal is one that the person wants and is willing to work toward achieving.
- M—It is *Measurable*. How will you know that progress is being made toward this goal? What observable changes will there be?
- S—It is *Specific*. Vague and general goals are harder to achieve. If there is a bigger long-term goal, one way to make it more specific is to identify the next step to take toward it.

One broad approach is to offer your client a menu of possible goals or topics. An advantage of a menu over open-ended discussion of needs is that you can quickly survey a range of possible goals that might not otherwise be considered. One simple format for this is a "What I Want from Treatment" questionnaire (see Box 7.3). The particular items on this questionnaire are not fixed. Rather it is a survey of things that a client *might* want from Phase 3 treatment. The menu can be as long or short as you choose, and can be tailored to your own particular setting and population. What we provide in Box 7.3 is just one example.

But to back up a step: Why ask at all about what the client wants? Why not just prescribe the goals of treatment or announce what the program's goals are for everyone? One obvious reason is that people's needs differ, even if a program happens to treat them all the same. If you personally or programatically cannot address some of the client's goals, you can at least link the client with other resources to help achieve them (see Chapter 8). There is also the pragmatic point that when it comes right down to it, no one but clients themselves *can* set their own goals. There is also the advantage that when people choose their own goals, they tend to be more motivated to pursue them.

There are various ways to present a client with a finite list of goals. What I Want from Treatment items could be placed instead on small cards, one to each card. The client then sorts these cards into stacks—perhaps Yes, Maybe, and No piles. For shorter menus, another approach is to use a single sheet of paper with a number of bubbles (circles or ovals) on it. Each bubble contains a possible topic for discussion, which in turn could lead

BOX 7.3. What I Want from Treatment

William R. Miller, PhD, and Janice M. Brown, PhD

People have different ideas about what they want, need, and expect from treatment. Please tell us what you hope to happen in your treatment here.

1. I want to receive detoxification, to ease my withdrawal from alcohol or other drugs.   Yes   No

2. I want to find out whether I have a problem with alcohol or other drugs.   Yes   No

3. I want to stop drinking alcohol completely.   Yes   No

4. I want to decrease my drinking.   Yes   No

5. I want to take medication that would help me to avoid drinking.   Yes   No

6. I want to quit smoking (tobacco).   Yes   No

7. I want to stop using other drugs.   Yes   No

8. I want to decrease my use of other drugs.   Yes   No

9. I want to learn more about alcohol/drug problems.   Yes   No

10. I want to learn how to keep from returning to alcohol or other drugs.   Yes   No

11. I want help in dealing with cravings or urges to drink or use drugs.   Yes   No

12. I want to know more about 12-step groups like Alcoholics Anonymous (AA)   Yes   No

13. I want to know more about mutual help groups other than the 12-step groups.   Yes   No

14. I need to fulfill a requirement of the courts.   Yes   No

15. I want to learn how to resist social pressure to drink or use drugs.   Yes   No

16. I want to find enjoyable ways to spend my free time without drinking/using.   Yes   No

17. I want to decrease the level of stress, tension, or anxiety in my life.   Yes   No

18. I want to improve my physical health and fitness.   Yes   No

19. I want help in managing my depression or moods.   Yes   No

(cont.)

This questionnaire is in the public domain and may be reproduced without further permission.

BOX 7.3. *(cont.)*

20. I want help in managing my anger.	Yes	No
21. I want to have healthier relationships.	Yes	No
22. I want to discuss sexual problems.	Yes	No
23. I want to learn better ways to express my feelings.	Yes	No
24. I want to learn how to deal with boredom or loneliness.	Yes	No
25. I want to decrease or prevent violence at home.	Yes	No
26. I want to find a job (or a better job).	Yes	No
27. I want to find a better place to live.	Yes	No
28. I want help with legal problems.	Yes	No
29. I want to feel better about myself, to have more self-esteem.	Yes	No
30. I want to discuss my thoughts about suicide.	Yes	No
31. I want information about or testing for HIV/AIDS.	Yes	No
32. I want information about or testing for other infections (like hepatitis, TB, STDs)	Yes	No
33. I want someone to listen to me.	Yes	No
34. I want to learn to have fun without drugs or alcohol.	Yes	No
35. I want someone to tell me what to do.	Yes	No
36. I want help in setting goals or priorities for my life.	Yes	No
37. I want to learn how to use my time better.	Yes	No
38. I want to talk about my past.	Yes	No
39. I want to learn how to use my time better.	Yes	No
40. I want help in getting more motivated to change.	Yes	No
41. I want my spouse (or someone close to me) to come to treatment with me.	Yes	No
42. I want my treatment to be short.	Yes	No

toward change goals (see Box 7.4). Note that there are also several empty bubbles on the page, and you can say something like this:

> "Here are some things that people sometimes want to improve or change in their lives. Or perhaps there are priorities on your mind that are not here at all. That's why there are some empty bubbles. Which of these (if any) are important to you, as things you might choose to work on?"

The same approach can be used to set the agenda for a particular session:

> "Here are some things that we could talk about today, or maybe what's most on your mind is something that's not listed here. That's why there are some empty bubbles, for anything else you might want to talk about. Where would you like to start?"

Abstinence and Moderation Goals

An enduring and often hotly debated issue in addiction treatment, particularly in the United States, regards what to do with clients who do not embrace a goal of total lifelong abstinence, but want to reduce their use. For the sake of simplicity, imagine that there is only one drug involved. You favor complete abstention and the client says absolutely not, but does want to cut down to a moderate, problem-free level. What would you do?

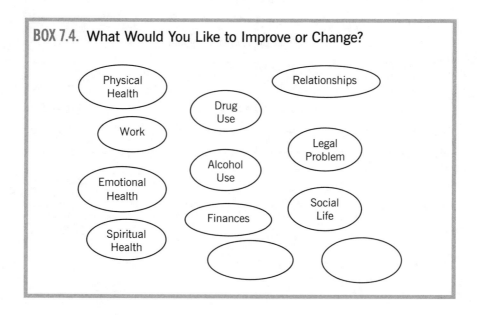

BOX 7.4. What Would You Like to Improve or Change?

1. Tell the client to try out self-control and come back when he is ready to abstain (Mann, 1950).
2. Explain why his goal is unrealistic, unachievable, and ill-advised, and push him to commit to abstinence (Milam & Ketcham, 1984).
3. Indicate that you are willing to work with him to reduce his use and see how it goes (Sanchez-Craig, 1996).
4. Say that you are willing to help him taper down toward an ultimate goal of abstinence (quitting "warm turkey" [Miller & Page, 1991]).
5. Encourage the client to at least try out a period of abstinence and negotiate an agreeable trial period (Meyers & Smith, 1995).
6. Explore the reasons for the client's preferences.

There are practitioners who do each of these things, and there is no one right answer for all situations. It depends in part on your own level of comfort with each of these options. One historic conception of substance dependence (discussed in Chapter 2) is that it involves a permanent loss of the ability to control one's own use, except via abstinence. Even within this view, however, there are many other nondependent people who, for example, drink too much and suffer adverse consequences. Few professionals object to screening for alcohol use in primary health care and counseling heavier drinkers to reduce their consumption (National Institute on Alcohol Abuse and Alcoholism, 1996, 2005). Some research-tested methods for doing so are described in Chapter 12.

Choosing Strategies

The next step in developing a change plan is to discuss possible steps or strategies to move toward each goal. These also should meet ARMS criteria, and it's usually good to have a time line attached to them. "By next week I will make an appointment to see my doctor." Considering the available options to move toward each goal, what is the person most ready, willing, and able to do? People who receive the treatment they prefer are more likely to stick with it and have better outcomes (Swift, Callahan, & Vollmer, 2011).

The change plan is a living document. Often a strategy is simply a next step in the direction of a change goal. As steps are accomplished, new ones take their place until a goal is reached. New goals may be added, and others modified. Involve your clients directly in preparing their own change plans, and gradually turn the whole process over to them to make the plan fully their own. It's often useful to prepare and provide a written change plan that can be easily modified. Erasable writing on heavy paper works; so do electronic documents.

Getting to "Yes"

Because the change plan is developed with and belongs to your client, she or he should be able to say "yes" to it. The basic question for the overall plan is: "Is this what you want to do?" For a more specific piece of the plan (like a task to be completed before next session), a better question is: "Is this what you're *going* to do?" If you sense reluctance, there is more work to do. What is the reluctance about? The importance and confidence rulers can be helpful here:

> "On a scale from 0 to 10, how *important* would you say it is for you to reach this goal, if 0 means not at all important and 10 means very important?"
> And on the same scale from 0 to 10, how *confident* are you that you can reach it, if 0 is 'I'm sure that I can't' and 10 is 'I'm sure that I can'?"

Sometimes reluctance reflects doubt about how important a goal really is, and sometimes it signals low self-efficacy to achieve it.

This issue of change planning raises some of the cardinal considerations in client–treatment matching. Who should do the matching? To what extent do clients set their own goals and get involved in choosing and designing their own treatment? What evidence-based knowledge do we have to inform the matching process? What attributes of treatments and of people are most important to consider in matching? How does one go about helping clients to find an optimal approach to recovery? And just how well does matching work, as compared with offering the same treatments to everyone? Those are central questions in this chapter.

CLIENT–TREATMENT MATCHING

It is a sensible idea that people do not all respond the same or best to any one particular treatment approach. One size does not fit all. A method that works very well for one person may be ineffective, unacceptable, or culturally inappropriate for another. As reflected in the chapters of Part III, the addiction treatment field is blessed with a menu of evidence-supported interventions, so that it is also possible to ask which of an array of potentially effective methods might be best for the particular person sitting in your office. It is an idea that can be traced right back to the beginning of systematic treatment for addictions, and is found in the classic writing of Bowman and Jellinek (1941). How should such matching occur?

Natural Matching

Wherever there are treatment options, some degree of natural matching is already happening. People vote with their feet. If they try a treatment program and it doesn't feel right, they are less likely to come back for a second visit. When they find a place or approach that suits them, they are more likely to stay. It's a bit like how churchgoers choose their home congregation, or how AA members find their home group. They shop around, in person or by telephone or computer, until they find one that they perceive to meet their needs, and where they feel at home. Being coerced into a particular program (e.g., by the courts) narrows the options, but even then there is a substantial degree of variation in attendance and compliance.

There are many important influences on natural matching, one of which is word of mouth. Deserved or undeserved, programs develop different reputations in the community, and people talk to each other about the options. There are practical considerations, such as relative cost, ease of access, length and type of commitment required, geographic accessibility, waiting lists, safety, and past experience. In a managed care context, only one or a few options may be covered by a particular health plan. Then there is the experience that people have during initial sessions. Early dropout is common in addiction treatment. Clients quickly develop a sense of the quality of the working alliance they would have with a counselor, and this perception affects the course and outcome of therapy. All of these influence the treatment options that clients choose for themselves.

Clinical Judgment

A second common source of matching is the clinical judgment of professionals. The judgment of an individual clinician is perhaps the most common way in which decisions are made about what treatment would be best for a particular individual. Many different factors might influence such decisions, including client characteristics and preferences, one's training and theoretical orientation, past experience, personal recovery history, program reputation and marketing, cost, location, health plan coverage, and interprofessional relationships and agreements. In one disconcerting study, however, there was little variability in treatment recommendations (Hanson & Emrick, 1983). Actors who presented with very different alcohol problem histories went to various alcohol treatment programs, asking for advice as to what approach would be best for them. The study was designed to discern what criteria were being used to match people to programs, but what it showed was that programs almost always recommended themselves regardless of a client's problems or severity.

BOX 7.5. Personal Reflection: On Giving People What They Want

I once worked with a hospital's psychiatry consultation liaison service. We would receive consult requests from the medical teams for patients who had been admitted to the hospital, and go to see them.

This particular consult request read, "Patient interested in abstinence from alcohol." I met with this middle-aged man for a little while, discussing what led him to this point and what types of help he might prefer on his path to recovery. After a long discussion, he decided that inpatient treatment was his preference. He liked the idea of being away from people who might encourage him to drink and from places where he would feel tempted. Access to residential treatment programs was very difficult, though, particularly for public programs. While he was still in the hospital we were able to get his name on a waiting list, but he wasn't able to transition directly into an inpatient program from the hospital. I was frustrated by this, knowing that he was ready and willing to make a change, and that the barrier was the unavailability of treatment.

A few days later, I was walking through the emergency department when I heard him call out my name from behind one of the curtains. I turned around and peeked in, wondering why he was back in the hospital. He had seemed to be one of the most highly motivated people I had talked to while on this rotation, and yet here he was back for an alcohol-related hospital admission. A few days after his prior discharge, he had gone sober to a local treatment program, where he was told that immediate admissions were only for people who were acutely intoxicated. "Basically," he explained, "they were telling me to come back when I was good and drunk!" Even though he had stayed sober during the days since he left the hospital, what he really wanted was the structure of a residential program. So he did what seemed logical: in order to show up at the treatment program drunk and thus get into treatment, he went to the liquor store and bought two fifths of vodka.

"So what happened?" I asked with interest.

"Well, I drank so much that I forgot to go back!" he replied.

—A. A. F.

Decision Rules

One way to reduce the arbitrariness of individual clinical judgment is to use a consistent set of decision rules. For example, both commonsense (Miller & Caddy, 1977) and data-based criteria (Miller & Muñoz, 2005; Miller, Zweben, DiClemente, & Rychtarik, 1992) have been suggested for advising people as to the likelihood of success with abstinence or moderate drinking goals in their particular case. The advantage of matching by such systems, of course, depends on the scientific validity of the decision rules.

Another approach is to develop decision rules based on the professional consensus of a group of experts in the field. The most common example of this in the United States is the Patient Placement Criteria of the American Society of Addiction Medicine (ASAM; Gastfriend, 2003). In the 1970s and 1980s, a majority of funds for addiction treatment in the United States were being spent on inpatient and residential treatment programs, typically of 28 days' duration (which was the maximum duration that most insurers would reimburse). As it became clear that the outcomes of inpatient programs were on average the same as those from less costly outpatient options (Institute of Medicine, 1990; Miller & Hester, 1986), third-party reimbursement for inpatient treatment was dramatically curtailed. In this managed care environment, a group of treatment program directors in northern Ohio convened to develop a consensus set of decision rules, called the Cleveland Criteria (Hoffman, Halikas, & Mee-Lee, 1987), to guide and defend placing people into specific levels of care. These were adopted and published by ASAM in 1991 (Hoffman, Halikas, Mee-Lee, & Weedman, 1991) and have been subsequently revised in increasingly complex systems (ASAM, 1996, 2001). Four levels of care are recognized, of increasing intensity and cost: outpatient treatment (Level I), intensive outpatient or "partial hospitalization" (Level II), residential/inpatient treatment (Level III), and medically managed intensive inpatient treatment (Level IV). Decision rules for placement are based on assessment of two medical and four psychosocial dimensions: (1) acute withdrawal potential and need for detoxification; (2) biomedical conditions and complications; (3) emotional, behavioral, and cognitive conditions or complications; (4) motivational readiness for change; (5) history of relapse and potential for continued drug use and problems; and (6) environmental support for recovery versus drug use. These data are combined by specified decision rules to arrive at a recommended level of care based on this consensus clinical judgment system.

Matching Algorithms

It is a nearly universal finding in psychological research that as clinicians we place far higher trust in our own clinical judgment than is warranted. Give accurate information for about 100 cases to a computer and also to a clinician and then ask each to make predictions about 100 new cases. It has been known for a long time that the computer is usually far more accurate in predicting diagnoses or outcomes (Wiggins, 1973). But what if the computer were given only a particular clinician's own judgments, rather than the actual truth about the 100 cases? In this case, the computer develops a mathematical model of the clinician's judgment. Then give a new set of 100 cases to both the computer and the clinician whose judgment it modeled, and once again the computer is likely to be more accurate! It has, in essence, abstracted the rules by which the clinician makes reasonably good judgments, and then applied them with perfect reliability (Goldberg, 1970).

Computer algorithms known as "expert systems" have been developed to improve the accuracy of many decision processes, from making medical diagnoses to flying aircraft. When your judgment tells you one thing and the computer tells you another, which should you trust? In most situations the computer is more likely to be right, but as clinicians we do overwhelmingly prefer to go with our own judgment.

Suppose that the outcome to be predicted is the risk that a driving-while-intoxicated (DWI) offender will repeat the offense. Computer algorithms can do a reasonably good job of predicting recidivism, given accurate data about the characteristics and outcomes of past cases (C'de Baca, Miller, & Lapham, 2001). The accuracy of such actuarial prediction programs is very likely to exceed that of nearly all clinicians, and yet these important public safety decisions continue to be made largely by clinical judgment.

Informed Self-Matching

Still another option is to involve clients in selecting and designing their own treatment. There are at least two possible advantages in doing so. First, people know something about which approaches are likely to be helpful, acceptable, and attractive for them. In oncology medicine it is normal good practice to give patients a fair description of the treatment options available to them and the most likely outcomes of each, and allow them to make an informed judgment as to what treatment they want. The same could surely be done with regard to addiction treatment options. The self-referral biases of treatment programs suggest that such matching ought to be done by an independent professional or agency not invested in particular choices (Martin, 1995), but the implementation of such a system can be both complex and expensive, as illustrated by the "core-shell" system experiment in Ontario (Weisner, 1995).

A second reason for informed self-matching is the motivational advantage of having chosen a course of action. When people perceive that they have freely selected, from among options, a particular product or course of action, they are likely to be more satisfied with and committed to it. There is evidence that taking active steps toward change increases the likelihood of successful change, no matter what the action happens to be. If what matters is that the client do *something* and stick with it, then it makes sense to allow clients to select that to which they will be most committed.

RESEARCH ON MATCHING PEOPLE TO TREATMENTS

A prerequisite for matching is the availability of different treatment options. Where there is only one option available, then there is no room or need for matching. Where different options are available, matching depends on knowing about the alternatives and who is most likely to benefit from each of them.

The earliest research relevant to matching asked, "Who responded best to Treatment *X*?" An implicit assumption here is that the treatments themselves are fixed and consistent, and the challenge is to identify those people who best fit into a particular approach. Over a span of decades, findings accumulated to suggest which clients might respond best to particular treatment methods (Miller & Hester, 1986).

The next generation of matching studies compared client responses to two or more different treatments. The usual purpose of these clinical trials was to evaluate the relative effectiveness of different treatments, but studies also began to include measures of client characteristics in order to determine whether different people had benefitted from each treatment. One study found, for example, that people who needed structure responded best to more directive therapists, whereas those who preferred less structure fared better with less directive therapists (McLachlan, 1972). Nevertheless, until the 1990s the data on matching consisted of a collection of isolated studies, most of which addressed a single client characteristic or treatment method, and most reports of matching were unreplicated.

A single basic prediction underlies the scientific validity of any system for matching people to different treatments: that those who are correctly "matched" should have better outcomes than do people who are "mismatched" according to the criteria. Research on matching came of age when this hypothesis began to be tested directly. Fortunately, it is not necessary to randomly assign people to be matched or mismatched to treatments in order to test this hypothesis. Such a design is logically equivalent to a normal clinical trial in which people are randomly assigned to different treatments (Miller & Cooney, 1994). As long as the criteria for matching are specified a priori (ahead of time, before looking at the outcome data), and the appropriate measures of client characteristics are obtained, virtually any matching hypothesis can be tested retrospectively within a clinical trial (Longabaugh & Wirtz, 2001).

Matching to Levels of Treatment Intensity

The ASAM criteria for assigning people to levels of treatment intensity (described earlier in this chapter and in Chapter 6) provide an example of the matching hypothesis. If these decision rules are valid, then patients who are correctly matched to level of treatment should have better outcomes than those who are given a lower intensity of treatment than that recommended by the criteria. Cases are "matched" when the assessed level of need (I, II, III, or IV) is the same as the level of treatment received. This creates four possible matched conditions and 12 possible mismatches. When a person receives a *higher* level of care than recommended by the criteria, the case is said to be *overmatched*. Conversely, when the level of care provided is *lower* than that recommended by the placement criteria, the case is said to be *undermatched*.

Studies of the validity of the ASAM criteria to date have been few and findings mixed. An early study of the Cleveland criteria (McKay, McLellan, & Alterman, 1992) found no significant differences in 6-month outcomes between matched and undermatched cases receiving outpatient treatment (Level II). In a complementary study of inpatient treatment (Sharon et al., 2004), only one significant outcome difference was reported between matched and mismatched groups: undermatched people at the highest level of severity (Level IV) had significantly more days of subsequent rehospitalization.

Potentially more informative are studies with clients in more than one level of care. One such study (Magura et al., 2003) followed people who were naturalistically (nonrandomly) assigned to Levels I, II, or III. Of the nine potential mismatches, only one affected outcomes ($p < .018$): People assessed at Level II fared better when receiving intensive outpatient (II) than regular outpatient treatment (I). In a controlled clinical trial (McKay, Cacciola, McLellan, Alterman, & Wirtz, 1997), no significant matching effects were found for medically stable people randomly assigned to Level II (day hospital) or Level III (inpatient) treatment for cocaine or alcohol dependence. A similar randomized trial (Angarita et al., 2007) reported only one significant effect: among overmatched patients (assessed at Level II but given inpatient treatment), those with comorbid mental disorders were more likely to be no-shows for treatment.

There are numerous methodological problems with such studies. Typically there are multiple potential mismatches, and a variety of outcome measures are assessed. When one outcome variable is related to one possible mismatch, its "significance" is dubious if there is no correction for the number of tests run. In most studies, the match that was found had not been predicted a priori but was found among multiple a posteriori tests, and the outcome variable showing a match is different in each study. None of the observed matches described above would be statistically significant if corrected for these factors. In sum, scientific evidence for the validity of ASAM's placement criteria is weak thus far. Certainly no robust outcome differences are being found or replicated for cases matched versus mismatched according to ASAM criteria.

Stepped Care

A simpler alternative to ASAM criterion-based matching is to follow the stepped care approach that is commonly used in medicine in the treatment of chronic diseases (e.g., Baker, Turner, Kay-Lambkin, & Lewin, 2009;

Sobell & Sobell, 2000). With Type 2 diabetes, for example, one might try first to
control blood glucose by a combination of
diet, exercise, and oral medication. If this

> Stepped care is commonly used in the treatment of chronic diseases.

is insufficient, medication might be changed or dosage increased. Insulin
could be initiated next, with hospitalization used only when there is a need
for acute stabilization of medically ill individuals.

The logic of stepped care is to offer the least intensive and intrusive
level of care that is likely to help. If one level of care is not sufficient to
resolve the problem, then the client is stepped up to the next higher level
of intensity. There are several advantages in this approach. One is a cost
advantage, in that less expensive options are the first line of defense. If
these are successful, then the more expensive level of care is not required
(and is more available for those who do need it). It is common for clients to
surprise us—to respond to lower levels of care than a clinician might expect
to work (Miller, 2000). It is easy to overestimate the amount of help that
clients will require. Another advantage is that lower levels of care are more
likely to be immediately available. When clients are placed on a waiting list,
the window of motivation for change may have closed by the time a space
opens up. Offering something immediately, albeit less intensive, can foster
improvement. When space opens in the higher intensity care setting, the client can be transitioned if that level of care is still required. In the meantime
you've been doing something helpful and supportive.

It is by no means a foregone conclusion that if one level of care fails,
only a higher level of care will work. In fact, there is no guarantee that
more intensive care will help. Another option is to try a different approach
at the same level of intensity, particularly if higher level options are not
available. A client who has not responded to a 12-step-oriented outpatient
program, for example, might be referred to a cognitive-behavioral outpatient approach. A more general principle is that if one approach hasn't been
working, *try something else.*

Matching to Type of Treatment

The level or intensity of treatment (e.g., outpatient, inpatient) tells nothing
about what treatment is actually being delivered in that setting. It has long
been believed that differing types of people would be likely to benefit from
different kinds of treatment.

Beginning in 1990, the National Institute on Alcohol Abuse and Alcoholism (NIAAA) funded what would be the largest controlled trial ever
conducted for alcohol treatment methods. This study, known as Project
MATCH, began only with a general concept of testing strategies for matching people with optimal treatment approaches. Based on a competition for
research concepts, nine clinical research sites were selected, spanning the

United States from coast to coast. Then began a collaborative process of designing and implementing a study to yield broad new knowledge about how best to match people to treatment methods (Project MATCH Research Group, 1993).

In the end, three treatment methods were selected, representing conceptually different approaches: 12 sessions of 12-step facilitation therapy (TSF; Nowinski, Baker, & Carroll, 1992), four sessions of motivational enhancement therapy (MET; Miller, Zweben, et al., 1992), or 12 sessions of cognitive-behavioral therapy (CBT; Kadden et al., 1992). Because it was unclear which personal characteristics would prove most important, the 1,726 participants completed extensive pretreatment assessment. Clients were then randomly assigned to one of the three treatment methods, and a priori matching hypotheses were formulated and tested (Longabaugh & Wirtz, 2001). The full story of Project MATCH is recounted in a single volume (Babor & Del Boca, 2003), summarizing findings from a series of published detailed reports (Project MATCH Research Group, 1997a, 1997b, 1998b, 1998c, 1998d).

As hoped, the three therapeutic methods produced, on average, excellent and equivalent outcomes, whether offered as outpatient treatment or as aftercare following intensive treatment. Furthermore, clients' outcomes were reasonably stable across 3 years of follow-up, with relatively little loss of posttreatment improvement. On one outcome measure—the percentage of clients who remained totally abstinent—the TSF group showed about a 10% advantage throughout follow-up.

Project MATCH was not primarily a horse race, however; the central interest was in matches between clients and therapies. Project MATCH revealed surprisingly few robust matches. Nearly all previously reported matching effects from single studies were not replicated in this multisite trial. Some reliable matches were found, however, suggesting clinical guidelines in choosing among these three treatment approaches:

• As predicted, clients whose social networks supported continued drinking rather than abstinence fared best in TSF therapy, an advantage that appeared only in the long run at 3-year follow-up. One clear reason for this is that clients became more involved in the fellowship of AA, which provided them with a strong social support network for abstinence. The key, then, appears to be for such clients to get involved in AA or another abstinence-supporting network *during treatment*, to compensate for the lack of support for sobriety among their own significant others. When clients' own social support networks favored abstinence, they fared at least as well in the other two treatments as in TSF.

• Some clients did better with MET. The clinical method of motivational interviewing (see Chapter 10) was designed to reduce client resistance and elicit intrinsic motivation for change. As predicted, more angry clients fared best with MET (Waldron, Miller, & Tonigan, 2001). Angry clients are more likely to offer resistance when directed to change, and resistance in turn predicts poorer outcomes. A year after treatment, there were also better outcomes in MET for clients who had presented with low initial motivation for change (Witkiewitz, Hartzler, & Donovan, 2010). Advantages of MET were not found for clients with low anger or high motivation.

• Clients with less concomitant psychopathology, whose problems centered mainly on alcohol, fared better in TSF therapy than in CBT. This was an unexpected and unexplained finding. Suffice it to say that the advantages of this AA-focused approach were clearest for clients with relatively few psychological problems.

• In aftercare, clients with more severe alcohol dependence also fared better in TSF than in CBT. In contrast, clients with less alcohol dependence had better outcomes with CBT than with TSF. This is consistent with the more severe picture of alcoholism that is presented in AA, whereby more severely impaired individuals might be expected to recognize themselves.

Subsequent analyses of the MATCH data have revealed matching effects not tested in the original trial. One study found that depressed clients had better outcomes (on drinking measures) when working with therapists who focused *less* on painful emotional material (Karno & Longabaugh, 2003). Regardless of the form of treatment they received (CBT, MET, or TSF), clients with concomitant depression fared significantly worse when treated by therapists with a high focus on negative emotional issues. In another analysis, Native American clients were found to fare significantly better in MET than with CBT or TSF, whereas such differences were not found for white and Hispanic clients (Villanueva, Tonigan, & Miller, 2007).

Matching to What?

Triage into different kinds of psychotherapy is only one kind of matching. Far less is known about how to match clients at other decision points such as group versus individual therapy or behavioral therapies versus pharmacotherapies. Guidelines for knowing when clients are likely to need detoxification are provided in Chapter 6.

There is another form of matching, however, that not only makes good clinical sense but also has strong empirical support. People who present for treatment of substance use disorders usually come with a host of other problems as well. Because health and social service systems are often frag-

> Sobriety was predicted by the extent to which clients had received the services they had said they wanted.

mented into specialty clinics, there is a tendency to focus addiction treatment solely on the use of alcohol and other drugs. It is now clear that clients will be more successful in recovering from addiction when their other needs are addressed as well (McLellan et al., 1998; McLellan et al., 1999). In one study (Brown & Miller, 1993), inpatients were given at admission a list of possible services (see Box 7.3) and asked which ones they wanted as part of their treatment. Then at discharge they were asked, via a parallel questionnaire, which services they had actually received. Sobriety at 3 months after discharge was predictable from the extent to which they had received the services they had said they wanted. The extent to which they had been given other services (which they had not asked for) was unrelated to treatment outcomes.

This is not to say that clinicians who treat addictions must also handle every other problem that clients present. What it does imply is the need to make sure clients are at least referred to the other services they need, and do connect with those services. If those additional services are provided at the same location (one-stop treatment), so much the better, but if not there are some simple ways to help people get to the services they need. One, of course, is knowledge about where specific services can be obtained. Community service directories are often compiled annually, and increasingly are available online. It also helps to know how best to access those services, and to have specific contact names. The likelihood of a client completing a referral is substantially increased if you place a call to the service agency while the client is still in your office, establishing a direct link and appointment (Kogan, 1957). These case management functions are discussed more fully in Chapter 8.

PRACTICAL GUIDELINES

Given the findings of research to date, what are some practical implications for matching clients to optimal treatments?

1. *Put client welfare first.* First of all, match treatments to people, rather than trying to make people fit into particular programs. The purpose here is to find the approach that is best for this particular person, which can conflict with a desire to fill certain beds or treatment slots.

2. *Offer a menu.* Provide clients with a variety of options, and provide the information they need to make informed choices. Make use of clients' own wisdom and preferences about what will work for them.

3. *Try something different.* If the person has tried a particular approach in the past without success, consider other options rather than more of the same.

4. *Attend to the person's larger needs.* Look beyond substance use problems, and connect the person with needed services.

5. *Practice appropriate humility.* Research clearly supports modesty regarding clinical judgment in knowing what is best for clients. Consider the possibility that "clients know best."

6. *Make use of available knowledge.* Nevertheless, there are findings to inform the matching process. For example, if the person has very little family and other social support for abstinence, consider mutual help programs as an enduring social support network (see Chapter 14). If motivation seems low and resistance high, consider a treatment approach to enhance motivation for change (Chapter 10).

7. *Consider collecting your own data.* While matching guidelines from other settings can be informative, consider the possibility of developing your own. If you have reliable information about what treatment people have received and about their outcome (such as recidivism data), you have the basics for developing data-based decision rules that work for your own client population (e.g., C'de Baca et al., 2001; Martin, 1995).

8. *Remember general factors.* There is considerable evidence that therapist and client factors have a greater impact on outcome than the particular treatment procedures used (Imel et al., 2008; Miller et al., 1980). Empathic listening, hope and optimism, treating clients with respect and honoring their autonomy will go a long way beyond the specific treatment methods you use. Similarly, there is much you can do to activate the client factors that promote change: hope, self-efficacy, motivation, and taking small steps. Don't get too invested in clients taking a certain path that you favor. It may be more important for them to do *something* to move in the right direction than to take the particular road you have in mind.

KEY POINTS

- Four phases of treatment are (1) palliative care, (2) stabilization, (3) rehabilitation, and (4) maintenance.

- A change plan involves negotiation of a client's goals and strategies for reaching them. A treatment plan is a subset of a change plan.

🖈 A variety of evidence-based treatment approaches are available from which to choose what best meets each person's needs.

🖈 There is a modest research base on what treatment approaches work best for whom.

🖈 People should be active participants in designing their own treatment, based on informed choice.

REFLECTION QUESTIONS

💬 How do you go about selecting the most appropriate treatments for the people you serve?

💬 In developing change plans, to what extent do you rely on clients' own wisdom and preferences about how to proceed?

💬 In the setting where you work, how might a stepped care approach be implemented, starting with briefer interventions and stepping up level of care as needed?

CHAPTER 8

Case Management

As we have emphasized, people seeking addiction treatment commonly have various problems accompanying their substance use such as employment, financial, family, physical, and emotional concerns (Siegel et al., 1995). Individuals with co-occurring disorders and life problems are not a subpopulation, but the norm in addiction treatment (see Chapter 18).

Historically, many addiction treatment providers have not responded adequately to these concomitant problems (Benshoff & Janikowski, 2000; Willenbring, 1996). Inadequate response may stem in part from a belief that substance use disorders represent the "primary" disease, the resolution of which will naturally result in improvement in other life areas (Siegel et al., 1995). Within this understanding, it would be irrelevant to focus on other problems because they are only secondary consequences of the primary disorder. Attempts to intervene with such practical and psychological problems, in fact, have even been construed as "enabling" or interfering with the recovery process. Allowing clients to experience these negative consequences of substance use, it has been argued, can enhance their motivation for change.

This is, in our view, a strangely punitive perspective. For what other chronic illness would one withhold treatment in order to sustain suffering in hopes of increasing motivation for change? Substantial evidence also seriously questions the validity of this perspective. Research indicates instead a complex or reciprocal relationship between substance use and sundry social, legal, and economic problems (Rose & Zweben, 2003; Rose et al., 1999). Alcohol or other drugs may be used to forget, avoid, or cope with very real problems of living that are still present in abstinence. Some people essentially self-medicate for emotional problems that could otherwise be effectively treated, and that continue or even worsen with sobriety (see Chapter 18). People who fall into addictive use of substances often have diminished capacities for self-regulation and coping with everyday hardships, even when sober (Brown, 1998). In others words, psychosocial problems may be a precipitant, consequence, and/or maintaining factor associated with substance use disorders, or may simply be coexisting conditions.

Furthermore, failing to address these concomitant problems during addiction treatment may place clients at increased risk for continuing or recurring substance use (Morgenstern, Hogue, Dauber, Dasaro, & McKay, 2009; Substance Abuse and Mental Health Services Administration, 1998; Willenbring, 1996). Some of the most strongly evidence-based treatment methods for substance use disorders do not focus primarily or exclusively on the addiction itself, but aim to improve quality of life and more general coping skills (Berglund et al., 2003; Miller & Carroll, 2006; Miller, Wilbourne, & Hettema, 2003). Ancillary services are often effective in producing positive change with individuals who need help with alcohol/drug problems. Clients who are more involved with medical and social services are likely to remain longer in addiction treatment and tend to have better posttreatment outcomes on social and psychological well-being as well as reduced substance use relative to those not receiving such services (Hesse, Vanderplasschen, Rapp, Broekaert, & Fridell, 2007; McLellan et al., 1999; Morgenstern et al., 2009; Siegal et al., 1996; Siegal, Li, & Rapp, 2002; Siegal, Rapp, Li, Saha, & Kirk, 1997; Sullivan, Wolk, & Hartman, 1992).

> Some of the most strongly evidence-based treatment methods do not focus primarily on the addiction itself.

In other words, case management (CM) is a vital component in addiction treatment, to help clients find, gain access to, and use supplemental services that will support their change in substance use. CM is an expertise in itself, and in this chapter we examine different models, identify active ingredients of CM, and review current research evidence. We give particular emphasis to practical issues of how CM can be effectively included in addiction treatment.

WHAT IS CM?

In general, CM is aimed at helping clients acquire resources to resolve their presenting problems. This is in contrast to treatment, where the focus is on producing interpersonal and intrapersonal change (Alexander, Pollack, Nahra, Wells, & Lemak, 2007; Rothman, 2003). CM is not an alternative or substitute, but rather an important complement for treatment, an approach that attends to matters or tasks that are *not* routinely dealt with in therapy (Hesse et al., 2007). Linking clients with needed services such as housing, economic, employment, and legal assistance facilitates the rehabilitation process (Rapp et al., 2008). Although some treatment methods such as the community reinforcement approach (Chapter 11) do give substantial attention to social work issues, most often CM services are not provided by clinical staff but by other professionals with particular expertise in CM. CM can be integrated within a particular organization such as a hospital or outpatient treatment center (as in a team approach) or can be a stand-alone service developed and jointly sponsored by several providers to link clients with appropriate resources (Vanderplasschen, Rapp, Wolf, & Broekaert, 2004).

There are several approaches to CM, including a traditional broker/ generalist model and more intensive interventions such as the strengths-based assertive community treatment (ACT) and clinical/rehabilitation approaches (Rapp, 2002; Rothman, 2003; Substance Abuse and Mental Health Services Administration, 1998; Test, 2003; Walsh, 2003). Differences between these models mainly deal with the number and kinds of services provided and the amount of emphasis placed on particular components. Some models focus primarily on assessment, information, and referral activities, whereas others (such as strengths-based models) place more emphasis on therapeutic skill and building a working alliance, providing information, and linking clients with suitable services. Nondegreed paraprofessionals are more likely to be employed as case managers in programs that are based on broker/generalist models than in those founded on a therapeutic strengths-based model of CM.

The ACT model is more comprehensive than a broker-generalist approach (Inciardi, Martin, & Scarpitti, 1996; Substance Abuse and Mental Health Services Administration, 1998; Test, 2003) and pursues a larger number and variety of goals. Unlike other CM models, ACT also advocates proactively for the establishment of new community resources as a response to the needs of clients in coping with problems of everyday living. ACT programs typically serve clients with both substance use disorders and concomitant serious mental health conditions. Such vulnerable groups particularly benefit from intensive CM and a wide variety of concrete resources to improve their functioning in the community, and flounder if left alone to deal with fragmented service systems (Ridgely, 1996; Shavelson, 2001).

RESEARCH ON CM

The evidence for including CM in addiction treatment is persuasive. Outcome studies show that people who are given CM stay in addiction treatment longer, are less likely to be readmitted to detoxification, and show greater improvement across a variety of life areas including substance use, employment, physical health, and legal problems, compared to those not receiving CM (Conrad et al., 1998; Cox et al., 1998; Kirby et al., 1999; Najavits, Weiss, Shaw, & Muenz, 1998; Siegal et al., 1995, 1996, 1997, 2002; Sullivan, 2003; Sullivan et al., 1992). What components of CM are particularly associated with these positive outcomes? CM appears to be more effective when there is a strong working relationship between client and manager, when needed services are more readily available and accessible, and when the case manager follows a more structured (e.g., manual-guided) approach. Also, the more time that is spent on CM core functions (like goal setting, case monitoring, client advocacy, and service coordination), the more positive the outcomes (Alexander et al., 2007; Morgenstern et al., 2008; Noel, 2006; Vanderplasschen et al., 2004). There are also some basic core competencies (such as motivational interviewing; see Chapter 10) for case managers. As with treatment services (Miller, Sorensen, Selzer, & Brigham, 2006), quality in delivering CM activities is supported by more thorough training, coaching and supervision, and by strong administrative support (Vanderplasschen, Wolf, Rapp, & Broekaert, 2007). Successful CM, of course, does depend on having available community resources for helping clients deal with their various problems (Walsh, 2003). Case managers are particularly likely to notice significant gaps in care, and to advocate for needed services.

Outcome evaluations of CM are challenging to conduct in real-life systems. The typical design compares usual care with or without additional CM services, and thus far it is not possible to conclude whether it was specifically the CM (rather than just additional time and attention) that resulted in better outcomes. There is also little information about the relative efficacy of different CM models. Another limitation of research to date is the lack of monitoring and quality assurance to ensure the fidelity of CM services delivered.

Illustrating this complexity, McLellan and colleagues (1999) studied the impact of CM services on client outcomes in eight addiction treatment programs. Because of the large volume of clients seeking services from these programs, not all could be given CM, and whether or not they received it was essentially due to "chance." This permitted a natural experiment of CM. Clients who had been given CM were compared with non-CM (NCM) clients on a variety of outcomes such as medical status, employment, family relations, and legal status. Two waves of clients were evaluated in this study: one at 12 months and the other at 26 months after CM was initiated in the treatment system. In Wave 1 few benefits of CM were found, but in Wave 2 CM clients fared significantly better than NCM clients with regard to drinking, drug use, psychiatric symptoms, and legal and employment issues. Differences on the Addiction Severity Index (see Chapter 5) were particularly large. The difference in outcomes might be explained by the fact that CM clients in Wave 2 made greater use of services than their counterparts in Wave 1. For example, in Wave 1 only 25% of the CM clients became involved with an employment specialist, whereas in Wave 2 the comparable figure was 52%. This was in turn attributable to the fact that more community services such as drug-free housing, employment, and training opportunities became available between the two waves. The case managers may also have become more skilled with experience.

CLIENT READINESS FOR CHANGE

An important consideration in developing and implementing CM plans is client *readiness* to seek services. How willing a client is to undertake various CM tasks depends on at least two factors: (1) their perceived *importance* of or need for the service and (2) their perceived *ability* to use the service (Zweben & Zuckoff, 2002). In other words, clients are most likely to use a service if they perceive it to be relevant to their personal goals, and if they believe that it is possible for them to access it (Siegal et al., 1996). Suppose you wanted to refer a woman who is in addiction treatment to a free shelter for victims of domestic violence. The woman is most likely to accept and complete the referral if (1) she believes that her violent partner has been a barrier to the changes she wants to make and it is important for her to be protected; and (2) if she believes that it is possible for her and her children to get to the shelter safely.

What might stand in the way of the first of these factors's perceived *importance*?

- *Need.* Clients may perceive that they do not really need the services.
- *Efficacy.* They may not believe that the services would help or work for them.
- *Relevance.* They may not perceive a relationship between the services and their substance use problems.
- *Priority.* They may see a need, believe the services would be helpful, and understand their relevance, but just have higher priorities right now.

And what might interfere with the second factor, perceived *ability?*

- *Practical obstacles.* Clients may feel obstructed by real-life factors (e.g., child care, safety, transportation, cost) that prevent them from seeking services.
- *Self-efficacy.* They may perceive that they are personally unable to do what is needed (e.g., don't have the skills, time, education).
- *Feeling overwhelmed.* They may in general be too demoralized to do it (depression, illness, demands, confusion, low self-esteem).

As in treatment (see Chapter 10), enhancing clients' readiness for change is part of the case manager's task and skill. With appropriate clinical strategies, it is possible to increase clients' acceptance of and engagement in services (Conrad et al., 1998). This is particularly important for individuals with substance dependence, who may not benefit from conventional CM approaches with a broker-generalist model (Substance Abuse and Mental Health Services Administration, 1998).

ASSESSING CM NEEDS OF CLIENTS

A useful tool is a services request form (see example in Box 8.1) on which clients can quickly indicate areas where they would like help. The form covers such matters as finances, child care, living arrangements, employment, medical, and behavioral health care. On this form clients are also asked to assign a priority rating (1–10) for each service. Having clients complete a services request form helps acquaint them with community resources that are available and could support their efforts to change addictive behaviors. It also provides information for completing a CM plan with specific goals and tasks.

A first step in CM is to identify broader goals and specific objectives. This in turn leads to a list of particular tasks to be completed by the client or case manager. What specific manageable steps could be taken to fulfill CM goals? Accomplishing small, practical steps enhances self-efficacy, which is an important component in building commitment to change. To illustrate, improving physical health could be identified as a broad goal, having a medical exam as a more specific objective, and component tasks that are steps in that direction could include locating a physician in the resource directory, making an appointment, arranging transportation, and keeping the appointment. Box 8.2 is an example of how CM can be used in ongoing practice.

FACILITATING THE REFERRAL PROCESS

It is common in addiction treatment that clients need ongoing encouragement, contact, and support to complete the tasks within a CM plan. This usually involves taking quite a proactive and assertive role to help clients take the steps they need. Sometimes counselors worry that their clients should "take responsibility" and do it on their own, but the plain fact is that proactive CM substantially increases the likelihood of getting there. Our inclination is to help clients get there as a first step. What will it take to do that? Sometimes what is needed is to meet them in the community and accompany them to social service agencies to obtain the needed resources

BOX 8.1. Services Request Form

(Please circle Yes, Maybe, or No for each)

Would you like assistance in any of these areas? If YES, mark with an X and indicate how important it is for you on a scale from 1 (least important) to 10 (most important).	If YES, Mark X	How Important? 1–10
1. Housing (place to live, landlord, etc.)		
2. Employment (finding a job, better job, etc.)		
3. Legal problems or advice		
4. Health care or medical problems		
5. Medications or managing medications		
6. Self-help or support groups		
7. Child care (or other dependent care)		
8. Parenting and family issues		
9. Obtaining or keeping benefits or insurance (disability, Medicaid, SSI, VA, etc.)		
10. Financial assistance (debt, budgeting, food stamps, welfare, etc.)		
11. Work or employment training		
12. School, education, GED, etc.		
13. Personal or family safety		
14. Mental health or psychological problems		
15. How I spend my free time		
16. Advocacy with another system		
17. Utilities (telephone, heat, water, etc.)		
18. Food		
19. Clothing and household needs		
20. Transportation		
Are there other areas (not listed) in which you need assistance? *Please write these below.*		
21.		
22.		
23.		

BOX 8.2. CM in Addiction Treatment: A Case Example

Sondra listed "job training" as a major priority on her services request form. Asked what her concerns were in this area, Sondra revealed that she had been haphazardly employed and that with better training, she hoped she might find steady employment. To understand and enhance Sondra's motivation for change, the case manager asked how getting assistance with this might help her, and specifically might support her intention to be free from drug dependence. She said that having stable employment would improve her financial situation, which in turn would allow her to move away from her current neighborhood which was "infested" with drug dealers and users. Living in this environment made it particularly difficult for her to remain drug-free. Because Sondra did not have specific ideas about a direction to pursue, the case manager suggested some career testing and counseling to discover where her skills and interests might best fit. She agreed, and accepted the referral. The case manager called the career counseling service while she was still in the office, and gave the phone to Sondra to make the appointment. Later, they met again to discuss what she had learned and to explore options for further education and training.

(Willenbring, 1994). It is also possible to enhance clients' own personal motivation to follow through, using some of the methods described in Chapter 10. For example, identifying areas of past successes, affirming strengths and current steps in the right direction, and generally supporting self-efficacy can be important in sustaining motivation (Najavits, 2002; Najavits et al., 1998).

FORGING A CONSENSUS

| Negotiate a change plan that your client will endorse, own, and commit to follow. |

The importance of client choice cannot be over-emphasized in facilitating adherence with CM plans. This involves negotiating a change plan that your client will endorse, own, and commit to follow. Clients tend to become disengaged from the change process when counselors push their own agenda rather than listening to and understanding the clients' goals (Cooney et al., 1995; Rapp, Kelliher, Fisher, & Hall, 1996). An important task, therefore, is to establish a consensus with your client on what life domains (e.g., medical, employment, leisure time, residential) need to be addressed, and in what order of priority. In using this consensus approach to develop CM plans, Siegal et al. (2002) found that two-thirds of CM objectives were completed across nine life domains. The more clients were involved and participating in planning, the more improvement occurred in family, employment, and overall psychosocial functioning along with a reduction in cocaine and marijuana use.

An interesting way to assess discrepancies between the client's perceptions and your own is for both of you to complete the services request form for the client, including priority ratings. This lets you identify differences in perceptions of what is needed and how important each issue is. You can then discuss these differences in priorities. Do they arise, for example, from different perceptions of how these areas impact alcohol/drug use? You can explore this in more detail using an assessment instrument such as the Inventory of Drinking Situations (IDS; Annis et al., 1987) or the Desired Effects of Drinking (DED) scale (Doyle, Donovan, & Simpson, in press) that can help to clarify CM needs. (See Box 18.1 in Chapter 18 for the DED scale.) These instruments provide relevant data on various events (e.g., mood disorder) that might serve as triggers (i.e., high-risk situations) in initiating drinking or other drug use.

In some cases, sharing relevant information may not be sufficient to resolve counselor and client differences regarding CM needs (Zweben & Zuckoff, 2002). Clients' reluctance about agreeing to or following through on a referral may be more related to an underlying fear of the consequences associated with change than a lack of awareness of their CM needs. For example, gaining steady employment may estrange clients from their familiar pastimes and companions, or enable separation for a spouse who had been previously unable to leave due to financial instability. Clients may also have real doubts about their own abilities to succeed in certain CM goals and the tasks that they require, and this can interfere with willingness to proceed.

Failing to detect and address such underlying motivational issues can increase the chances of treatment dropout (Zweben & Zuckoff, 2002). These adherence problems require more than merely sharing information. The next section describes several motivational strategies that can be helpful here (Miller & Rollnick, 2002; Miller, Zweben, et al., 1992; Zweben & Barrett, 1997).

MOTIVATIONAL STRATEGIES TO STRENGTHEN ADHERENCE

Motivational Interviewing

A variety of methods from motivational interviewing (see Chapter 10) can help move toward a consensus CM plan. Empathic, reflective listening (Chapter 4) helps both you and your clients understand their misgivings or reluctance about pursuing particular goals or tasks. It can also be useful to normalize counselor/client differences in perception—explaining that this is quite common and arises from differences in perspective and interpretation. It is important here to recognize, acknowledge, and honor clients' own perspectives and autonomy, their right and ability to make their own choices.

Decisional Balance

Another possible tool is to construct a decisional balance, exploring the pros and cons, the "good things" and "not so good things" about pursuing a particular goal or task (Janis & Mann, 1977). This gives clients the freedom to express their reservations and also give voice to possible advantages and benefits. What, for example, does the client perceive as the pros and cons of arranging child care in order to attend treatment and pursue job training? Ask first about the downside, the disadvantages, and then the possible benefits of a particular CM task. Such a discussion may increase a client's willingness to follow through.

Delaying a Decision

It can be helpful to remember and acknowledge that a decision doesn't have to be made right away. Particularly when clients seem to be reluctant to commit, invite them *not* to decide now, but to continue talking about it in future visits. This is better than forcing the client to make a premature decision or agreement to please you, and then later save face by not returning for future appointments (Zweben, Bonner, Chaim, & Santon, 1988). Clients who are confronted with decisions that conflict with their own current beliefs and attitudes may be better prepared to act favorably on them at a later time. Pressing for an immediate commitment is more likely to engage resistance. Another advantage of this approach is that it allows the client time to gain additional information and support from significant others about undertaking the various tasks (Cooney et al., 1995).

Refocusing

Despite your efforts, some clients might continue to have strong reluctance about accepting or carrying out a particular CM task or referral. Instead of continuing to press, shift the focus to a goal or task that is more acceptable to the client. What *is* the client willing and interested to do? Success with these less ambivalent tasks can pave the way later to discuss other goals and tasks.

Developing Proximal Goals

Accomplishing even a minor goal can help build self-efficacy, which is important for improving motivation. Break down a broader goal into more specific short-term component tasks that can be accomplished. What would be a first step in the right direction? Perhaps it is asking to use a neighbor's phone to arrange a baby-sitter for a medical appointment. If the client does not seem confident, it can be helpful to role-play a conversation, to practice the skills needed to complete a particular task (Rapp, 2002; Sullivan, 2003). You might, for example, first model how to call a social service agency to ask for an immediate appointment. Then have the client try it out, and give positive feedback on what he or she is doing right.

Problem-Solving Obstacles

In preparing a client to undertake a referral or other task, consider possible obstacles that might occur after leaving your session. You could ask *"What might happen to prevent you from doing this?"* If the client is uncertain or unable to identify potential obstacles, you might suggest some possibilities (transportation, waiting lists, lack of child care, unexpected illness) and ask how she or he might respond to those if they arise. Also normalize such setbacks so that there is no shame should the client be unable to carry out a task (Zweben & Zuckoff, 2002). Respond to nonadherence or setbacks with problem solving. What went wrong? What can you and the client do to make it work next time? Again emphasize personal choice, that if they find one referral source to be unsatisfactory, you will explore other options to try (Siegal et al., 1996). In this way you can reduce the danger of the individual avoiding you or dropping out if she or he is unable to carry out a particular task.

Use of Written Materials

Written materials can also be useful in helping clients to understand and think further about CM needs and tasks (Najavits, 2002). These might be brochures or downloads from possible referral agencies that describe location, services, a contact person, fees, insurance coverage, and the duration of waiting period for the initial appointment. You can review such pamphlets with clients, asking them to consider the pros and cons of particular services. Taking written materials home also allows clients to share and discuss the information with significant others.

Importance of Follow-Up

A vital component of CM is proactive, assertive follow-up on your clients' progress at subsequent sessions, or via other contact between sessions. This communicates that you care and are available and willing to help and support them. Checking in during or between sessions allows you to intercede if there are obstacles to progress. You can initiate these contacts, or arrange for your clients to contact you with progress reports by telephone,

BOX 8.3. Is There a Role for the Significant Other in CM?

As head of social work at a large agency in the 1980s I often advised practitioners to involve the significant other (SO) in helping clients address everyday problems associated with their substance use such as managing finances or inadequate housing. My advice was met with mixed results. Some social workers preferred to work with the client alone (in part, because it's easier!). Not unexpectedly, most practitioners chose the spouse as the SO, many of whom were overwhelmed with the stress and hardships of living with a partner who is drinking excessively or using drugs. As a result, many of these SOs were not very supportive and helpful in the planning process.

As I gained experience in addiction treatment, I realized that involving an SO could be more beneficial if you choose the appropriate person. The SO you are looking for does not have to be a spouse or live-in partner, but an individual who is strongly committed to the relationship, is interested in promoting positive change, and whose support is highly valued by the client. This could certainly mean involving the spouse if she or he meets these criteria, but it might also be a friend, employer, sponsor, clergy, or relative.

How do you go about finding such a person? Take some time early on to consider whether there is a supportive SO in the client's social network. Ask clients whether there is anyone around whom they see often, has an interest in their sobriety, and might be willing to attend sessions with them. When there is doubt as to whether the proposed SO is actually supportive of sobriety, my experience is that it's best not to invite that person, since he or she could even undermine the client's efforts to change (Zweben, 1991).

If you identify such a person and the client agrees, you can invite the SO to join in some or all of the sessions. How many sessions SOs attend will depend on their availability and how helpful they prove to be in the CM process. Depending on the person selected, SOs can be helpful in a variety of ways. Based on their knowledge of and relationship with the client, SOs can offer constructive feedback on the client's plans, identify potential obstacles, suggest options to facilitate sobriety, and provide practical and moral support.

It is important to coach the SO about how best to participate in sessions—for example, how to make suggestions without the client feeling ganged up on or controlled. Ultimately it is the client who decides what to change, no matter how much the SO (or you) might like to make that choice. Help SOs to understand that change does not always come quickly and that it is normal for the client to experience "ups and downs" before positive change is sustained. This can help keep the SO from jumping in and eliciting resistance when the client appears reluctant to change.

—A. Z.

voice mail, or electronic messages. If the client is to contact you, set up a reminder system for yourself so that you notice if you don't hear back as expected. The overall goals of the follow-up are to provide support, monitor progress toward CM goals, and assist in developing alternative goals and plans when obstacles are encountered.

Ask what has happened since your last contact in terms of completing agreed-upon tasks toward CM goals. For some clients, it is helpful to have them keep a log of particular tasks (e.g., job interviews) completed. Affirm all efforts that are made toward CM goals, even if they did not have the intended outcome (Sullivan, 2003). Some clients enjoy planning for a particular reward after completing an agreed-upon task. Remain supportive and nonjudgmental even if the client has not finished task assignments (Zweben & Zuckoff, 2002). If a client has not completed a task assignment, explore briefly what interfered with getting it done. Ask the client to take you through the step-by-step process of what interfered with completion of a particular task (e.g., logistics, low self-efficacy or motivation, unclear assignment, and poor social support). This can help you to anticipate and plan together how to respond to such obstacles in the future. For example, for one client the obstacle to AA meetings might have been a practical problem of arranging child care (logistics). Another might lack the confidence to attend AA sessions (low self-efficacy). A third client might be unclear about the location of meetings he or she had planned to attend (unclear assignment).

When client motivation or confidence is shaky, it can be helpful to involve a significant other (Meyers & Smith, 1995; Zweben & Barrett, 1993). This can be useful not only in bolstering the clients' confidence but in providing constructive feedback on the task assignment as well. When breaking down goals into component tasks, follow up as each successive task is completed and agree on a next step, staying engaged until the goals have been met. It is possible for CM follow-up to continue after an episode of formal treatment has been completed. This helps not only in pursuing CM goals, but in detecting early a need to resume treatment (see Chapter 19).

KEY POINTS

🔖 CM helps clients access resources for resolving the practical problems that often accompany addiction.

🔖 Psychosocial problems may be a precipitant, consequence, and/or maintaining factor in substance use disorders.

🖈 Addressing these concomitant problems *during* addiction treatment facilitates recovery.

🖈 Therefore, CM is a vital component in addiction treatment, to help clients find, gain access to, and use supplemental services that will support their change in substance use.

🖈 Beyond a traditional broker/generalist model, there are also more intensive CM models that integrate a higher level of therapeutic skills.

REFLECTION QUESTIONS

Q Within the population you serve what are the most common concomitant problems?

Q How can the people whom you serve gain access to a case manager?

Q If specialist CM is not accessible to your clients, how can you include this service in the care you give them?

PART III

A Menu of Evidence-Based Options for Addiction Treatment

S ome good news you can share with your clients is that the addiction field has come a long way in developing effective treatments. As recently as the 1960s, there were essentially no evidence-based treatment methods, none that were well supported by clinical trials, although the mutual help network of AA was already well established. Programs experimented with dozens of different treatments, some of them quite bizarre by modern standards (White, 1998; White & Miller, 2007). Some claimed to be the best or only route to recovery. Over the ensuing decades there has emerged an enormous literature on the effectiveness (and ineffectiveness) of various treatment methods, with over a thousand published clinical trials for substance use disorders. It has never been the case that there is one superior approach for everyone. Instead we are blessed with a menu of different treatment options with good evidence of efficacy, so that if one method is not working there are others to try. Long-term survival and recovery rates after addiction treatment compare quite favorably with those for other chronic diseases (McLellan et al., 2000). Part III provides just such a menu of evidence-based treatment methods. Each chapter describes the basics of an approach and the current state of scientific evidence, with references for readers who want to learn more about it. We begin with *brief interventions* (Chapter 9), usually involving one to four contacts. There is solid evidence that relatively brief counseling, at least of certain types, is far better than doing nothing at all or placing people on a waiting list. Brief intervention is feasible even within the time-pressured context of ongoing health care and social service systems. We describe in practical terms what seem to be the key ingredients of effective brief intervention.

Chapter 10 extends this discussion to the broader issue of enhancing motivation for change. Whereas once clients were blamed for being unmotivated, there are now effective methods to address this important aspect of change. One of these is the clinical style of *motivational interviewing*, which can be used as a stand-alone brief intervention, a prelude to treatment, or a platform for ongoing consultation. Another broad clinical method with good evidence of efficacy across substance use disorders is the *community reinforcement approach* (Chapter 11), which focuses on tipping the client's everyday balance of positive reinforcement in favor of sobriety. Also, there is strong evidence for the usefulness of teaching *behavioral coping skills* that a client can use in everyday life. These include general *social and assertiveness skills* (Chapter 12) and *relationship skills* for strengthening family and other close ties (Chapter 13).

What about the long-standing 12-step programs such as AA (and NA, CA, etc.), and other mutual help networks? Chapter 14 offers practical recommendations for how to integrate *mutual help group* involvement with treatment, and describes *12-step facilitation therapy*.

There has at times been a strong bias against using any medications in the treatment of substance use disorders, and not without reason. Isn't that fighting fire with fire? Yet certain medications, when well managed, do significantly improve treatment outcomes. Chapter 15 addresses the various uses of medications that directly target alcohol/drug use, which tend to be specific to the target problem drug, although some that were originally developed to address one class of drugs turn out to be useful in treating another as well. Medications for concomitant disorders will be discussed in Part IV, which covers other clinical issues in addiction treatment.

CHAPTER 9

Brief Interventions

Throughout this book we describe people with addiction problems as a diverse population with varying levels of severity, and advocate a continuum of services that are responsive to these various severity levels. In describing a menu of treatment options, we begin in this chapter with relatively brief and low-cost interventions. These began as opportunistic interventions, particularly in health care settings where people being seen for medical problems were screened for heavy drinking and alcohol-related problems. A positive screen (see Chapter 5) would trigger a brief intervention, even though the patient was not seeking consultation in regard to alcohol (Bien, Miller, & Tonigan, 1993; Dunn, Deroo, & Rivara, 2001; Fleming & Manwell, 1999). Such brief interventions have since been applied to address the use of tobacco (Colby et al., 1998; Glasgow, Whitlock, Eakin, & Lichtenstein, 2000) and other drugs (Bernstein et al., 2005; Marijuana Treatment Project Research Group, 2004; Marsden et al., 2006), and expanded for use in a wide range of settings including primary care clinics, social service agencies, emergency rooms and trauma units, employee assistance programs, public schools, child protection services, criminal justice facilities, and college health services (Miller & Weisner, 2002; Moyer, Finney, Swearingen, & Vergun, 2002; Rollnick, Butler, & Miller, 2008).

In other words, alcohol and other drug problems have come to be seen as public health issues that should be addressed far beyond the bounds of specialist addiction treatment. Most people with substance use disorders never get to specialist treatment, but do turn up regularly in health care, social service, employee assistance, and correctional systems. Such systems are now using brief on-site interventions as an alternative or to facilitate referral to specialist addiction treatment (Babor & Higgins-Biddle, 2000;

Institute of Medicine, 1990; National Institute on Alcohol Abuse and Alcoholism, 2005; National Institute on Drug Abuse, 2010).

Along with such opportunistic applications, brief interventions are also being included in the continuum of addiction treatment services. One reason is that a sizeable proportion of patients complete only one or a few visits in specialist treatment, so brief interventions are front-loaded to ensure that these people are given something useful even if they subsequently drop out. Happily, such up-front brief interventions also appear to improve retention. Immediate brief intervention is a preferable alternative to just placing clients on a waiting list and is more likely to activate the person's own change resources (e.g., Harris & Miller, 1990; McHugh et al., 2001). Finally, brief intervention can be regarded as the entry point of stepped care, whereby the person is initially given short-term treatment. Many people respond relatively quickly to addiction treatment, whether it is of shorter or extended duration (e.g., Anton et al., 2006; Project MATCH Research Group, 1998a). Those who do not respond favorably to brief intervention can then be offered additional treatment (Bischof et al., 2008; Smith et al., 2001). This chapter discusses the use of brief interventions for substance use problems in both generalist and specialist contexts.

WHAT IS BRIEF INTERVENTION?

Brief interventions usually comprise one to four visits, which may vary in length from 10 minutes to an hour or longer. Within this span of time, many different approaches could be taken. What, then, are the components of effective brief counseling? A review of this literature (Bien, Miller, & Tonigan, 1993; Miller & Sanchez, 1994) pointed to six common elements found in effective brief interventions for alcohol problems, summarized by the mnemonic acronym FRAMES:

> F: *Feedback* to the client of personally relevant information about his or her drinking and its consequences.
>
> R: An emphasis on the client's personal *responsibility* for change—that it is up to the individual to decide and choose what, if anything, to change.
>
> A: Clear *advice* from the provider recommending behavior change.
>
> M: A *menu* of options from which to choose, if the client should decide to pursue change.
>
> E: An *empathic* counseling style (Chapter 4) that is respectful and supportive, listening to the client's own concerns and perspective.
>
> S: Encouragement of *self-efficacy*, that the client could be successful in changing.

These components are not specific to alcohol, of course, but are more general elements of a brief counseling approach to facilitate change. It recognizes the client's autonomy, honoring personal choice and options. Clear advice is given within this context, that the person is (necessarily) free to follow or not. It focuses on the client's personal reasons for change, both through individual feedback of assessment findings and by listening to the person's own motivations (Chapter 10), and it offers hope and encouragement.

The choice of change goals and approach is a process of negotiation. In addition to possible treatment options, clients can be offered evidence-based self-help materials (Apodaca & Miller, 2003) or encouraged to become involved in mutual help groups in the community (Chapter 14).

By virtue of their brevity, brief interventions typically focus on enhancing clients' motivation and mobilizing their own resources for change (DeShazer et al., 2007; Viner, Christie, Taylor, & Hey, 2003). The essential goal is to activate the person's own self-regulation processes (Baumeister, Heatherton, & Tice, 1994; Brown, 1998; Vohs & Baumeister, 2010). Motivational interviewing (Miller & Rollnick, 2002)—a person-centered counseling method to enhance personal motivation for change—may be particularly useful when the primary obstacle to change is the client's ambivalence (rather than a lack of resources or skills). From a transtheoretical states-of-change perspective (see Chapter 5), the goal is to help the person move from contemplation (ambivalence) to preparation and action (DiClemente & Velasquez, 2002; Tomlin & Richardson, 2004). This counseling style is described in more detail in Chapter 10.

Brief intervention is a form of treatment, and for some clients it may be all that you have time to offer, or need to. It is clear that even a single session of the kind of brief counseling described above is significantly more effective than no treatment at all (Bien, Miller, & Tonigan, 1993; Dunn et al., 2001; Moyer et al., 2002), and often yields surprisingly similar outcomes to those from more extended treatment (Chapman & Huygens, 1988; Edwards et al., 1977; Marijuana Treatment Project Research Group, 2004; Project MATCH Research Group, 1998b; UKATT Research Team, 2005). Such brief intervention can also serve to enhance motivation, retention, and outcomes in subsequent treatment (Dench & Bennett, 2000; Zweben et al., 1988).

> Brief intervention is a form of treatment, and for some clients it may be all that you have time to offer, or need to.

Relatively brief counseling regarding substance use can be implemented in various contexts and for different purposes. A brief intervention may be *freestanding*, a single event offered as opportunity affords in hope of enhancing motivation for change. Similarly, brief motivational counseling can be offered in an *initial session* with the intention of strengthening motivation, retention, and adherence in subsequent treatment contacts. A brief substance use intervention can also be *embedded* within treatment that is focused primarily on other topics. This can range from a few minutes taken within a primary care visit to an alcohol/drug-focused session or two within an ongoing course of counseling.

EVIDENCE FOR THE EFFICACY OF BRIEF INTERVENTION FOR SUBSTANCE USE DISORDERS

Earlier studies on the efficacy of brief intervention focused mainly on people with alcohol-related problems. Interventions delivered opportunistically in primary care settings were found to reduce drinking and facilitate openness to additional services. More recent studies have shown that brief intervention can reduce drinking in postpartum women seen in obstetrical practices (Fleming, Lund, Wilton, Landry, & Scheets, 2008), diminish illicit drug use among patients seen in medical clinics (Bernstein et al., 2005; Madras et al., 2009), reduce heavy drinking and marijuana use among young adults seen in emergency departments (Magill, Barnett, Apodaca, Rohsenow, & Monti, 2009), decrease pathological gambling (Petry, Weinstock, Ledgerwood, & Morasco, 2008), and reduce problem drinking among college students (Baer, Kivlahan, Blume, McKnight, & Marlatt, 2001; Walters, Bennett, & Miller, 2000). In short, there is substantial evidence that brief interventions can influence addictive behaviors across a wide array of settings.

This is not to say, of course, that brief intervention is all that our clients need. More intensive treatment may yield better outcomes sooner, reducing the period of risky use (Moyer et al., 2002; O'Malley et al., 2003; Project MATCH Research Group, 1998c). Some studies have pointed to better long-term outcomes with more intensive treatment (Alterman et al., 1994, 1996; Burke, Dunn, Atkins, & Phelps, 2004). Two studies aimed at reducing HIV risk-taking behaviors among injecting drug users showed that more intensive cognitive-behavioral intervention yielded greater benefits than a brief motivational intervention (Baker, Heather, Wodak, Dixon, & Holt, 1993; Baker, Kochan, Dixon, Heather, & Wodak, 1994). In a rigorously designed multisite trial (Marijuana Treatment Project Research Group, 2004) both two-session and nine-session treatments were more effective in reducing marijuana use compared to the delayed treatment control. The nine-session treatment included motivational interviewing, cognitive-behavioral therapy, and case management. The nine-session intervention, however, produced superior outcomes compared with the two-session motivational treatment in terms of reduction in marijuana use up to 12 months after treatment, and the authors noted that reductions in the nine-session intervention were more clinically meaningful.

There are then perhaps two broad service delivery lessons to be learned from the brief intervention literature. One is that we may overestimate the level of service that many clients need. There is a natural tendency for behavioral health professionals to assume that more is better in terms of our services. The good news here, in an environment where need far exceeds availability of services, is that we may be able to serve more people well by building in effective brief intervention at the very front end of treatment, which is often dominated by administrative tasks and assessment. A second broad take-home message is to adjust service delivery to clients' needs (Chapter 7). For a certain proportion, a briefer motivational intervention is sufficient, increasing the availability of more intensive services for others who need them. As discussed in Chapter 7, such a "stepped care" approach is common in health services.

BRIEF INTERVENTION AS A TREATMENT ADHERENCE STRATEGY

As mentioned earlier, brief intervention has also been used as a preparation for additional addiction treatment, which may involve either pharmacological or behavioral interventions, to facilitate adherence to the substance use treatment. The idea here is to prime client motivation for, retention in, and adherence to treatment in order to improve outcomes.

There is strong evidence for the efficacy of adding such front-end brief motivational preparation for treatment (Bien, Miller, & Tonigan, 1993; Zweben & Zuckoff, 2002). Connors, Walitzer, and Derman (2002) found that clients randomly assigned to a pretreatment motivational interview had better attendance rates and drinking outcomes than those assigned to either a role induction interview or no-treatment control condition. Early randomized trials found that the addition of a brief motivational intervention roughly doubled the rate of abstinence following outpatient (Bien, Miller, & Boroughs, 1993) and inpatient treatment for alcohol dependence (Brown & Miller, 1993). Another early study found improved motivation and attendance with a motivational brief intervention (relative to an educational control condition) in a methadone maintenance clinic (Saunders, Wilkinson, & Phillips, 1995). Similar findings have emerged in medication trials. Pettinati and her colleagues developed and tested a repertoire of adherence strategies for medical management of naltrexone treatment for alcohol dependence (Pettinati, Volpicelli, Pierce, & O'Brien, 2000; Pettinati et al., 2004, 2005). Other trials, however, have not found the expected benefit from pretreatment interventions targeting retention and adherence (e.g., Carroll et al., 2006; Dench & Bennett, 2000; Donovan, Rosengren, Downey, Cox, & Sloan, 2001; Miller, Yahne, & Tonigan, 2003). The factors that account for such large variability in effectiveness of brief interventions remain to be clarified.

BRIEF INTERVENTION AND HARM REDUCTION

People coming for general health care and social services are often reluctant to discuss or change their use of alcohol or other drugs. They are seeking help for other health and social problems, and even though substance use may play a salient role in these presenting concerns, they may not think of themselves as having "a problem" in this area. They may not yet have expe-

> Attempts to pressure people into changing their alcohol/drug use are likely to engender resistance.

rienced serious adverse consequences, and thus may feel little pressure to change their substance use. Attempts to pressure such people into changing their alcohol/drug use are likely to engender resistance (see Chapters 10 and 16) and can jeopardize one's professional relationship with and retention of clients. A primary goal in harm reduction (which is discussed in more detail in Chapter 19) is to maintain contact and relationship with people who are at risk, both to reduce those risks and to keep the door open for further treatment, even though they are not currently seeking help for substance use disorders.

Opportunities for repeated brief interventions arise when people return for health and social services in relation to problems that arise. Over time, it is often possible to help clients see the connection between their substance use and the concerns that bring them in for services. Windows of opportunity open up. Often the first opportunities are for small steps in the right direction, targeting behaviors that pose the highest risk for harm to the client or others. There is an obvious parallel here to stepped care, offering help with whatever steps the person is willing to take. It is not necessary to wait passively for willingness to arise. A motivational counseling style can enhance readiness for change, even in brief contacts (see Chapter 10).

An example of a harm reduction effect comes from a study by Peter Monti and his colleagues (Monti et al., 1999). Adolescents seen in an emergency service following an alcohol-related injury were randomly assigned to receive a brief motivational interview focused on drinking or standard medical care. Both groups significantly reduced their drinking following the alcohol-related event, with no between-group difference. However, those in the standard care condition were four times more likely to be drinking and driving during follow-up, compared with those receiving the brief intervention.

FURTHER CONSIDERATIONS

Dose–Response Effects of Brief Intervention

As stated earlier, brief interventions vary widely in "dose"—from one to four or more sessions that can range from a few minutes to an hour or more. Does dose matter? There is some indication that a single interview is not as effective as more than one contact (Burke, Arkowitz, & Menchola, 2003; Longabaugh, Woolard, et al., 2001; Stout, Rubin, Zwick, Zywiak, & Bellino, 1999). Some of the classic studies demonstrating the efficacy of brief interventions in health care settings involved repeated visits over time (Burke, Arkowitz, & Menchola, 2003; Chick, Ritson, Connaughton, Stewart, & Chick, 1995; Kristenson, Ohlin, Hulten-Nosslin, Hood, & Trell, 1983; Wallace, Cutler, & Haines, 1988).

In essence, repeated brief contacts can be thought of as case monitoring, or a form of aftercare (Stout, Rubin, Zwick, Zywiak, & Bellino, 1999). This is familiar and standard practice in the treatment of chronic medical conditions. At each visit, the person's current status and progress are monitored, and adjustments in treatment or lifestyle are considered if warranted. Continued contact with care (rather than discharge from treatment) is a goal.

Combining Brief Interventions and Pharmacotherapies for Alcohol Problems

Recent advances in medication development may have important implications for managing substance use disorders within primary health care systems. Several pharmacotherapies have a solid base of evidence for efficacy (see Chapter 15). Such studies have typically combined pharmacotherapy with some form of brief counseling to facilitate medication adherence and to enhance treatment outcomes (Anton et al., 2006; Carroll, 1997b; Mason & Goodman, 1997; O'Malley et al., 2003; Pettinati et al., 2004). These counseling strategies were specifically designed for settings in which substance use problems are addressed within the context of delivering medical services. Naltrexone in particular has been found to significantly improve outcomes (relative to placebo) when added to brief counseling for alcohol dependence, and even the placebo effects of taking medication can improve outcome substantially (Anton et al., 2006).

All these findings support combinations of pharmacotherapy and brief counseling as a viable model for treating substance use disorders beyond a specialist care context, making services available to a wider range of people (Willenbring & Olson, 1999). This is important within the current trend toward reduced availability of speciality addiction treatment programs (McLellan, 2006). Addressing addictions through broader health care and social service systems is a way to provide care to those who cannot or will not access specialist treatment (Miller & Weisner, 2002; Weisner, Mertens, Parthasarathy, Moore, & Lu, 2001). Substance use disorders are already disproportionately represented in health care and social service settings, contributing to and exacerbating treatment of the problems presented in these contexts. Given the already busy workloads of physicians, it may be more feasible for brief interventions to be provided by nurses or behavioral health specialists working in health care clinics (Ernst, Miller, & Rollnick, 2007), using medical management protocols that have been developed and tested in clinical trials (Pettinati et al., 2004). On-site provision of addiction counseling in primary care and family practice settings seems a sensible way to treat alcohol/drug use as health behavior, address patient reluctance to seek specialist care, and assist medical staff with concerns about prescription drug misuse and dependence.

While there are many efficacy studies of pharmacotherapies and brief counseling, there have been fewer effectiveness trials to test these interventions in real-world settings outside the carefully controlled conditions of clinical studies. Certainly there is enough research to be confident that brief interventions *can* be effective in ongoing service systems, yet important questions remain to be answered. What amounts and kinds of training are needed for providers to learn and competently deliver brief interventions? What doses and types of brief intervention are most likely to work in particular service contexts? What differentiates providers who are more versus less effective in delivering brief counseling? Can we know ahead of time which people are likely to respond to brief intervention, and who will need more intensive treatment? How should brief interventions be adapted to serve particular subpopulations? How might we reach a still broader population with brief interventions (e.g., via web-based approaches; Clark, Gordon, Ettaro, Owens, & Moss, 2010; Hester, Delaney, Campbell, & Handmaker, 2009).

WHY DO BRIEF INTERVENTIONS WORK?

The brevity and content of the FRAMES interventions described in this chapter don't correspond well to popular notions of what it takes to change addictions. There is no skill training, contingency management, personality or cognitive restructuring, confrontation, induction to mutual help networks, or working through transference. How is it that even a brief counseling event of this kind can trigger a change in an addictive behavior that has been in place for years and has often persisted despite adverse consequences? Brief interventions don't always work, of course, but why do they work at all?

One plausible explanation is that they impact motivation for change and, more specifically, that they trigger normal self-regulation processes (Brown & Miller, 1993; Miller, 2000). The underlying question in behavioral self-regulatory systems is, to oversimplify a bit, like that of a thermostat: Is a change needed? These systems are constantly "on" during waking hours, and even to some extent while asleep (Vohs & Baumeister, 2010). There is a constant stream of information coming in through sensory channels and interpreted through perceptual systems. This information (how it is) is constantly compared with norms or expectations (how it should be), scanning for discrepancies that may signal the need for a change. In driving an automobile, for example, one scans the road ahead for anything that requires slowing down, turning, stopping, and the like. An object coming in on a collision course from the periphery captures the attention, triggering an evaluation of whether a course correction is needed and of the options available (see Box 9.1). The same self-evaluation process is in constant operation, scanning for whether a change in behavior is needed. The most commonly stated reason for the lack of change in addictive behavior is something like "I didn't think I had a problem" or "I didn't think I needed to." No problem, no change.

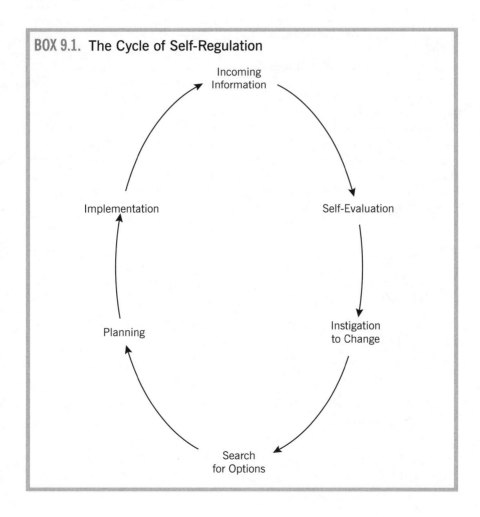

BOX 9.1. The Cycle of Self-Regulation

Incoming Information

Self-Evaluation

Instigation to Change

Search for Options

Planning

Implementation

When a meaningful discrepancy receives attention, however, there is an instigation to change and a search for options: "What could/should I do?" If an option appears reasonable and doable, behavior may change. The person tries it out to see how it works. This in turn provides new information that is evaluated, and the loop continues until the discrepancy is satisfactorily resolved. The elements of FRAMES—those that seem to be present when brief interventions work—make sense in this regard. The person receives feedback (sometimes in comparison to norms) in an empathic counseling style that decreases defensiveness and lets the information in. Personal responsibility and freedom of choice are emphasized ("If it's going to change, I have to do it"), along with gentle advice. A menu of options is described, with encouragement of self-efficacy ("I can do it").

If such triggering of self-regulatory processes is a key step in changing addictions, then the data and clinical experience regarding brief intervention make more sense. Until there is instigation to change, no self-regulation efforts are likely to occur (a condition sometimes called "denial"). When something does trigger a discrepancy ("How it is isn't how I want it to be"), then behavior change is more likely. Since *self*-regulatory processes are triggered, nothing more may be required. This also makes sense of why substantial behavior change is often observed quite early in the course of addiction treatment. People with addiction problems, however, often show significant neurocognitive impairment in various components of this self-regulatory process (Brown & Miller, 1991), so it also makes sense that they may need additional help putting self-controls into place. In any event, it appears to be important to address clients' motivation for change, the topic to which we now turn in Chapter 10.

KEY POINTS

- Brief intervention for substance use is often effective and is a reasonable first step within a stepped-care approach.

- Immediate brief counseling is preferable to placing people on a waiting list.

- Brief intervention can be freestanding, an initial session, or embedded within treatment for other issues.

- There is an opportunity for brief intervention whenever people with substance use disorders seek health or social services for other concerns.

- Common elements in effective brief intervention are individual Feedback, emphasis on personal Responsibility, Advice to change, a Menu of options, an Empathic counseling style, and support for Self-efficacy (FRAMES).

REFLECTION QUESTIONS

Q Where in your community are people with substance use disorders already receiving health or psychosocial services? How might brief interventions be integrated into these services?

Q Sometimes providers believe that if you only have a short time, you just have to tell people what to do. Suppose you had only 10 minutes to counsel someone regarding his or her drinking, smoking, or other drug use. How would you use the time?

Q How do you explain the fact that such brief interventions are often effective in changing substance use patterns that have been ongoing for a long time? What do you think is happening?

CHAPTER 10

Enhancing Motivation for Change

Once upon a time it was believed that if clients weren't motivated enough for change, then there was nothing you could do. "Come back when you're ready to change" was common advice. If people didn't respond well to treatment, it was chalked up to their poor motivation.

That view is no longer tenable or professionally responsible. It is clear that motivation is not a stable trait people carry around with them, but rather a dynamic process that has everything to do with interpersonal interactions. That makes it part of our clinical task to enhance clients' motivation for change, instead of blaming them for not having enough of it.

One of the earliest clues for this perspective came from studies in the 1950s and 1960s searching for the client dropout profile. Personality measures were administered to predict which people were going to drop out of treatment early. If those likely to drop out could be identified, then programs could either not waste their time with them, or could take extra steps to prevent attrition. It turned out, however, that there was no dropout personality profile. Instead, it appeared that a good predictor of dropout was the counselor to whom the client had been assigned. Some counselors had very low dropout rates, whereas others lost many clients early on. One study even found that referral completion rate could be robustly predicted from a doctor's *tone of voice* when talking about "alcoholics"—the more anger in the doctor's voice tone, the less likely his or her patients were to enter treatment (Milmoe et al., 1967).

Subsequent research has confirmed that regardless of the type of treatment for addiction, it makes a difference *who* delivers it. The particular clinician to whom a person is assigned can be the difference between clients getting worse or getting better (McLellan, Woody, Luborsky, & Goehl, 1988; Valle, 1981). Even when treatment is manual-guided and standardized, client outcomes are significantly and sometimes substantially linked to the therapist who delivers them (Luborsky et al., 1997; Luborsky, McLellan, Woody, O'Brien, & Auerbach, 1985; Miller et al., 1980; Project MATCH Research Group, 1998d).

To be sure, clients do present with a wide range of beginning readiness for change. As we discussed in Chapter 7, the transtheoretical stages offer a way of understanding how far along a person is at any given time with regard to making a particular change. The transtheoretical model, in fact, was a significant factor in the addiction field's change of heart and mind regarding client motivation. Once it becomes clear that clients are at differing points of readiness, then it follows naturally that they need different kinds of help in order to move along toward change:

> Clients who are at differing points of readiness need different kinds of help.

- *Precontemplation*: At this stage, the first step is to *become* ambivalent, to begin wondering whether a change may be needful and beneficial.
- *Contemplation.* For people in contemplation, the key is to help them resolve their ambivalence in the direction of change.
- *Preparation.* Once the balance has begun to tip in the direction of change, the person goes though a stage of preparation. The important process here is to help the person develop, accept, and commit to a plan for change.
- *Action.* Next comes implementation of the plan. In the action stage, the task is to help people carry out and stick with their efforts long enough to bring about change. The remaining chapters of Part III are particularly focused on effective methods for helping clients in the action stage.
- *Maintenance.* It is human nature to fall back into old and familiar ways. The challenge here is to maintain those initial changes. That is the subject of Chapter 19.

The present chapter is focused primarily on how to help people who are in the precontemplation, contemplation, or preparation stage, who are not yet quite ready for action. There is, it turns out, much one can do to help them. Enhancing motivation for change is often the first task that faces those who treat addictions. Just helping people to advance one stage (e.g., from precontemplation to contemplation) increases the likelihood of eventual behavior change (Heather, Honekopp, Smailes, & UKATT Research Team, 2009).

FIVE DIMENSIONS OF MOTIVATION

Consider what constitutes motivation for change. There are, of course, many different kinds of motivation; it is not monolithic. One clinical study administered a wide variety of measures of motivation to a large sample of people entering treatment for substance use disorders (Miller, Yahne, et al., 2003). There was no single underlying factor of motivation. Instead, most measures were at best modestly correlated with the others, even though all of them ostensibly measured motivation for change. There is, it seems, no single entity here.

Substantial help came from a psycholinguist colleague, Paul Amrhein, who has devoted his career to studying the language of motivation. Drawing on natural language that people use to talk about their motivations, he identified five categories with distinctly different meanings (Amrhein, Miller, Yahne, Palmer, & Fulcher, 2003):

- *Desire.* People talk about *wanting* to change, *wishing* they could change. Such language reflects one's degree of desire for change. Of course desire language can also apply to the status quo: "I really *like* marijuana and I don't *want* to give it up."
- *Ability.* Second, there is the person's perceived ability to change. People say that "I *can*" or "I *could*" quit. Motivation involves, in part, a person's perceived ability (self-efficacy) to change (Bandura, 1997).
- *Reasons.* Third, people express reasons to make (or not make) a change. These are the pros and cons, the specific perceived advantages and disadvantages of change. A list of reasons does not, however, mean that the person experiences a *need* to change.
- *Need.* And so, fourth, people verbalize their level of need to change (or not to do so). "I've *got* to do something!" "I really *should* quit." "I don't *have* to quit." The language of need is a general imperative. It expresses a degree of urgency (or lack thereof). Listen a little longer and you may hear particular reasons behind the need.
- *Commitment.* Finally, there is specific language that signals the level of commitment to change. "I *will* go to an AA meeting this week." "I *guess* I will." "I *promise.*" Amrhein found that of the five, only this one type of client speech actually predicted subsequent drug abstinence: commitment. To say that one *wants* to, or *could*, or has *reasons* to, or *needs* to do something is not in itself to make a commitment. However, expressions of desire, ability, reasons, and need did increase the likelihood of commitment and subsequent change.

Interestingly, Amrhein did not find a meaningful separate category of readiness. While people do talk about being ready to change, it seems to be a reflection of the other five categories of motivation above (Amrhein, 1992; Amrhein et al., 2003).

So, what are the clinical implications of this research on motivation? First, it is helpful to explore and have your clients express these various kinds of motivation for change. (Some specifics for doing this are described later in this chapter.) In what ways do they *want* to change, and to continue using? (It is not, of course, inconsistent for a person to both want and not want something simultaneously—that is the nature of ambivalence.) How *able* would they be to make a change, if they decided to do so? What *reasons* do they have for using and for quitting or cutting down? And to what extent do they *need* to change (or continue) their substance use?

Second, Amrhein's findings indicate that *any* of these avenues can lead to commitment and change. One does not need to have all of them, just enough of them. A client may, for example, decide to change based on reasons and need, even though it is not what he or she wants to do. Work with the motivations that you have.

Third, commitment is an important step (see Box 10.1). Talking about desire, ability, reasons, and need is a good start, but you're less likely to see

---

BOX 10.1. Levels of Commitment

There is a natural language that signals how ready a person is to change. The following are examples of words that people use to signal their level of commitment:

Stronger Commitment			Weaker Commitment	
5	**4**	**3**	**2**	**1**
I guarantee	I am devoted to	I look forward to	I favor	I mean to
I will	I pledge to	I consent to	I endorse	I foresee
I promise	I agree to	I plan to	I believe	I envisage
I vow	I am prepared to	I resolve to	I accept	I assume
I shall	I intend to	I expect to	I volunteer	I bet
I give my word	I am ready to	I concede to	I aim	I hope to
I assure			I aspire	I will risk
I dedicate myself			I propose	I will try
I know I will			I am predisposed	I think I will
			I anticipate	I suppose I will
			I predict	I imagine I will
			I presume	I suspect I will
				I contemplate
				I guess I will
				I wager
				I will see (about)

change until the person signals some level of commitment to do so. Commitment seems most similar to what is generally meant by being "ready" for change.

Finally, remember that all five of these types of motivation are a matter of degree. One could have a lot of reasons and need for change, a moderate level of desire, and very little confidence or self-efficacy. This also highlights that knowing the level of one type of motivation does not in itself reveal a lot about the others. Listen to your client's language along these five dimensions for indications of motivational levels (Rollnick, Miller, & Butler, 2008).

WORKING WITH LESS MOTIVATED CLIENTS

Precontemplation

In imagination, at least, the most daunting motivational challenges are presented by people in the precontemplation stage. They see no reason or need and have zero desire for change. These are, it would seem, the most difficult or impossible people to help.

However, clinicians seldom see people who are truly in precontemplation. Those whose motivational level is absolute zero rarely appear in a treatment center. Even coerced clients, we find, have usually experienced enough adversity in their lives to be at least somewhat ambivalent about his or her substance use. If you tell someone in precontemplation that you are concerned about his or her substance use, his or her reaction is more likely to be surprise or puzzlement than defensiveness and anger. A high degree of defensiveness bespeaks ambivalence, not precontemplation.

Suppose, however, that you do encounter people genuinely in precontemplation. It might happen, for example, if one screens in health care settings for indications of heavy drinking. In such a setting, one might identify people who really are drinking too much by objective standards, but who have never really considered the possibility. Precontemplation might also be found in subcultures where substance dependence is normative. What then?

A good goal here is to move people ahead one stage, into contemplation. Some straightforward health information may begin to plant doubts. Personal feedback may be persuasive. Don't expect instant miracles. You have done well to start the decisional balance moving, to plant the seeds of ambivalence and contemplation, leaving the door open for future discussion (Rollnick et al., 2008).

Sometimes the term "precontemplation" is also used for other motivational states. It is common, for example, that after a person takes action and fails to maintain the change, there is a period of demoralization during which the person is not considering renewed action. This is quite a different situation from the person who has never considered change in the first place. The obstacles are more likely to involve low confidence in ability to change, that is, low self-efficacy. The challenge is still to move the person along to once again contemplate, prepare for, and take action toward change. This particular situation is addressed in Chapter 19.

Contemplation: The Dynamics of Ambivalence

If they are not in precontemplation, who then are these highly resistant, defensive, angry clients of counselors' nightmares? We find most often they are in contemplation. They are people who have within themselves *both* sides of an argument. They like what they are doing, and they also don't, at least to some extent. In some ways they don't want to change, and in other ways they do. They have mixed motives.

What happens if someone (including a counselor) points out to such a person that he or she has a problem and needs to do something about it? Most likely the person will respond with the other side of his or her ambivalence, sometimes vehemently. An angry defensive response suggests that you have touched a sensitive nerve connected to underlying ambivalence. People are, after all, most stung by those accusations that contain some grain of truth. Argue for change, and it is natural for an ambivalent person to argue against it. It's human nature. In a way, you are acting out the person's ambivalence.

Unfortunately, American addiction counselors during the 20th century were often trained that interpersonal dynamic signaled denial which in turn called for confrontation (i.e., more vehement argumentation from the counselor). The result with ambivalent people is quite predictable: they usually dig in, and act out the other side of their internal conflict.

That might be harmless enough—a kind of psychodrama—except for the fact that people get committed to that for which they argue. When clients are caused to argue against change, they become more committed to the status quo and are less likely to change. It is when they give voice to their own intrinsic motivations for change, the positive side of the argument, that they become more committed to change and actually do it. We will return to the problem of how to respond effectively to resistance in Chapter 16. For now we focus on the positive side of motivation.

Motivational Interviewing

So how does one respond, as a counselor, in order to evoke from clients their own motivations for and commitment to change? That is a central aim of *motivational interviewing* (MI; Miller & Rollnick, 2002; Naar-King, & Suarez, 2011). It is not a simple technique, but a complex counseling style that requires some time to learn (Madson, Loignon, & Lane, 2009; Mitcheson, Bhavsar, & McCambridge, 2009). Happily, once you know what to look for, your clients become your best teachers. When a client expresses motivations for change (desire, ability, reasons, need, and commitment), you know you're headed in the right direction. Client resistance, in contrast, is a signal to change how you are responding (see Chapter 16).

Fundamental to MI are the client-centered counseling skills described in Chapter 4, particularly accurate empathy (reflective listening). In MI, these skills are applied in a consciously strategic manner, to move in a particular direction (toward change). Remember the OARS? Ask open questions that evoke the client's own motivation for change:

> "How might you *like* for things to be different?" (Desire)
> "If you did decide to quit, how *could* you do it?" (Ability)
> "What *reasons* might there be for you to make a change?" (Reasons)
> "How *important* is it for you to do something about your cocaine use?" (Need)
> "What do you think you'll *do*?" (Commitment)

When you hear such "change talk"—the person's own expressed motivations for change—reflect and affirm it. Each time the client expresses a desire, ability, reason, or need for change, it is as if they are offering you a flower. Collect the flowers, and periodically offer them back to the client in short summaries, like a bouquet:

> "So you don't like having the courts and probation officer butting into your life, and your drug use has caused some troubles with your girlfriend. In fact, you're worried she might leave you if things don't change. And you think you waste too much money and time on drugs. What else?"

When MI is going well, clients hear themselves expressing their own motivation for change, then hear you reflect it back to them, then later hear it all again drawn together in your summaries. This is the process that clients often have difficulty doing on their own. Ambivalent people often think of one reason for change, then a reason for not changing, then feel stuck and stop thinking about it. In MI you help people keep moving in the same direction and thus find their way out of the forest.

More than 200 clinical trials of MI have been published, many reporting significant beneficial effects across a broad range of problem behaviors, with some of the strongest evidence being in the area of addictive behaviors (Burke et al., 2003; Dunn et al., 2001; Hettema et al., 2005; Martins & McNeil, 2009). It is also clear, however, that the effectiveness of MI can vary widely across programs and clinicians providing it (Ball et al., 2007; Project MATCH Research Group, 1998d; Winhusen et al., 2008). This suggests that MI is sensitive to the manner and context in which it is being delivered. In this regard, it is important to understand the "active ingredients" of MI and what aspects of it are most important in delivery. Closer counselor adherence to and skillfulness in the prescribed style of MI predict greater client change in addictive behaviors (Daeppen, Bertholet, & Gaume, 2010; Pollack, et al., 2010).

Miller and Rose (2009) described the evolution of MI and proposed a research-based theory of its efficacy emphasizing two components: a *relational* and a *technical* component. The relational component focuses on the therapeutic relationship and working alliance between counselor and client, with particular emphasis on accurate empathy (see Chapter 4). The technical component focuses on specific aspects of client speech (e.g., change talk) that the MI provider is to recognize, evoke, and strengthen (Glynn & Moyers, 2010; Rollnick et al., 2008).

Regarding the relational component, Miller and Rollnick (2002) described an underlying "spirit" of MI comprising of three broad themes. First MI is *collaborative*, a partnership in which clients are recognized as experts on themselves. It is also *evocative*, calling forth the client's own insights, motivations, and resources, rather than trying to install things that the client is presumed to be missing. The basic assumption is not "I have what you need," but rather "You have what you need, and together we will find it." MI spirit communicates *acceptance*, respecting and supporting the clients' *autonomy*, their power and right to make decisions about their own lives and behavior. In this way, MI is consistent with *self-determination theory* (Deci & Ryan, 1985, 2008) and its emphasis on transforming external into internal motivation (Markland, Ryan, Tobin, & Rollnick, 2005; O'Toole, Polling, Ford, & Bigelow, 2006). MI helps clients to adopt new behaviors by linking change with internal motivational processes, including an enhanced sense of self (*autonomy*), a belief that change is within their own reach (*competency and self-efficacy*), and having a voice in the decision-making process (*relatedness of choice*) (O'Toole et al., 2006; Wild, Cunningham, & Ryan, 2006; Zweben & Zuckoff, 2002). In essence, MI is mobilizing the client's own wisdom, motivation, and resources for change (Faris, Cavell, Fishburne, & Britton, 2009). Relatedly, the spirit of MI also includes *compassion*, a fundamental commitment to the client's welfare as first priority.

In technical approach, MI differs dramatically from historic addiction counseling methods in which the counselor is the expert and authority, a highly authoritarian style involving closed questions, confrontation, teaching, and persuading, and in general pursuing topics of interest to the counselor rather than the client. Such strategies are inconsistent with MI and tend to evoke resistance and nonadherence that in turn are associated with lack of behavior change (Karno & Longabaugh, 2005; Miller, Benefield, & Tonigan, 1993). In contrast, MI practices are essentially client-centered and nonauthoritarian, entailing open questions, affirmation, and reflective listening. MI specifically focuses on motivational language, evoking client change talk and commitment. This is linked to cognitive and social psychological research showing that overt verbal expression of commitment to a specific plan increases the likelihood of change (Gollwitzer, 1999; Gollwitzer & Schaal, 1998). Client change talk is significantly strengthened by MI (Glynn & Moyers, 2010; Gaume, Bertholet, Faouzi, Gmel, & Daeppen, 2010; Miller et al., 1993; Moyers & Martin, 2006) and has been shown to predict substance use outcomes not only in MI (Amrhein et al., 2003; Moyers, Miller, & Hendrickson, 2005) but in cognitive-behavioral and 12-step facilitation therapies as well (Moyers et al., 2007).

Why does evoking client change talk promote actual behavior change? It's not that chanting "I will change" a hundred times is going to make it happen. The original theory of MI (Miller, 1983; Miller & Rose, 2009) involves developing discrepancy, a perceived inconsistency of current behavior with the client's own goals and values (Apodaca & Longabaugh, 2009). Hearing oneself voice the arguments for change is one way in which discrepancy emerges. Another path toward discrepancy comes from personal feedback.

> Hearing oneself voice the arguments for change is one way in which discrepancy emerges.

Developing skillfulness in MI, as in any complex skill, typically requires some coaching and feedback based on observed practice (Miller,

---

BOX 10.2. Personal Reflection: A Rough Start

Wouldn't you know. My very first client during graduate training was transgendered. She called me prior to the intake to inform me of her recent surgery. I was nervous enough about doing my first session, compounded with wondering how I was going to react: "What if I stare inappropriately or say something dumb?"

The first thing she asked during the interview was, "Do I freak you out?" I had two options. I could pretend and say, "Nah, I've seen everything," but the truth was that my exposure to diverse populations was pretty limited, so I responded honestly saying, "I'm not freaked out; I respect your courage for making a decision that makes you happy and I just want to understand."

A few days after this session I received a handwritten letter in the mail. She wrote, "Thank you for meeting with me. I appreciated that you showed an understanding of who I am. That made me feel good. Thank you for being so real." I have kept that letter because I never want to forget the importance of collaboration—drawing the person out in a way that creates discovery and movement rather than making assumptions about who someone is because of their particular ethnicity, religion, or sexual preference. Clients are experts on themselves and, given the opportunity, will share what we need to know to understand and help them.

—A. A. F.

Yahne, et al., 2004). A variety of resources are available to support learning of this clinical method (e.g., Rosengren, 2009; see *www.motivationalinterview.org*).

Assessment Feedback

It can also be interesting and motivating to receive credible, accurate information about oneself. Why are bathroom scales found in so many homes? Feedback tells you how you're doing, and whether you need to make a change.

Many counselors and programs have clients complete some form of assessment at the beginning of treatment (see Chapter 5). The Addiction Severity Index, for example, is widely used in U.S. addiction treatment and is now required in many states (McLellan et al., 1992). Ideally, such assessment is done because it provides useful information about the individual person.

If this is so, then why not share that information with the client? Personal feedback has been found to motivate change in substance use when presented in an informational and nonconfrontational manner that does not evoke defensiveness (Agostinelli, Brown, & Miller, 1995; Miller et al., 1993; Palfai, Zisserson, Saitz, 2011). This need not require a long time. Just present the findings, particularly in relation to norms from a general or clinical population. Where does the client stand on this measure, relative to other people? The dimensions could include level of use, severity of problems and dependence, physical health, and risk factors. Providing assessment feedback in combination with the clinical style of MI is what constitutes *motivational enhancement therapy* (MET; Miller, Zweben, et al., 1992).

It is also possible to offer an evaluation checkup for people who are not seeking treatment. We advertised to the community a drinker's checkup for people who would like to find out whether their alcohol use is harming them (Miller & Sovereign, 1989; Miller, Sovereign, & Krege, 1988). The advertisement specified that it was not part of any treatment program, that participants would not be labeled, and that they were free to use the information (or not) as they saw fit. This approach attracted drinkers who were 3–5 years earlier in the development of alcohol problems, relative to people entering treatment programs. Most of them had never sought any form of help for their drinking, but the checkup caught their attention. Why had they not sought help? In essence they didn't think that they needed it. They didn't view themselves as alcoholics or problem drinkers, and thought that their drinking wasn't all that serious. Why, then, did they come in for a checkup? They thought that they might have problems with alcohol, might be alcoholic, might be harming their health, and were concerned with some of the things happening in their lives with regard to alcohol. In short, they were in early contemplation, ambivalent enough to come for a checkup, but not (yet) considering formal treatment.

The checkup offered them a fairly comprehensive evaluation of their alcohol and other drug use, consequences, dependence, and risk factors, and some early indicators of alcohol's effects on the brain and liver. Then they returned for a single session to receive their feedback, and had follow-up interviews for 1 year afterward. A few sought formal treatment, but most did not. Nearly all, however, significantly changed their drinking, on average reducing their drinking by half (Miller et al., 1993).

Working through Family and Friends

Every addiction counselor and program receives them: desperate phone calls from people concerned about a loved one's substance abuse. They have tried everything to get their loved one to seek help, but to no avail. The problems continue to mount, and they want to know what to do. How should you respond?

Three approaches have been relatively common in North America:

1. Tell them that the drinker/drug user has to be the one to take the initiative, and to have the person call when he or she is ready.
2. Refer the caller to Al-Anon for support.
3. Arrange for an "intervention" in the original style of the Johnson Institute in which the person is confronted by family and others with the consequences of his or her substance abuse and urged to seek treatment.

Here is what is known about each of these three approaches.

1. *Wait for the substance user to get ready.* Predictably, when the caller is told that the drinker/drug user has to be motivated enough to make the call him- or herself, it's unlikely to happen. Sometimes the family will increase their pleas or pressure, but fewer than 10% of the identified patients (IPs) call back.

2. *Refer to Al-Anon.* It is clear that participating in Al-Anon can be helpful and supportive to the concerned significant other (CSO). The CSO may show reductions in physical symptoms, depression, and stress, and general improvement in personal well-being. That is good in itself, but it does not directly address the reason for the CSO's call. Participants in Al-Anon are usually advised that they are powerless to influence the drinker, to detach, and to desist from efforts to change their loved one. It is unsurprising, then, that while the CSOs themselves improve, only about one in

eight of their IPs may get into treatment within a year (Miller, Meyers, & Tonigan, 1999).

3. *Conduct an "intervention."* What happens when the family is counseled to prepare for a confrontational meeting with the IP? Early reports indicated that when the family went through with the full intervention, a high percentage of their loved ones were persuaded to enter treatment. It is also the case, however, that even with highly skilled counselors, the vast majority of families decide not to go through with the confrontational family meeting. This was the principal reason why, in a randomized trial, only 30% of families counseled in this way succeeded in getting their loved one into treatment (Miller, Meyers, & Tonigan, 1999).

Community Reinforcement and Family Training

An alternative to these three approaches grew out of the community reinforcement approach (CRA) to addiction treatment, which we will discuss more generally in the next chapter (11). Because it is designed to motivate treatment engagement, this application of CRA is included in this chapter. In the first clinical trial of this community reinforcement and family training (CRAFT) method, 64% of IPs entered treatment for their alcohol problems (Miller, Meyers, & Tonigan, 1999). As indicated above, the comparable figures were 13% with Al-Anon facilitation counseling, and 30% with the Johnson intervention. In a parallel study, 67% of drug-abusing IPs were engaged in treatment within 6 months (Meyers, Miller, Smith, & Tonigan, 2002). Other studies have yielded similar success rates with CRAFT and closely related approaches (Barber & Gilbertson, 1997; Meyers, Miller, Hill, & Tonigan, 1999; Sisson & Azrin, 1993; Thomas, Santa, Bronson, & Oyserman, 1987).

The crux of CRAFT is teaching family members that they *can* make a difference; and teaching them how encourages CSOs that they can make a difference by teaching them specific ways in which to use the considerable social incluence they do have (Meyers & Wolfe, 2004; Smith & Meyers, 2004). In particular, CSOs are taught how to provide positive reinforcement for abstinence and to avoid inadvertently reinforcing the loved one's drug use. CSOs are also prepared to watch for windows of motivational opportunity and how to encourage their loved one to seek help at those times. When the IP finally does agree to seek help, it is important that treatment be readily accessible. When a new window of readiness opens, it is no time to place someone on a waiting list.

> The crux of CRAFT is teaching family members that they *can* make a difference, and teaching them how.

Some of the basic principles of CRAFT are common sense when viewed from the perspective of reinforcing the right stuff:

- Do not buy or otherwise provide the IP's alcohol/drugs, or provide money that can be used to buy them.
- Do not protect the IP from the natural negative consequences of substance use.
- Give positive feedback and reinforcement when the IP is not using.
- Schedule time and activities together that compete with ordinary periods of drinking or drug use.
- Withdraw from the IP and be careful not to provide reinforcement when he or she is using.

Engaging the IP in treatment is not the only possible benefit of the CRAFT approach in working with families. The family members themselves tend to become more hopeful, and show significant improvement in depression, anxiety, and physical symptoms. The IP's substance use has also been found to decrease when family members change their patterns of reinforcement, whether or not the IP enters treatment (Sisson & Azrin, 1993).

As with MI, CRAFT is not easily learned simply by reading about it. Guidelines in implementing CRAFT are available both for counselors (Smith & Meyers, 2004) and family members (Meyers & Wolfe, 2004), but we recommend obtaining specific training to gain competence in using these methods.

Removing Obstacles

Finally, you increase the chances that clients will take steps toward change by removing practical obstacles that stand in their way. When you want to refer a client to another professional or program, make the call while the client is still in your office and set up an appointment (Chapter 8). Facilitate transportation to treatment or aftercare appointments, and minimize the distance that the client needs to travel. In one study, the best predictor of aftercare attendance was simply the distance from the client's home to the treatment center (Prue, Keane, Cornell, & Foy, 1979). Provide bus tokens or taxi fares. Consider home visits. Although addiction counselors have traditionally worked from their offices, social workers are quite accustomed to going where their clients live, and AA members regularly make 12-step calls. Make it *easy* for the client to do what he or she needs to do. Sometimes such facilitation is pejoratively called "enabling," but in fact it is good practice. The pejorative meaning of *enabling* is doing that which makes it easier for the person to continue his or her substance use. Facilitative actions do precisely the opposite: they make it more likely that the person will take needed steps in the right direction, and taking active steps is one of the best predictors of behavior change.

KEY POINTS

🖈 Client motivation for change is a good predictor of behavior change and is highly responsive to counseling style.

🖈 Depending on their initial level of readiness for change, clients need different approaches.

🖈 MI is a collaborative and evocative counseling approach helpful in promoting motivation for change.

🖈 CRAFT is a highly effective method for helping families engage a loved one in treatment.

🖈 Some simple steps to remove practical obstacles can also enhance change.

REFLECTION QUESTIONS

🗩 What do you believe is most important to help people with addiction become more motivated for change?

🗩 What has been standard practice where you work when a concerned family member calls for help regarding a loved one who refuses treatment?

🗩 What are the pros and cons of making home visits to provide care for addiction?

CHAPTER 11

A Community Reinforcement Approach

There are at least two striking facts about the community reinforcement approach (CRA). The first is that it is one of the most strongly supported addiction treatment methods in terms of evidence of efficacy. The second is that for a long time, relatively few addiction treatment professionals had ever heard of it.

CRA: THE BIG PICTURE

> In order to give up drug use, the alternative needs to be more rewarding.

Central to CRA is the principle of positive reinforcement: that when a behavior leads to rewarding consequences, it is likely to be repeated. The underlying perspective of CRA is relatively simple: in order for a person to give up a significant reinforcer such as drug use, the alternative needs to be more rewarding. That is, life without drugs needs to be better than a life of drug use.

There is good reason for CRA's focus on positive reinforcement rather than negative consequences. Indeed, if suffering and punishment cured addiction, there would be far less of it. Most of the people we see for treatment have experienced substantial, sometimes astonishing levels of adverse effects of drug use: family, health, financial, social, legal, and/or psychological problems. It is a central puzzle of addictions why these behaviors persist despite such high levels of negative consequences. In his history of Australia, Hughes (1987) described the willingness of convicts to incur beatings, torture, and even the threat of execution in order to obtain tobacco and alcohol. Attempts to punish away substance use are notoriously ineffective and can even backfire.

There is no mystery, though, as to why drugs of abuse are reinforcing. Laboratory animals will self-administer nicotine, cocaine, heroin, and amphetamine without further encouragement, with drugs often taking precedence over primary reinforcers such as food and sex. Certain animal strains also show strong preference for alcohol, whereas others avoid it. All of these drugs in some way access the brain's central reinforcement systems that signal "Do that again!" (Koob, 2005). Beyond this direct reinforcement, which often occurs within minutes or even seconds of drug administration, there can also be powerful psychosocial reinforcers for drug use. Other real or imagined effects of drugs can also be desirable, such as relaxation, suppression of memories, sexual facilitation, and feelings of well-being or power. Family and friends may encourage substance use, and help to insulate the user from its negative consequences. Drugs are problematic precisely *because* using them activates positive reinforcement. One need not look much beyond basic principles of learning to understand how and why people become addicted to such drugs (Logan, 1993).

CRA fundamentally seeks to increase positive reinforcement for sobriety and to undermine the rewards associated with drug use. The CRAFT approach, discussed in Chapter 10, includes teaching family members how to avoid inadvertently reinforcing substance use. CRA can also incorporate certain medications that interfere with the usual positive consequences of drug use (see Chapters 3 and 15), such as those that block receptor systems (e.g., naltrexone) or impose adverse effects (e.g., disulfiram; Azrin, 1976). Reducing sources of positive reinforcement for drug use is one avenue toward change.

The primary focus in CRA, however, is not on suppressing use, but rather connecting the person with natural alternative sources of positive reinforcement that do not involve substance use, and ideally are incompatible with it. In short, the goal is to help people construct a life that is joyful, rewarding, and meaningful without using drugs.

As we will review later in this chapter, CRA has been used effectively in both residential and outpatient settings, with adolescents and adults, with homeless individuals, and for dependence on alcohol, heroin, cocaine, and multiple drugs. In outpatient contexts, the special procedures of CRA typically require between 6 and 18 sessions. Often CRA begins with motivational counseling to enhance the person's readiness for change (see Chapter 10).

CRA PROCEDURES

CRA draws on a menu of procedures that are used flexibly, as appropriate to the individual's situation. Therefore the length and content of CRA treatment are not prescribed. For some people, a few of the procedures may suffice to establish and maintain sobriety. For others, more extensive life changes are needed.

Functional Analysis

One defining characteristic is that CRA begins with a careful *functional analysis* of drinking or drug use, examining both the antecedents and the consequences of substance use. With regard to antecedents, when is the person most likely to use (or use to excess)? Are particular times of day, days of the week, feelings, places, or companions particularly associated with use? Sometimes the use of one drug triggers the use of another. Smoking and drinking are often closely linked, for example, and resumption of cocaine use frequently occurs in the context of drinking alcohol. One way to assess antecedents is to ask about the person's "triggers" for drinking or drug use. In group counseling, we often generate a list of such triggers, writing them on the left side of a board or paper.

With regard to consequences, the interest here is particularly in the positive, rewarding consequences of use. "What do you *like* about alcohol?" or "What do you hope will happen when you use marijuana?" Here again one can generate a list, either in individual or in group counseling. We do this on the right side of the board or paper.

Next it can be helpful to make connections between these two columns: the point is that drugs are often used to get the person from one state (the trigger situations) to another (the consequences). This can be illustrated by drawing lines from each element in the left-hand list, to a corresponding goal in the right-hand list. Each item may have more than one partner in the other list. It also happens that there are items in one list that do not seem to have a partner in the other, in which case it is usually possible to fill in a missing component. Box 11.1 provides one example of a list that might be generated by a group.

After creating and discussing the list of triggers and consequences, brainstorm alternative ways of getting from one point to another, or to cope in a manner that does not require the use of drugs. These are, in essence, "new roads" (Miller & Pechacek, 1987). As long as a person has only one way (a drug) to get from point A to point B, he or she is by definition psychologically dependent on the drug for coping. An important goal of functional analysis is to identify how the person has been using drugs, the functions that they have served, and then to find new ways to serve those needs.

As you consider alternative behaviors, it can also be useful to do a functional analysis of these as well. When, where, and with whom is the person most likely to engage in these alternative behaviors? What are the possible positive consequences? This process emphasizes that the person is already engaging in some positive activities that do not involve substance use.

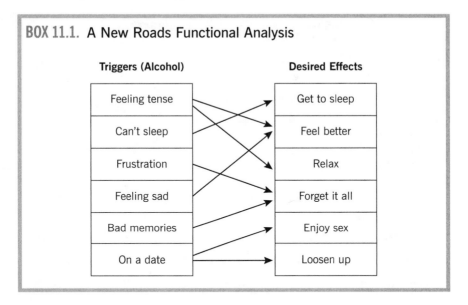

BOX 11.1. A New Roads Functional Analysis

Triggers (Alcohol)   Desired Effects

Feeling tense	Get to sleep
Can't sleep	Feel better
Frustration	Relax
Feeling sad	Forget it all
Bad memories	Enjoy sex
On a date	Loosen up

Happiness Survey

In considering alternative sources of positive reinforcement, one useful tool is a happiness or life satisfaction survey, which is another characteristic procedure in CRA. This is a simple list of life areas that the person rates from 1 (completely unhappy or dissatisfied) to 10 (completely happy or satisfied). The scale might look like the one shown in Box 11.2, although the specific items can be adjusted to your own setting and population.

Areas of dissatisfaction that are identified on this form can become goals on a treatment or case management plan, as areas to strengthen in positive reinforcement. "My drinking" or "my drug use" can also be included on this survey, to gain a sense of the person's current satisfaction or dissatisfaction with substance use.

Sobriety Sampling

One sound motivational principle in counseling is not to ask clients to do something that they are unwilling to do. This is not to say you should approve of the status quo, but before you ask a client to do something, you should assess and work on the person's motivation to

> One sound motivational principle in counseling is not to ask clients to do something that they are unwilling to do.

do so (Chapter 10). If a client is unwilling to consider long-term abstinence, the method of successive approximation is one way to proceed. What step

---

BOX 11.2. Current Happiness Scale

My work or education	1	2	3	4	5	6	7	8	9	10
My financial situation	1	2	3	4	5	6	7	8	9	10
My social life	1	2	3	4	5	6	7	8	9	10
My family life	1	2	3	4	5	6	7	8	9	10
My love life	1	2	3	4	5	6	7	8	9	10
My spiritual life	1	2	3	4	5	6	7	8	9	10
My friends	1	2	3	4	5	6	7	8	9	10
My spouse/partner	1	2	3	4	5	6	7	8	9	10
My personal freedom	1	2	3	4	5	6	7	8	9	10
My emotional life	1	2	3	4	5	6	7	8	9	10
My overall happiness	1	2	3	4	5	6	7	8	9	10

---

in this direction might the client be willing to take? That is the basic idea behind the CRA method of sobriety sampling (Meyers & Smith, 1995). In essence, the counselor and client negotiate a period of abstinence that the client is willing to try.

Start by clarifying the advantages of being drug-free for a period of time. Perhaps it has been some time since the client has experienced sobriety, and this is a chance to experience what it is like. It can demonstrate to others the person's desire to change, and decrease immediate levels of interpersonal conflict. Following principles of MI (Chapter 10) it is better to elicit the positive benefits of sobriety from the client rather than presenting them yourself.

A period of sobriety also quickly clarifies the ways in which the client has become dependent on substance use for coping, for a sense of well-being, and for managing symptoms. If the trial period of sobriety proves challenging, the specific difficulties that are encountered can be quite instructive.

The point is to negotiate an initial trial period of abstinence that seems manageable, and to which the client will agree. It might be a specific number of weeks, or even days. Remain in close contact with your client during this period, particularly during the first few days. If there is indication of physical addiction and the possibility of serious withdrawal (e.g., from alcohol or sedatives), the client will need close monitoring during early abstinence (see Chapter 6). Even if the client's long-term intention is to cut down rather than abstain (see Chapter 12), there are good reasons for a trial period of abstinence at the outset (Miller & Muñoz, 2005; Sanchez-Craig, 1996).

Monitored Medication

For certain drugs of abuse, there are medications available to help in maintaining abstinence (see Chapter 15). Disulfiram (trade name Antabuse), for example, when taken daily induces discomfort and illness only if the person drinks alcohol. It thus serves as a significant deterrent to alcohol use, which may also help the person to refrain from other drug use (e.g., cocaine or other stimulants) for which drinking is a trigger (Carroll, 1999; Carroll, Nich, Ball, McCance, & Rounsaville, 1998; Carroll et al., 1993). Another drug, naltrexone (trade name Revia), effectively binds opioid receptors, blocking the desired effects of heroin, and also apparently reduces the reinforcing effects of alcohol.

One limitation on the effectiveness of these medications, of course, is that clients discontinue them, or are reluctant to take them in the first place. MI (Chapter 10) can be used to strengthen motivations for a trial period of such medication, similar to the strategy of sobriety sampling. Many clients find, for example, that they experience little or no desire to drink when they know that they have taken disulfiram. Taking such medications can also demonstrate commitment to one's probation officer, family members, and loved ones.

CRA includes another procedure that can be quite effective in maintaining adherence: supportive monitoring by a loved one of the client's medication taking. The loved one is given brief training in how to administer the medication in a way that ensures it is taken (Azrin, 1976; Meyers & Smith, 1995). The client and loved one agree to a specific time when they will be together to complete the daily routine. The loved one's role is not that of an enforcer, but rather a reinforcer, providing appreciation, support, and encouragement for the client's continued commitment to change as demonstrated by taking the medication. There is a further agreement that if either party declines to participate in the daily routine, the other will contact the counselor promptly. (Given the half-life of most medications used in this way, this immediate contact gives you a chance to intervene before substance use resumes.) Although medication is not an essential part of CRA (Meyers & Miller, 2001), this procedure can be quite helpful in getting clients through the more difficult early weeks of abstinence.

Use of Time

A diagnostic aspect of substance dependence is that it consumes large proportions of a person's time. Substance-dependent people spend a lot of time obtaining, using, recovering from, and coping with the consequences of using drugs. Consequently, when drug use stops, they find that they suddenly have a lot of time on their hands. It is important to anticipate this problem and help your clients plan for positive alternative ways to use their time.

A prime goal, of course, is to have the person spend time in activities that bring positive reinforcement without substance use. What brings this person joy? A general guideline is: do things that you enjoy, and do them with or around other people who are not drinking or using drugs. To be sure, enjoyable solitary activities are also fine, but there is added value in having fun with others that is not associated with substance use.

Clients may at first be at a loss to think of ways for spending time and having fun that don't involve biochemistry. Here it can be useful to have a menu at hand. There are various long lists of possible reinforcers available (e.g., Lewinsohn, Muñoz, Youngren, & Zeiss, 1992; Miller, 2004), or you can construct your own. In cities, the newspapers often print a weekly list of local groups, activities, meetings, clubs, and entertainment. The key is to help your clients identify activities that they do enjoy, have enjoyed, or might enjoy, and then to start sampling them. Help clients as well with the follow-through process, perhaps by connecting clients with contact people who can help them get acquainted and be comfortable with initial experiences.

Interpersonal Relationships

Close relationships can be a primary source of positive reinforcement (and also, of course, of stress and conflict). Because interpersonal relationships so importantly influence both substance use and sobriety, CRA includes helping clients to develop and strengthen relationships that will support sobriety. This involves two common components of cognitive-behavioral relationship counseling: strengthening positive communication and problem-solving skills, and participating together in enjoyable activities that do not involve substance use (see Chapter 13). Having both the client and the SO complete the same happiness survey (see Box 11.2) allows you to compare their areas of satisfaction and dissatisfaction, providing areas for focus in communication training and problem solving. There is a particular focus on increasing positive communications such as compliments, appreciation, affection, and pleasant surprises, and decreasing negative communication patterns such as nagging, criticizing, threatening, and blaming.

Job Finding

Nathan Azrin, who introduced CRA, also developed effective methods for helping clients to become employed or find a more rewarding job (Azrin & Besalel, 1982). This has become a key component of CRA, and with good reason. Stable employment is a strong predictor of sobriety. Counseling methods for helping clients find rewarding employment are described in Chapter 12.

Sobriety Skills

Abstinence is the absence of a behavior. It is, in a way, doing nothing, not responding. Displacing a previously preferred behavior, however, usually requires some particular skills, which your clients may need some help developing.

Refusal Skills

One set of skills has to do with turning down opportunities for substance use. A person recovering from substance dependence will surely continue to have many such opportunities, and by experience will be particularly attuned to cues that signal availability. Sometimes the refusal of temptation just involves avoiding high-risk situations: driving past the bar rather than stopping in; choosing an alternative route that does not pass through prime drug-dealing territory.

At other times, specific interpersonal skills are needed to refuse drinks and drugs that are directly offered. A previous connection may try actively to recover a lost customer by offering free or inexpensive drugs. Friends who are themselves heavy drinkers or users may, for a variety of reasons, pressure the person to resume use. It is important to anticipate these nearly certain situations, and help your clients prepare for them.

The usual approach is to prepare and practice a sequence of responses that escalate as needed, depending on the aggressiveness of the person offering (Monti et al., 2002). The overall pattern here is persistently repeating the refusal while adding further communications as necessary. The first line of defense is a simple "No thank you" refusal, which often is sufficient. When a friend persists, for example in offering a drink, suggesting a specific alternative is a second possibility: "No thanks, but let's have coffee." An effective third step is to state one's refusal firmly and then change the subject: "I told you no! Now let's talk about something else." A further escalation, seldom needed, is to begin questioning the motives, needs, friendship, or integrity of someone who continues pushing so aggressively: "Hey! Why is it so important to you that I drink? Now stop it and be my friend."

Instead of just talking about these strategies, it is important to practice them in session. First, after explaining the basic principles, have the client pressure you as others may pressure him or her, and model effective refusal responses at each level. Then reverse roles. Have the client coach you on the people and strategies he or she is likely to encounter, and let the client portray them in a role play first while you demonstrate assertive refusal skills. Then you take the role of someone putting on pressure, and gently shape the client's refusal skills, reinforcing the good aspects of responses and suggesting additional refinements.

Coping Skills

As discussed above in the "new roads" analysis, it is common for people to use psychoactive drugs as a coping strategy. When people abstain, they will continue to encounter situations that require coping, and may not have effective alternative responses. This often becomes apparent during the early weeks and months of sobriety. In essence, the general strategy is to strengthen the client's skills for coping with expected and unexpected situations that could trigger resumed use. This is the principal focus of Chapter 12.

Motivational Incentives

Contingency management (sometimes called motivational incentives) is another method for reinforcing change. What would happen if you could offer positive incentives for abstinence? Suppose, for example, that you could pay a drug-dependent person to refrain from using drugs? Could and would they do so?

Regardless of the drug in question, the answer is clearly "Yes." Many studies dating to the 1970s convincingly demonstrated that even severely alcohol-dependent people can voluntarily reduce or refuse available alcohol in response to a wide variety of incentives including money, access to social interaction, and an enriched environment (Heather & Robertson, 1984). Illicit drug use is similarly responsive to external contingencies (Higgins & Silverman, 1999; Stitzer, Petry, & Peirce, 2010), and behavioral economic theory is clarifying the determinants of the choice to use or not use psychoactive drugs (Vuchinich & Heather, 2003). Contingency management has also been used successfully to improve retention and outcomes in smoking cessation programs for people in recovery from other substance use disorders (Dallery & Raiff, 2011; Hunt, Rash, Burke, & Parker, 2010).

Clearly, then, it is possible to pay people to refrain from drug use, and such contingency management has been combined with CRA. Steve Higgins and his colleagues, for example, have effectively modified drug use in cocaine-dependent people through financial incentives for urine-verified abstinence (Higgins & Katz, 1998). Similar success has been shown in reinforcing abstinence from heroin (Higgins & Abbott, 2001). Contingency management can also be used on its own, apart from other CRA procedures.

Limitation of resources is one obstacle to this approach, although immense amounts of funding are certainly expended in unsuccessful social attempts to control drug use. The amount of payment that is required to establish abstinence may be relatively modest, compared with the costs of repeated treatment or institutionalization (Sindelar, Olmstead, & Peirce, 2007). Social and professional attitudes about paying people to remain abstinent can also represent obstacles.

The general principle, however, is clear and important. It is quite possible to provide positive incentives that compete successfully with the choice to continue using drugs (Petry et al., 2005; Stitzer et al., 2007). This is in contrast to the general failure of punishment to suppress drug use once it is established. The broader clinical implication is to seek methods to increase positive reinforcement for sobriety, and to decrease reinforcement for drug use. This might be done through any source of significant positive reinforcement for the individual: family, social services, employer, friends, and social support systems. Think creatively about how to reinforce "the right stuff" rather than relying on aversive control. That is fundamental to the CRA.

> Positive incentives can compete successfully with the choice to continue using drugs.

Practicalities

As is apparent by now, CRA involves a menu of procedures that are used flexibly to address the needs of each individual. It makes no sense to construct a one-size-fits-all CRA program in which all clients are given the same skill training, job club, relationship counseling, monitored medication, and so forth. The question is, What will it take *for this client* to tip the balance of reinforcement away from drug use and toward sobriety? A few components are offered for all clients in CRA: motivational counseling, a sound functional analysis, and clear goal setting (e.g., sobriety sampling). Beyond that, CRA relies on the creativity of the counselor to choose, from a menu of procedures, those most likely to solve problems and address needs of the individual client (Meyers & Smith, 1995; Miller, 2004).

There is, in CRA, a strong emphasis on encouragement and positive reinforcement during the process of counseling itself. The counselor is characteristically upbeat and affirming, acknowledging any and all efforts that the client makes to move in a positive direction. Timeliness of response is also important. When a window of opportunity opens and a client is ready to move, the counselor is ready to go. Motivation does not wait for waiting lists. Similarly, if a spouse or client calls to say that they have missed the daily medication monitoring routine, the counselor tries to see them that day or the next. A little attention right away can avert the need for much more treatment later.

THE EFFICACY OF CRA

There is strong evidence that CRA not only works, but adds significantly to the effectiveness of approaches with which it has been compared. A series of studies found CRA to be more effective than treatment as usual for alcoholism in both inpatient (Azrin, 1976; Hunt & Azrin, 1973) and outpatient settings (Azrin, Sisson, Meyers, & Godley, 1982; Miller, Meyers, Tonigan, & Grant, 2001). Other studies have found large effects for CRA with homeless adults and youth (Slesnick, Prestopnik, Meyers, & Glassman, 2007; Smith, Meyers, & Delaney, 1998). Four trials have shown CRA and contingent voucher payments for abstinence to be significantly more effective than traditional approaches in treating cocaine dependence (Higgins et al., 1991, 1993, 1994, 1995; Higgins, Wong, Badger, Haug Ogden, & Dantona, 2000). Opioid-dependent patients treated by CRA also showed better outcomes than those in usual treatment on measures of detoxification completion and abstinence from heroin (Abbott, Moore, & Delaney, 2003; Abbott, Waller, Delaney, & Moore, 1998; Bickel, Amass, Higgins, Badger, & Esch, 1997). Subsequent studies have found a CRA-based method to be substantially more effective in engaging "unmotivated" adolescent and adult drinkers and drug users in treatment through unilateral intervention with loved ones, as compared with traditional methods for working with family members (Meyers et al., 1999, 2002; Miller, Meyers, & Tonigan, 1999; Waldron, Kern-Jones, Turner, Peterson, & Ozechowski, 2007). A community-based effectiveness study showed similarly high rates of engagement when implementing CRAFT outside the conditions of a controlled trial (Dutcher et al., 2009). Studies have also evaluated self-help (Manuel et al., in press) and computer-based delivery of CRA-based methods (Brooks, Ryder, Carise & Kirby, 2010). Treatment outcomes have been specifically linked to the delivery of CRA procedures: the more CRA treatment procedures used, the greater the change in substance use (Garner, 2009).

KEY POINTS

🖈 CRA helps people rearrange their lives so that sobriety is too good to give up.

BOX 11.3. Personal Reflection: Evidence-Based Treatment

When I go to my primary care doctor or other health care providers, I expect them to be keeping up with new research in their field and to provide me with current science-based advice and treatment. I certainly experienced this in facing a life-threatening illness. One of the earliest things I did after diagnosis was to read the clinical trial literature on the outcomes of the various treatments that were available to me. None of my doctors found this threatening; in fact they encouraged me to do so. To my eyes as a patient, a 5% difference in outcomes looked pretty large, whether or not it was statistically significant.

How odd it is that this same standard has only recently been applied to the treatment of addiction, which is definitely a life-threatening condition! There is a long history of "one approach fits all" in this field, that approach being whatever the provider happened to have learned or experienced. Impassioned debates have raged between different "schools" of thought as to which is the one correct (or at least superior) perspective. These generate more heat than light.

I am just as concerned about the cynical view that it doesn't really matter what treatment method is used—that all treatments are equally effective. (Imagine being told this if you went for cancer treatment!) To be sure, the specific treatment method used is not the *only* thing that influences outcome. Client characteristics and efforts matter, and as emphasized in prior chapters, counseling *style* (such as empathy and basic kindness) can have a larger impact than specific treatment techniques. Nevertheless, having for three decades reviewed all clinical trials for alcohol problems, I simply cannot agree that one treatment method is as good as any other (Miller, Wilbourne, et al., 2003). We really ought to be using what research tells us is most effective.

Yet implementing and monitoring evidence-based treatment is no simple matter (Miller, Zweben, et al., 2005). As most states have begun to *require* the use of science-based treatments, the tendency has been to develop a list of treatments that are "in" versus "out." The criteria for and selection of which treatments are "in" can be a highly political process, and there is pressure to approve a relatively long list of alternatives that meet some minimum standard, rather than focusing on those with strongest evidence.

Quality control in the delivery of evidence-based counseling methods is also challenging. I once gave a talk at a regional conference in Albuquerque on the current state of outcome research, concluding with a list of treatment methods having the strongest evidence of efficacy. A week later one of the local residential treatment programs ran a newspaper ad claiming that they were offering everything on my list, even though to my knowledge no one on their staff had received specific training in any of them. Without quality control, the requirement to use a specific list of methods may change only the self-report of what is being provided. Yet how does one audit the quality of talk therapy that occurs behind closed doors?

Furthermore, retraining in new evidence-based treatment methods requires significant time and resources. It is a reasonable question to ask whether the cost of retraining staff will be offset by a significant improvement in outcomes. Just attending a continuing professional education workshop is unlikely to yield much real change in practice, although it may convince participants that they now are delivering this new method (Miller

(cont.)

& Mount, 2001; Miller, Yahne, Moyers, Martinez, & Pirritano, 2004). The requirement to use new methods should be accompanied by resources to learn them.

The key, I think, is to find a middle way between simple-minded unfunded mandates of brand-name therapies and giving up on evidence-based treatment. Clearly we ought to be teaching the most effective treatment approaches to the next generation of providers from the very beginning. There have been experiments with paying for good outcomes, and leaving it up to the providers to figure out how best to do that—a situation that tends to create sudden interest in evidence-based treatment methods. We also need to pay attention to who is providing treatment and how, since there is clear evidence that this strongly influences client outcomes. The best path is unlikely to be simple, but we owe it to our clients to get it right.

—W. R. M.

- CRA focuses on positive reinforcement for positive alternatives to substance use.

- Contingency management is also an effective tool for reinforcing sobriety, which can be combined with CRA.

- CRA has been supported in every clinical trial in which it has been tested to date. In all of these studies, CRA was competing with bona fide treatment as commonly provided in community programs, which is a stringent test of efficacy.

- CRA has worked with particularly difficult-to-treat populations: those refusing to seek treatment, the homeless, adolescents, and people with cocaine, heroin, and polydrug dependence.

REFLECTION QUESTIONS

In your own community, what activities are available that are not associated with substance use?

Why is positive reinforcement more effective than punishment in changing addictive behaviors?

How comfortable are you with sobriety sampling when clients are not ready to commit to long-term abstinence?

CHAPTER 12

Strengthening Coping Skills

One way to make sense of substance abuse is to think of it as a coping strategy. The "new roads" analysis introduced in Chapter 11 (see Box 11.1) makes this explicit, seeking to understand how a person has been using chemicals as a vehicle, to move from one place (usually an undesirable one) to another. A person using a particular drug may be seeking, for example, to forget, to relax, to get to sleep, or to feel better.

This is not, of course, an uncommon use of drugs. Public airwaves and print media are filled with advertisements for over-the-counter or prescription medications to alleviate all manner of symptoms and improve life quality. An implicit message is that one need not tolerate discomfort even for brief periods: Take something! The "self-medication" hypothesis of drug abuse is precisely that people are "taking something" in order to feel better by treating symptoms and discomfort. Sometimes what the person is seeking to self-treat is an underlying condition such as bipolar disorder or attention deficit disorder. For others, drugs are used to cope with or avoid everyday emotions, frustrations, and challenges. The same can be true, of course, for other addictive behaviors that do not even involve the use of a drug, such as pathological gambling.

A common theme in cognitive-behavioral treatment of addictions is to teach clients the coping skills that they presumably lack, so that they need not rely on chemicals or addictive behaviors in order to handle the expected and unexpected challenges of life. Marlatt placed particular emphasis on this skill-building approach in his original "relapse prevention" model for treating addiction (Cummings, Gordon, & Marlatt, 1980; Marlatt & Donovan, 2005). With new skills in place, the person is better able to adjust to life's challenges and is not psychologically dependent on drugs for coping.

This skill-enhancing emphasis is entirely consistent with the CRA described in Chapter 11.

There is good reason for focusing on clients' coping skills. A return to using alcohol or other drugs often occurs in situations where other coping skills were needed (Marlatt, 1996). The risk of resumed use is not particularly related to exposure to high-risk situations per se, because virtually everyone who has been treated for alcohol/drug problems will encounter many such situations. Rather what predicts sustained sobriety is the person's capacity for dealing with life's challenges, particularly with coping strategies that do not involve avoidance (Miller et al., 1996). Avoidance of high-risk situations is useful in early sobriety, but in the longer run one needs positive coping skills (Monti et al., 2002).

THE EVIDENCE BASE

Clinical research has provided strong support for the value of a skill-enhancing approach. Most trials have evaluated skill training as an addition to treatment as usual, which is a fairly rigorous test of efficacy. In this value-added design, the new method that is being tested has to produce improvement above and beyond that resulting from normal treatment practices. In essence, this kind of clinical trial answers the practical question, "Is it worth my time and effort to add this new method onto what I'm already doing for my clients?" From studies of coping skill training, the answer has rather consistently been "Yes"—that there is significant added value above counseling as usual (Miller, Wilbourne, et al., 2003; Miller, Zweben & Johnson, 2005).

In Project MATCH (see Chapter 7), cognitive-behavioral skill training (CBT; Kadden et al., 1992) was also compared head-to-head with two other well-supported treatment methods: 12-step facilitation (TSF) and motivational enhancement therapy (MET). During the 12-week treatment phase, clients receiving CBT or TSF showed quicker reductions in their drinking as compared to those in MET. Once treatment had ended, however, all three therapies yielded similar (and substantial) benefit through 3 years of follow-up on the study's main outcome measures (Babor & Del Boca, 2003).

A skill-enhancing approach is not, however, incompatible with other treatment methods such as TSF and MET. In the subsequent COMBINE study, CBT and MET were merged with encouragement to attend mutual help groups, forming a "combined behavioral intervention" (Longabaugh et al., 2005; Miller, 2004) that significantly improved client outcomes (Anton et al., 2006). Enhancing clients' coping skills is not the entire answer in treating substance abuse, but it is one very useful tool to have at hand.

Skill training is one treatment method that can be offered quite well in group format. Clients can benefit from each others' range of skills and ideas, and also learn vicariously as each group member develops new ways for living drug-free. There is efficiency of scale in teaching new material to a group, rather than to one individual at a time (see Chapter 20). Furthermore, groups offer more opportunities to practice new skills with a variety of individuals in a supportive atmosphere during the learning process.

> Skill training is one treatment method that can be offered quite well in group format.

WHAT SKILLS?

What skills, then, should one focus on in treatment? It makes little sense to have the same standard skill-training package for everyone because people enter treatment with very different sets of skills. Some clients already have sufficient ability in managing their own mood states, for example, while for others this ability is underdeveloped. Some already have good jobs, whereas others need skills for finding and keeping employment. We therefore recommend having a menu of skill-learning options available, from which clients can choose the areas that are most likely to be beneficial to them.

Part of the clinical challenge here is in identifying skills that need to be strengthened in order to help your clients live fulfilling and addiction-free lives. Sometimes these are rudimentary but important life skills: how to use public transportation, prepare meals at home, or open a bank account. This is an area where volunteers can be meaningfully involved in helping clients to learn basic life skills out in the real world.

Nevertheless, there are a few major psychosocial skill areas that often need strengthening among people entering addiction treatment. Four in particular have been well researched: job finding, social skills, emotion regulation, and self-control. In each of these areas there are also specialized training resources for clinicians and for clients.

Job Finding

Employment is a strong predictor of sobriety. Despite seemingly positive response during a treatment episode, clients are much less likely to remain drug-free if they are unemployed. Discharging a client to unemployment is an invitation to failure.

> Discharging a client to unemployment is an invitation to failure.

Helping people to find a job may not seem like it is part of addiction treatment and should be someone else's responsibility. Yet experience with the CRA (Chapter 11) shows that it can be done as part of treatment. Referring out to an employment agency always runs the risk of clients not getting there or having insufficient patience to get through the bureaucracy. Getting (and keeping) a job involves particular strategies and social skills, which may not be offered in traditional employment agencies.

Help with job-finding skills can be included in individual or group counseling. Some common and effective components to include are help in preparing an effective résumé, advice on how to dress and present oneself for interviews, asking friends and relatives to alert them to job leads, taking the initiative to contact potential places of employment, rehearsing job interviews, and completing applications for available positions. Treatment programs can also set up an ongoing "job club" program, usually operated each morning. The basic idea here is that finding a job is itself a full-time job that requires substantial devoted effort. Unemployed clients come to the job club daily to learn some of the above-described skills and to devote time to contacting potential employers, calling friends and relatives for leads, and completing applications. The job club facilitator coaches clients on interviewing skills, listens in on cold contact calls, and provides resources. Then in the afternoon each day, clients visit potential employers and go for interviews. Clients keep coming to the job club daily until they get a job.

Social Skills

Perhaps the strongest evidence for enhancing coping skills comes from studies of social skill training. The emphasis here is on strengthening clients' abilities to form and maintain rewarding drug-free social relationships (Monti et al., 2002).

Like employment, the client's social support network is a strong predictor of posttreatment sobriety. Those who have a strong social network in support of sobriety are significantly more likely to achieve it. Those whose friends and family support continued drinking or drug use are at much higher risk, and in essence need to develop new social networks (Longabaugh, Wirtz, et al., 2001; Longabaugh et al., 1998). As discussed in Chapter 11, some of this change involves engaging the client in new networks that support sobriety, such as 12-step fellowships or religious congregations.

> The client's social support network is a strong predictor of posttreatment sobriety.

Some clients, however, may not have developed the social skills they need to enter and succeed in normal social networks. If their family and current friends support substance use, they are also likely to benefit from preparation to respond in new ways to social temptations, particularly when old networks cannot be completely avoided.

Regarding the first of these tasks, preparing clients to develop new positive social relationships, research and clinical resources have focused particularly on communication skills. The concept of *assertive communication* represents a middle ground between two extremes: passivity and aggression (see Box 12.1). When operating in a passive mode, people sacrifice their own needs by giving in, not expressing themselves, and stuffing their feelings and reactions. Giving other people what they want does tend to please them, but it comes at a cost if this is the person's consistent coping style. In essence, the person's own needs are not met, and there is little genuine two-way communication and negotiation. At the other extreme of aggression, people demand and coerce in order to meet their own needs at the expense of others. This tends to yield some immediate gratification but sacrifices relationship, engendering resentment and hostility.

Assertive communication honors and balances one's own needs with those of others. Feelings, requests, and feedback are not suppressed, but rather are expressed in a way that respects others, thus inviting and fostering relationship. This is a delicate balance, and one that varies substantially across cultures. An appropriate assertive response within one culture or subculture, for example, may constitute an aggressive and socially inappropriate response in another, or passive and ineffectual behavior in yet another. The point is to help clients recognize this search for middle ground in communicating, and to differentiate effective assertiveness from passive and aggressive responses in their own social contexts. This is a process in which group counseling can be particularly useful. Some basic tips for assertive communication are offered in Box 12.2.

Other basic social skills can also be strengthened. The ability to listen to others and reflect back the meaning that one heard (Chapter 4) is useful not only for counselors, but in social relationships more generally. Sometimes nonverbal communication skills need strengthening as well, such as maintaining an appropriate level of eye contact.

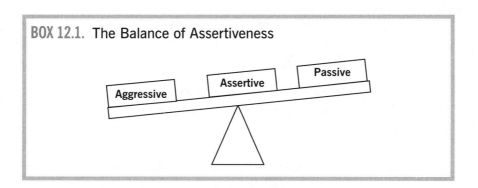

BOX 12.1. The Balance of Assertiveness

Aggressive   Assertive   Passive

BOX 12.2. Basic Tips for Assertive Communication

1. **Use an "I" message.** When you are expressing yourself—your thoughts, feelings, opinions, requests—begin with the word "I" rather than "You." By starting with "I," you take responsibility for what you say. Statements that start with "You" tend to come out as more aggressive—blaming, threatening, and so on.

2. **Be specific.** Address a specific behavior or situation and not general "personality" traits or "character." A specific request, for example, is more likely to result in a change, whereas general criticism is unlikely to improve things.

3. **Be clear.** Say what you mean. Don't expect the other person to read your mind, to just "know" what you want or mean. When you make a request, make it clear and specific. When you respond to a request, be direct and definite. "No, I don't want to do that" is clearer than "Well, maybe … I don't know." Your facial expression and body language should support your message. Speak loudly enough to be easily heard and use a firm (but not threatening) tone. Look the person in the eye (not at the floor). Don't leave long silences.

4. **Be respectful.** Don't seek to intimidate, win over, or control the other person. Speak to the person at least as respectfully as you would like to be spoken to. If you have something negative or critical to say, balance it with a positive statement before and after. Recognize that people have different needs and hear in different ways. In conflict situations, take partial responsibility for what has happened and is happening.

ASSERTIVE COMMUNICATION IN CONFLICT SITUATIONS

Three Parts of an Assertive Message

1. Describe the behavior.
2. Describe your own feelings or reactions.
3. Describe what you want to happen.

When Receiving Criticism

1. Keep cool; avoid escalation.
2. Listen carefully; show that you understand the other's perspective.
3. Correct any misunderstandings.
4. Take partial responsibility and apologize when appropriate.

When Giving Negative Feedback (Constructive Criticism)

1. Keep calm; don't speak in anger or hostility.
2. Choose the right time and place.

(cont.)

BOX 12.2. *(cont.)*

3. Be specific; describe behavior and don't blame.
4. Check out misunderstandings.
5. Use "I" language.
6. Take partial responsibility and offer to help, as appropriate.

When Asking for Change

1. Describe what the person is doing—the specific behavior that you would like to change.
2. Describe your own feelings or reactions using an "I" message.
3. Describe what you would like to happen.
4. Take partial responsibility or offer to help, as appropriate.

When it comes to dealing with old relationships that support substance use and afford temptation, assertive communication skills can also be quite useful. Drink- or drug-refusal skills may need strengthening. "Just say no" sounds like simple advice, but in fact it can be useful to practice specific ways in which to do so (Kadden et al., 1992; Monti et al., 2002).*

Emotion Regulation

People who have difficulty with self-regulation of emotions are also at higher risk for alcohol/drug problems. Their mood may shift quickly among fear, anger, and despair. Skills in self-soothing, in calming oneself down when emotions flare, may also be shaky. When such is the case, it may be tempting to use alcohol or illicit drugs to regulate emotions.

A good first step is to help clients understand what emotions are and how they occur. One useful heuristic for this is the "STORC" model that describes a cycle:

- Situation—the stimuli or antecedents in the person's environment
- Thoughts—how the person interprets and thinks about the Situation
- Organism—what happens physically in the body
- Response—what the person does
- Consequences—what happens as a result, which in turn changes the Situation

---

*The specific procedures for teaching coping skills can themselves fill a book, and guidelines are available in both the public domain (Kadden et al., 1992; Miller, 2004) and copyrighted volumes (Monti et al., 2002).

An optimistic aspect of this model is that it places experienced emotion in the context of the environment and the person's behavior, and it suggests multiple points in the chain where changes are possible (Miller & Mee-Lee, 2010b). People can change aspects of their situation (e.g., by avoiding certain places or people), modify how they think about and interpret it (a focus of cognitive therapies), alter how they react physically (by learning relaxation skills or adjusting medication), change how they respond, or take steps to affect the consequences they experience.

Self-monitoring is a common step in learning emotion regulation skills. A STORC diary (see Box 12.3) can be used to analyze situations in which significant emotions arose. When a significant feeling arises (usually recorded in the organism column), what was the situation in which it occurred, what were the person's thoughts and interpretation, what did he or she do (response), and what were the results (consequences)? Making a change at any step in the STORC chain is likely to affect other parts of the cycle.

Managing moods is one common issue in addiction treatment, perhaps especially so for women, who have a higher incidence of concomitant depression. What is it about the person's situation that might be contributing to depression (e.g., very little positive reinforcement)? Does the person have thinking patterns that are often associated with depression, and might these be changed via cognitive therapy (Beck, Wright, Newman, & Liese, 2001; Miller, 2008b)? Might meditation (Aron & Aron, 1980; Bien & Bien, 2002, 2003; Marlatt & Marques, 1977) or a medication (see Chapter 18) be appropriate to alter the underlying physiology (organism)? How is the person responding that might exacerbate depression (e.g., excessive sleeping and withdrawing)? Is depression being reinforced in some way (consequences) in the person's social environment?

Similarly anger management is a common addiction treatment issue, more often for men than for women. What are the situational factors, the stimuli that seem to trigger anger? What are the thought patterns that exacerbate and maintain anger and resentment? (Anger is an emotion that needs constant cognitive fueling.) What is going on in the person's organism, his body, when anger flares? Might relaxation skills or breathing exercises interrupt this, and might a psychiatric evaluation for medication be appropriate? Is the person using stimulants (like caffeine, nicotine) that are likely to increase autonomic arousal? How does the person respond when angry, and what alternative responses are available? Are there payoff consequences for the person's aggression (like he gets what he wants)? Again, making changes at any of these links in the chain may affect the whole cycle. You can help clients to learn these skills in individual or group counseling (Nay, 2004).

BOX 12.3. STORC Self-Monitoring

Situation	Thoughts	Organism	Response	Consequences
Where was I? Whom was I with? What was going on?	What was I thinking? Or what *must* I have been thinking?	What was I feeling? What was happening in my body?	What did I do? How did I respond?	What happened? What was the result?

Behavioral Self-Control

A fourth evidence-based skill set that can improve outcomes is addressed by *behavioral self-control training* (BSCT). This method generally involves teaching people some common principles of learning (such as positive reinforcement) and self-control and how to use these principles to manage their own behavior. BSCT has often been used to help people make changes in their own substance use (Hester, 2003), but the same approach can be applied more generally to self-change (Bandura, 1997; Baumeister et al., 1994).

Some common components of BSCT include setting clear and specific behavior change goals, and self-monitoring to keep careful records and raise awareness of behavior and progress. Change is often broken down into small steps in the right direction, and the principle of positive reinforcement can be applied to reward completing these steps. Small changes may be made in the target behavior, and alternative responses learned and practiced.

The most common use of BSCT in the addiction field has been in helping people with alcohol problems to moderate or stop drinking (Miller & Muñoz, 2005; Sanchez-Craig, 1996). BSCT strategies have also been applied to help clients learn how to cope with cravings and urges, and more generally to maintain treatment gains and prevent a return to prior substance use (Kadden et al., 1992; Marlatt & Donovan, 2005; Miller, 2004; Monti et al., 2002). People seem to be able to learn and use these skills not only with the help of a counselor, but also working on their own with self-help guidelines in book (Apodaca & Miller, 2003) or computer-based formats (Bickel, Christensen, & Marsch, 2011; Hester & Delaney, 1997; Hester et al., 2009).

Urges and Cravings

Another element in skill training focuses on coping with cravings and urges to use alcohol or other drugs (Kadden et al., 1992; Miller, 2004; Monti et al., 2002). A few basic perspectives can be helpful to clients who are troubled by urges to use:

- Urges are common during recovery and are not reason for alarm or an indication of failure. You are not helpless when they occur, and need not respond by using.
- Urges are not random or mysterious; they tend to occur in particular circumstances. It is possible to learn from them.
- Urges are temporary. The common fear is that cravings will grow steadily until it becomes unbearable, but in fact it usually peaks after a few minutes and then dies down like a wave on the ocean.

"Urge surfing" (Marlatt & Donovan, 2005) is riding it out until it subsides rather than falling into the wave.

- Giving in to urges strengthens them; riding them out weakens them.

Keeping records of urges and the circumstances in which they occur can help to demystify them, and may also suggest additional coping strategies. This can be done on an index card or sheet of paper with four columns:

- The date and time the urge occurred
- The situation in which it occurred: where, with whom, what was happening, and so on
- The strength of urge, rated on a 0–10 or 0–100 scale
- How you responded to the urge

This is essentially a functional analysis of urges and cravings: what happened just before and after they occurred. Remember that the "situation" need not be something happening in the environment. It can be an internal like a memory, emotion, or physical sensation.

As the circumstances associated with urges become clearer, a next step is to develop coping strategies. There are four basic alternatives (Miller, 2004):

1. *Avoid.* Reduce exposure to the situations that trigger urges to use. If seeing other people using triggers cravings, avoid such situations. If having alcohol around the house increases urges to drink, get rid of it. Avoidance of high-risk situations is particularly useful early in the recovery process.
2. *Escape.* It is not possible to avoid all problematic situations. A second strategy, when encountering an urge-exacerbating situation, is to leave it, to get out of the situation as soon as possible. Brainstorm with clients what situations might occur and how they could remove themselves from the risk.
3. *Distract.* Remember that urges are time-limited and tend to subside if they aren't indulged. When avoidance or escape isn't feasible, find an enjoyable distraction to surf through the urge. What could your client do in this situation that would take his or her attention away from the urge?
4. *Endure.* Then there are some situations that can't be avoided or escaped, and where distraction isn't possible or helpful. Here people need strategies to get through until the urge subsides. Some possibilities are talking it through with someone, mindfully observing the urge until it passes, calling someone for help in getting through

it, and taking along a reminder of the importance of sobriety (e.g., a photograph or an AA coin).

DO CLIENTS REALLY LEARN NEW COPING SKILLS?

The usual rationale for coping skill training is straightforward: that clients will learn new skills that they did not previously possess, and subsequently apply them in their lives to successfully manage their own behavior. Does this actually happen? Morgenstern and Longabaugh (2000) reviewed research studying the extent to which clients had actually acquired the intended skills, and the relationship of this learning to treatment outcome. Their findings were surprising. In some studies, clients did not learn the intended coping skills, but the treatment nevertheless worked. In other studies, clients did acquire some coping skills, but the extent to which they had done so was unrelated to outcome. In another, although client coping skills did predict better outcomes, clients had not learned them in treatment (Litt et al., 2003). In other words, although coping skill training is a treatment approach with good evidence of efficacy, it may not work for the presumed reason, by teaching clients new skills! A more recent study, however, did find that improvement in clients' coping skills after cognitive-behavior therapy (CBT) predicted longer posttreatment abstinence (Kiluk, Nich, Babuscio, & Carroll, 2010).

What, then, might be happening in skill training that seems to improve treatment outcome?

One possibility is that focusing on coping skills may increase self-efficacy, that is, people's belief that they are capable of making the intended change (Bandura, 1997). This may mobilize skills that they already possess, which they then use to move toward change. The same optimism regarding the client's capability for change is also being communicated by the counselor who is teaching coping skills, and that belief is contagious. The therapist's belief that a client will succeed in recovery has a way of becoming a self-fulfilling prophecy (Leake & King, 1977).

KEY POINTS

🖈 Alcohol and other drugs are sometimes used for coping and to get from one (usually undesirable) state to another.

🖈 CBTs are generally designed to teach self-management skills for successful living without substance use.

🖈 Job finding, emotion regulation, social skills, and assertiveness skills are among those commonly addressed in addiction treatment.

🖈 Behavioral skill training can also focus directly on self-regulation with regard to substance use, urges, and cravings.

🖈 Increased self-efficacy may also underlie the well-supported efficacy of CBTs.

REFLECTION QUESTIONS

💬 In your experience, what are some of the most common ways in which people use alcohol and other drugs for coping?

💬 What life skills do you think are most helpful for people in moving from addiction to sobriety?

💬 If someone needs to develop a particular social skill for drug-free living, how might you best help him or her to strengthen it?

CHAPTER 13

Involving and Working with Family

There is a long history of focusing on the individual in addiction treatment. The person with a substance use disorder comes for treatment alone, either in individual sessions or attending a group of other people with similar problems. Sometimes there has been a "family night" for educating concerned significant others (SOs), but treatment has usually focused largely on the individual with "the problem."

This is understandable from the clinician's perspective. Including an SO in treatment sessions adds a whole new layer of complexity. You have to manage not only the individual client, but also the family member and the dynamics of their relationship as well. Furthermore, many providers of addiction treatment have had little or no training in couple or family counseling. Some systems even preclude reimbursement for conjoint sessions.

Yet there are good reasons to include a client's SO in addiction treatment and it is quite feasible to do so (Magill et al., 2010). First of all, research shows that doing so can significantly increase the individual's chances of recovery, at least if an evidence-based approach to couple counseling is used. Sometimes the SO has a substance use problem of his or her own. Addiction is also hard on family members and relationships, and timely attention to these issues can prevent a host of problems later.

RECOVERY AND RELATIONSHIPS

In 12-step meetings it is common to hear about relationships breaking up during the first year of recovery. This is a disturbing message and, for those sitting in a meeting and contemplating a change in their substance use, it could even be a deterrent. Imagine if part of the informed consent process for individual treatment were a caution against the "side effects" of recovery: *Warning: Sobriety may be harmful to your relationships.*

Yet it's true, and maybe it should be part of the consent process for those who engage in treatment that does not include the SO in a meaningful way. In addition to the anecdotal accounts circulating among recovery groups, research has shown that a disproportionate number of relationships do end *after* addiction treatment (O'Farrell & Fals-Stewart, 2006).* Why is this so? Substance use and related consequences are tremendous stressors in a relationship. If the substance use is a primary source of conflict between a couple, shouldn't the relationship become stronger once stable abstinence is achieved?

Of course, substance use is likely not the only source of conflict in a relationship. Even when the substance use itself is removed, there may be other problems that linger or rise to the surface. Perhaps the couple grew apart during the time the person was actively using or in treatment, for even if the relationship preceded the development of addiction, it can be hard to remember what it was like before. Perhaps one or both decided that the relationship was no longer worth the investment and trouble of working through disagreements. It is also possible that the SO may not be ready to set aside past hurts and move forward. Conflicts that had been buried or avoided for years may be a dam of frustration and resentment that opens up once the person is sober. A situation in which a recovering individual comes home to an SO ready with a laundry list of complaints and with built-up contempt could lead to a cascade of conflict and relationship distress (Gottman, 1994). Newfound sobriety also can require a redistribution of power and roles within a relationship, with the recovering person ready and expecting to resume functions that had been taken on by the long-suffering partner.

It is worth saying here that most relationships do stabilize or improve rather than deteriorate once addiction is treated. Nevertheless, relationship problems persist or get worse often enough that it is definitely worthwhile to focus on improving relationship quality when treating addiction.

There is another piece of the puzzle surrounding the association between relationships and substance use: in research examining the main reasons why people *resume* substance use, interpersonal conflicts with an SO have been a frequent precipitant (Barber & Crisp, 1995; Hunter-Reel, McCrady, & Hildebrandt, 2009; Maisto, O'Farrell, Connors, & McKay, 1988). It is a destructive cycle. Relationships seem to be at risk for break-

---

*Tragically, claims of falsification of data were made against Dr. Fals-Stewart before his untimely death. Aware of this concern, we checked the veracity of research in which he collaborated and have been assured that the studies we cite were properly conducted, supervised, and verified by senior colleagues and the research team.

ing up during the recovery process and, at the same time, conflicts within relationships can endanger someone's ability to maintain sobriety. Modifying the cautions against the potential side effects of recovery, the warnings might read: *Warning: Sobriety may be harmful to your relationships ... and your relationships may be harmful to your ability to maintain sobriety.* To be most effective, then, it seems important to address not only the individual's substance use, but also the relationship in ways that are more conducive to stable recovery.

This is also consistent with the broader approach to conceptualizing addiction presented in Chapter 2 and throughout this book. Rather than viewing addiction just as an individual pathology, many factors influence whether a person will develop and maintain addiction, and changes in these factors can positively or negatively influence the likelihood of recovery. Relationship conflict appears to be one of these significant factors.

In sum, substance use disorders clearly affect both the individual and the family members with whom the person lives. Family relationships, in turn, can support or hinder recovery. By concurrently addressing both addiction and family functioning, outcomes for both can be significantly improved. You can increase the chances that a person's significant relationship(s) will favor rather than undermine recovery.

> By concurrently addressing both addiction and family functioning, outcomes for both can be significantly improved.

A HISTORY OF IDEAS ABOUT FAMILIES AND ADDICTION

It has long been recognized that addiction and family disturbance occur together, but *why* is this so, and what are the implications for treatment? There is an interesting history of guesses about the link between addiction and the family, leading to dramatically different implications for intervention (McCrady, 2006). Early writings on this subject typically focused on men with alcohol problems and their wives, and the implicit underlying question was, *"What is going on with these women?"* Various ideas have been proposed over the years.

Spouse and Family Pathology

The *disturbed spouse hypothesis* was that these wives had deep-rooted personality problems themselves as a result of developmental disturbances in childhood. Based on clinical impressions, this psychodynamic hypothesis arose around the 1940s and speculated that these women sought out alcoholic husbands in order to fulfill their own unconscious needs. One account, for example, described them as aggressive, domineering women who married in order to mother or control a man, and who therefore had an investment in the continuation of his drinking (Futterman, 1953). It would be expected, therefore, that a man's attempt to quit drinking would be undermined and sabotaged by his wife. Anecdotes (e.g., of a wife buying alcohol for her sober husband) were used to exemplify and support this view, and the term "enabling" came to be associated with family behaviors that promote the continuation of addiction. Related to the pathological spouse hypothesis was the belief that if the husband sobered up the wife would decompensate (Edwards, Harvey, & Whitehead, 1973). The logical intervention, given this view, would be individual psychotherapy for the spouse, focused on alleviating her personality disturbance and her need for her partner to remain addicted.

A similar proposed solution to this puzzle is the *disturbed family hypothesis*, often linked to family systems theory (Bowen, 1991; Shorkey & Rosen, 1993). Here the pathology is not attributed to an individual spouse, but rather to dysfunctional patterns of family interaction. The problem is seen as residing within the family system itself. Each member of the family has a particular pathological role that maintains the equilibrium of the system. As a unit, the family system works to preserve these roles because of the familiarity and comfort of knowing what to expect from each family member. Imagine a mobile hung over a baby's crib. Changing any one element unbalances the whole. Each family member represents a piece of the mobile that, by interacting in a particular way, helps to keep the whole system balanced. The addicted person occupies an important role within the system, crucial to the family's identity and self-regulation. In this view, the family would be expected to sabotage recovery. From a family systems perspective, enabling behavior would serve to restore the status quo and prevent deterioration of the family (Rotunda, West, & O'Farrell, 2004). The book *Games Alcoholics Play* (Steiner, 1984) described in detail such self-maintaining family dynamics, with supporting anecdotes. The logical intervention within this view would be therapy for the entire family in order to change its pathological interaction dynamics.

This view of family members as having unique independent pathology reemerged in a new but closely related form in the 1980s: the *codependence hypothesis* (Wegscheider-Cruse, 1990; Woititz, 1984). In this view, addiction is a "family disease" wherein both the addicted person and his or her family members are afflicted with complementary and interlocking illnesses. The term "codependence" was coined to describe the personality pathology of family members, which was alleged to be a separate disease that predates and exists apart from the loved one's substance dependence. As with earlier psychodynamic views, codependence was attributed to early childhood factors such as poor parenting, attributable perhaps to addiction in the prior generation, and was thought to share certain features of an addictive personality (Cermak, 1991). A wide variety of symptoms of codependence included continual emotional pain, inability to recognize one's needs and illness and ask for help, a high tolerance for inappropriate behavior, and compulsive dishonesty and pretending (Carruth & Mendenhall, 1989). Codependence was also said to have a definable course of deterioration mentally, physically, psychologically, and spiritually. Physical consequences of codependence were thought to include gastrointestinal problems, ulcers, high blood pressure, and even cancer, so that left untreated, the outcome of codependence would be death. Schaef (1986) wrote that the codependent person often dies before the addicted person. (We know of no sound evidence for this.) It would follow from this view that family members would also need separate treatment to overcome their disease of codependence. In essence, the codependence/family disease perspective represented a blending of disturbed spouse and disturbed family hypotheses.

All of these hypotheses posit the existence of pathology that is independent of and complementary to the loved one's addiction. They predict that certain relationships between behavior will be observed, and as such they are scientifically testable hypotheses. Within these views, the normal outcome of a person sobering up through individual treatment should be *increased* pathology in either the spouse or the family as a whole. The disturbed spouse and codependence hypotheses also predict the presence of stable and measurable personality disturbance in the spouse or other family member, independent of the loved one's drinking or drug use. None of these hypotheses has been supported by the weight of research evidence (Hurcom, Copello, & Orford, 2000; Paolino, McCrady, & Kogan, 1978). As we stated earlier, if you have to guess what will happen in a family when an addicted member sobers up, you can bet that things will get better rather than deteriorate. The typical outcome is that even if only individual addiction is treated, other life problems will tend to improve (Miller, Hedrick, & Taylor, 1983). There are exceptions, of course. Some problems and families do get worse, and it happens often enough to deserve clinical attention, but this is the exception rather than the rule. Furthermore, there is no scientific evidence that there is "something wrong" with the spouses or family members of people with addiction—that they tend to have any stable and unique personality patterns or problems of their own.

> There is no scientific evidence that there is "something wrong" with the spouses or family members of people with addiction.

Family Adjustment Model

Where did the field go so wrong in stigmatizing already-suffering family members? There is usually at least a kernel of truth from which mistaken ideas are grown. That kernel here seems to be the observation that spouses

> ### BOX 13.1. Personal Reflection: Am I Crazy?
>
> She came into my university office visibly upset. "The department secretary told me that you know something about addictions," she said, and I invited her to sit down. She explained that her father had recently been admitted to a local residential treatment program. "After I left home about 12 years ago, he started drinking more, and when he retired it really got bad." Two weeks into treatment, a counselor from the program called her to ask if she could come to family night in order to support her father's recovery. "I said of course I would, and I went last night. Some of the counselors took me aside, surrounded me, and told me that I have a fatal disease called codependence, and that people who grow up with an alcoholic are just as sick as he is." They described the symptoms to her, a few of which seemed to fit, but she protested that in general she felt normal and was quite happy with her life. "Then they told me that people who are codependent don't know what normal is, and this proved that I have it. I explained that Dad wasn't drinking much when I was still living at home, but they told me it didn't matter, and I definitely need treatment or I'll mess up my own kids. Am I crazy?" After talking with her a while longer, I explained that there had been an attempt to insert a diagnosis of "codependence" into the DSM, but the American Psychiatric Association had rejected it for lack of scientific evidence. I thanked her for being willing to help her father, and reassured her that I saw no reason for concern about her own mental health. She was clearly comforted to learn that she was not "crazy" or "terminally ill" herself.
>
> —W. R. M.

and other family members often *do* show high levels of emotional distress. But *why* is this so? Long ago Joan Jackson (1954) proposed a different solution to the puzzle: that the psychological disturbance and behavior of spouses represent understandable reactions and adaptive attempts to cope with the progressive deterioration of their partners' substance dependence. This *stress-coping hypothesis* posits that what appears from the outside to be aberrant behaviors of a spouse or other family member represents a normal adjustive reaction to the addictive behavior of their loved one. Within Jackson's perspective, behaviors stigmatized as "enabling," such as buying alcohol or other drugs for the person to use, or protecting the loved one from negative consequences, are understandable attempts to adjust to and cope with the chaos of addiction.

How would one help within this perspective? Certainly emotional support is in order for the family during the process of treatment, but family members can also play an important role in supporting recovery. One evidence-based approach here is to help SOs to distinguish between actions that favor recovery and those that favor continued use and addiction (Meyers et al., 2002). In essence, you teach the family to reinforce sobriety. It is common to advise family members to refrain from doing things that make use easier or reinforce it (sometimes called "enabling" behavior). But just as important if not more so is for the family to provide positive reinforcement for sobriety, for nonuse and alternatives to use (Meyers & Wolfe, 2004). This is part of the CRAFT method, described in Chapters 10 and 11, that has also been used effectively to engage reluctant loved ones in addiction treatment.

Al-Anon: Loving Detachment

Like other 12-step programs, Al-Anon (and Alateen for younger family members) does not endorse any particular theory of the etiology of addiction or related family problems. Although substance dependence is described as a "family disease" because it adversely affects those close to the person, family members are clearly not blamed or held responsible for their loved one's addiction. Meetings are free of charge, anonymous, and widely available. Separate "Nar-Anon" meetings are available in many areas for those whose loved one is involved with illicit drugs, although many such family members also attend Al-Anon and Alateen.

The response that is advocated in Al-Anon and Alateen meetings is "loving detachment" (Al-Anon Family Group Headquarters, 1976). The spouse or family member is encouraged to give up attempts to influence his or her loved one's drinking or drug use, accepting his or her own powerlessness to control the addiction, and to instead look for strength and support from other members. In the Al-Anon program, members are instructed to focus on themselves and their own well-being to reduce emotional distress and improve their coping skills.

Given the teaching that family members are powerless to influence addiction, the Al-Anon program does not usually focus on encouraging or facilitating the loved one's abstinence, or even on improving family relationships. Each individual is encouraged to focus on what he or she needs to do to improve his or her own life. Given this, it is not surprising that family involvement in Al-Anon has not been found to facilitate the loved one's seeking of treatment. Studies have found, however, that family members themselves who are receiving "Al-Anon facilitation therapy" to facilitate their involvement in Al-Anon do significantly reduce their emotional and physical distress and improve their coping (Miller, Meyers, & Tonigan, 1999).

Chicken and Egg: The Cycle of Substance Use and Relationship Distress

The causal connections between substance use and relationship distress are complex. The negative effects of substance use can produce relationship problems. Stress from relationship problems in turn can trigger or exacerbate substance use. Each affects the other in a destructive cycle. Consider these three scenarios and the interlocking chain resulting from each person's actions:

> A couple gets into a disagreement about whether the man was flirting with a waitress during dinner. The fight escalates and the woman accuses the man of cheating. Though they had already shared a bottle of wine at dinner, once home the woman retreats to her bedroom where she takes several painkillers and drinks another bottle of wine as a way to soothe herself and forget the upsetting thoughts.

Couple problems → increased use

> A man tells his wife that he is too hung over to go to work and too sick to even call in to his employer. Realizing that he will be fired if he has another unexcused absence, and that they won't be able to pay their monthly bills without his income, she calls his employer to say that he has the flu and won't be coming to work that day. She then fixes him breakfast in bed, gets the children ready for school, and before leaving for work leaves a note on the counter telling him that she hopes he feels better soon and that she loves him very much. He spends the day in bed drinking and watching television.

Increased use → caretaking, affection → more use

> A man returns home from a 30-day inpatient treatment program. Pleased with his new sober state, his wife begins talking to him about all of the things she has been angry about for years that he was never sober enough to hear in the past. It seems to him that each day she criticizes him about how he let her down, and he wonders if she was keeping a journal with detailed documenting of every minor thing he had ever done wrong in their relationship. After 3 weeks of what seems like endless shaming, he begins using again. With his resumed use, the woman stops airing her complaints for fear of violent consequences.

Recovery begins → increased conflicts → drug use →
decreased conflict

In other words, relationship conflict and substance use can be a self-sustaining cycle, and it is not crucial to decide which is causing the other. Identifying a person to blame is not fruitful, although distressed couples sometimes want you to do so. The point is to interrupt the cycle and start it turning in a positive direction.

THE EVIDENCE FOR FAMILY-INVOLVED TREATMENT OF ADULTS

> Addiction treatment including the person's SO results in more abstinence than does individual treatment.

Studies indicate that addiction treatment including the person's SO results in more abstinence than does individual treatment (McCrady & Epstein, 1996). Behavioral couple therapy (BCT) is the treatment method with the strongest research support for its efficacy in treating addiction in adults. A meta-analysis concluded that overall, BCT produces better outcomes than individual-based treatment (Powers, Vedel, & Emmelkamp, 2008). In addition to increased rates of abstinence, BCT leads to better relationship functioning, defined as lower risk of separation and divorce, compared to typical individual-based treatment, and reduces social costs, domestic violence, and the emotional problems of couples' children (Fals-Stewart, O'Farrell, & Birchler, 1997; McCrady, Epstein, Cook, Jensen, & Hildebrandt, 2009; O'Farrell, Murphy, Stephan, Fals-Stewart, & Murphy, 2004; Sayers, Kohn, & Heavey, 1998; Schumm, O'Farrell, Murphy, & Fals-Stewart, 2009). BCT can also improve adherence to recovery medications such as disulfiram (Azrin et al., 1982) and naltrexone (Fals-Stewart & O'Farrell, 2003).

There is surprisingly little evidence for involving the entire family unit in treatment. Rather, the treatments that work seem to focus on involving the spouse (O'Farrell & Fals-Stewart, 2006) or other concerned family member (Donohue et al., 2009; Smith & Meyers, 2004). With adolescents, there is strong evidence for involving the parents or caregivers, as we will discuss later in this chapter. We will now discuss a specific approach of spouse-involved treatment for adults.

WHAT IS BEHAVIORAL COUPLE THERAPY?

Behavioral couple therapy (BCT) is designed for married or cohabitating couples in which one person is seeking help for addiction. The primary goals of BCT are to include the SO in treatment as a way to increase and reinforce behaviors that support abstinence and long-term recovery and also improve the couple's overall relationship quality. Recovery is promoted with a contract that involves both members of the couple in a daily ritual to celebrate and reinforce abstinence. Relationship improvement is promoted primarily by (1) increasing shared positive activities, and (2) improving the couple's communication skills and decreasing hurtful interaction patterns. BCT is based on each partner's commitment to do what he or she can to improve the relationship.

BCT is a comprehensive treatment package that includes behaviorally oriented couple sessions in addition to whatever other individual counseling and group therapy sessions are provided. Thus BCT can be offered as an important adjunct to other services available in your treatment setting. A couple can begin BCT soon after the person with addiction seeks help and has completed detoxification, if necessary. BCT can easily be integrated with programs that emphasize 12-step, cognitive-behavioral, or pharmacotherapy approaches.

In its full traditional form, BCT consists of 12–20 weekly couple sessions, each of which lasts 50–60 minutes. Sessions tend to be moderately to highly structured, with the counselor setting the agenda at the outset of each meeting and giving the couple homework assignments between sessions. Though effective, this intensity of treatment can be prohibitive for some settings and populations. Consequently, a brief couple therapy was developed and tested in comparison to standard BCT or individual-based therapy. This briefer six-session BCT had posttreatment and 12-month outcomes that were equivalent to those for standard BCT and were still superior to those for individual treatment (Fals-Stewart & Lam, 2008). Thus it appears possible to reduce the intensity and cost of implementing BCT without undermining efficacy.

Typically the initial BCT sessions focus on establishing a recovery contract to support abstinence and to decrease couple conflicts about past or possible future substance use. Once abstinence and attendance at BCT sessions have stabilized, the counselor adds relationship-focused interventions to increase positive activities and improve communication. Finally, when abstinence has been maintained for 3–6 months, the counselor plans for continuing recovery to prevent or minimize a return to use (see Chapter 19) and fades the frequency of BCT sessions. There are four key objectives of BCT (O'Farrell & Fals-Stewart, 2006): (1) engaging the couple (2) supporting abstinence, (3) improving the relationship, and (4) continuing recovery. Later in this chapter we provide more detail on these four objectives.

Who Is Appropriate for BCT?

Clinical trials typically impose certain restrictions on the characteristics of people who can enter the study. These limitations impact the *generalizability* of findings. For example, BCT trials have been restricted to couples in which only one person in the relationship had a substance use disorder. Would BCT also work if both partners have alcohol/drug problems? It's unclear so far, although given the strength of research support for the efficacy of BCT with other couples it is certainly worth trying. But within the constraints of research to date, what is known about the characteristics of people for whom BCT is indicated?

Participants in studies that support BCT's efficacy have typically been couples who are married or cohabiting for at least a year and are willing to work together to see if their relationship can be improved. Although BCT was designed for couples experiencing significant relationship distress, there is also evidence that it can be useful even when the couple is getting along well (McCrady & Epstein, 1996). If relationship distress is not an issue for a couple, including the SO in treatment is still a useful way to support the partner's treatment gains (see Chapter 11). Studies to date have also required that the person entering addiction treatment be willing to accept at least a temporary goal of abstinence as a prerequisite for BCT. Finally, BCT studies have typically excluded couples in which either partner has a major mental disorder such as schizophrenia.

Does this mean that BCT is ineffective for other kinds of couples? Not at all. It simply means that research thus far has focused on currently cohabiting couples without other major psychiatric disorders who are willing to commit to treatment, and that is where we know that BCT is effective. Results from a pilot study indicated that behavioral family counseling, an adaptation of BCT involving family members other than the spouse, was effective in reducing substance use and improving treatment retention (O'Farrell, Murphy, Alter, & Fals-Stewart, 2010), but the preponderance of evidence is for involving the spouse or partner. The absence of BCT studies with the particular kind of couple you are treating is not a reason to prefer another treatment method for which there is little or no evidence of efficacy at all. Lacking research with clients having particular characteristics, you are still probably best off starting with evidence-based treatments that have worked with other types of clients.

Are there, then, contraindications to BCT? The primary reasons why BCT may not be appropriate for a couple relate to legal and safety issues. Domestic violence is more common in addiction treatment populations, and for this reason you need to be aware and take steps to protect each person's safety. Some concerns are more clear-cut; for instance, if there is a restraining order stating a couple may not have contact with each other, then these individuals should not be seen together in therapy unless an exception is granted and both are willing. Less clear-cut are situations in which there is a history of intimate partner violence. On the one hand, there is strong evidence supporting the efficacy of BCT with couples who have a history of partner violence (O'Farrell et al., 2004; Schumm et al., 2009). However, if there is an acute risk for domestic violence that could cause serious injury or be potentially life-threatening, then couple treatment can be unwise. It's a professional judgment call. Fals-Stewart and Kennedy (2005) offered five exclusion criteria that indicate an acute risk of severe violence:

1. One or both partners report a fear of injury or death
2. A history of violence has resulted in an injury requiring medical attention in the past 2 years
3. Violence has been threatened or inflicted using a weapon such as a knife or gun

4. One member of the couple expresses fear in participating in couple treatment because of concern that violence may occur
5. One member of the couple expresses desire to leave the relationship due to the degree and severity of partner aggression.

Learning BCT

Compared to individual therapy, couple therapy is challenging because there is now a third person in the room requiring your attention. It can be a struggle to empathize equally with both partners and form a strong therapeutic relationship with both people, yet this is important in order to avoid one person feeling like you are "ganging up" and taking sides. BCT requires clear structure and control over the sessions to maintain a focus on the goal of therapy, which is to address the substance use first and foremost, and prevent interactions in session that are further hurtful. As discussed earlier, the use of substances can lead to a great deal of anger and resentment in the relationship. The couple should be aware of what the BCT sessions entail; sessions are not an opportunity to vent and ruminate, something they might expect from stereotypes of "couple therapy." Rather, the goal of this treatment approach is to change ways that the couple should communicate and act toward each other from this point forward. Structuring sessions so that couples know the expected content and type of information that should be shared is a way you can maintain control over the session.

This takes time and practice. BCT is not readily learned by reading about it, and plenty can go wrong in couple sessions. As with other evidence-based treatments discussed in this book, we recommend both initial training and some ongoing feedback and coaching based on observed practice. That's what it takes to really learn most any complex skill. Is it worth it to take the time and expense of obtaining such training for treatment staff? We believe that the increased benefit of involving SO in treatment more than justifies learning BCT.

Four Goals of BCT

Whether using the full BCT or the shorter six-session version, there are four main goals to accomplish. The first is to build motivation for engaging in BCT and to discuss the BCT approach with the couple. Following engagement, the next treatment goal is to have the client achieve and maintain abstinence by implementing the recovery contract, teaching refusal skills, deciding together how to deal with stressful life situations without substance use, and addressing how the significant other can support abstinence. The third goal is to have the couple improve the quality of their relationship by working with them to increase positive and rewarding activities and behaviors, decrease negative interaction patterns, and learn skills for positive communication and resolving conflicts within their relationship. The final goal is to work with the couple to tailor a plan for continuing recovery following initial treatment. The continuing recovery plan may involve check-in visits with you and/or plans to continue activities practiced during treatment. Within these four goals, there is a great deal of flexibility in which methods you will use and in the type of skills training that would be most useful to the couple.

BCT techniques all follow a typical behavioral training format (see Chapter 12). When teaching each skill, you first describe the skill to the couple during the session, giving a rationale for why this approach is effective. Second, you show how to effectively use the skill through modeling. For example, in practicing drink refusal skills you would role-play as the client; making eye contact and saying "no" in a clear, firm, unhesitating voice, escalating refusal responses as needed. The third step is to have the couple practice the skill in-session while you offer positive reinforcement and coaching to give feedback on areas needing improvement. The couple is then instructed to practice this skill at home. When the couple returns, you review their real-world practice and offer further coaching and practice for areas that were difficult.

Engaging the Couple

None of this couple work is possible, however, unless you first engage them in treatment. To work with a couple, you must first receive permission to contact the spouse (see Chapter 22 on ethics for limits on confidentiality) by talking with the client who is seeking/in treatment. In this initial conversation, explore the person's thoughts about including his or her SO in the treatment process. Though many are happy to do so, it is also common for people to express fears and concerns about including their loved one in treatment. When these fears are shared, reflect the concerns to show understanding.

The process of engaging the SO in the therapy process can be broken down into smaller more manageable steps. The person doesn't need to swear permanent abstinence from all substances or definite long-term commitment to the relationship. It's very normal to have mixed feelings about such big long-term decisions. All that is needed in these early sessions is the willingness to explore things further in joint sessions.

After this initial conversation and permission, talk directly to the SO to invite him or her for a joint interview to discuss treatment planning and explore the possibility of BCT. O'Farrell and Fals-Stewart (2006) recommend calling the spouse while the client is with you, so the client can hear exactly what you say to the SO as a way to build trust. This also facilitates scheduling of the joint interview since everyone can give their availability and find a mutually convenient time. If the client has already expressed interest in BCT, the SO can be invited to learn more about the BCT program and find out if it is a good fit for both partners. If ambivalence is high regarding BCT, you can invite the partner to meet with you and the client to discuss treatment planning and to share his or her insights about the substance problem. We do not, of course, recommend pushing a particular treatment on a person; if someone is adamant that he or she is not interested in BCT, there are many other options; pursuing a treatment plan that the person is enthusiastic about is a much better strategy.

The next step is to meet with the couple and gain their commitment to trying BCT. In what is known as the *joint couple interview* (an initial session that does not assume further meetings as a couple), the goal is to establish rapport and determine if the couple is interested in and appropriate for BCT. Remember that the couple does not need to be experiencing serious relationship problems to be appropriate candidates; rather, the SO's involvement can be framed as a way to work together to promote recovery for the person seeking treatment. BCT is presented as an option during this session, seeking the partner's input in finalizing the treatment plan.

If the couple decides to try BCT, treatment orientation begins at the next couple session. During this session there is an initial assessment on domains relevant to BCT, including alcohol and drug use by the client and SO, relationship stability and commitment, relationship violence, and reasons for seeking help at this point in time. As discussed in Chapter 5, assessment should be personalized to key areas for the person seeking treatment as ways to inform and individualize the intervention. Even though BCT has been highly structured in the order of the sessions and the homework assignments, deciding which aspects of BCT get more emphasis than others is a matter for your clinical judgment. Also individually tailored are recommendations for adjunctive support such as mutual help meetings (Chapter 14), urine drug screens or breath tests, and recovery medications (Chapter 15). Provide the couple with information on the structure of BCT and the importance of completing assignments between sessions. Ask the couple also to make four promises to each other for the course of treatment (O'Farrell & Fals-Stewart, 2006), designed to begin BCT in a positive way: (1) not to threaten separation, (2) to refrain from violence and threats of violence, (3) to focus on the present and future, and (4) to actively participate in all sessions and complete home assignments.

Supporting Sobriety

It is possible that couples may be having little contact with each other and frequent arguments at the time they begin BCT. The recovery contract encourages the couple to talk together in a positive way every day about abstinence and recovery, and to avoid negative interactions. Use the above-described sequence of explaining, modeling, practicing in session, and then practicing in the real world. Explain the recovery contract, show the couple how they might make this a positive experience for each other, have them practice in session, and then have them try it out for a week. There are six possible components that can be included in the recovery contract: the trust discussion, medication to aid recovery, self-help involvement, urine screens or breath tests, other weekly activities to support recovery, and a calendar to record progress. Only two of these are essential: the trust discussion and the record of progress. The other components may or may not be included, based on the needs and willingness of the couple.

The first part of the daily recovery contract is the *trust discussion*. Each day, at a specific agreed-upon time, the client initiates this brief discussion. In the trust discussion, the client states his or her intent not to drink or use drugs that day, in the same tradition of the 12-step "one day at a time" (Alcoholics Anonymous World Services, 2001). The SO then expresses encouragement and support for the client's efforts to stay abstinent, and the client thanks the SO for supporting his or her efforts. To prevent substance-related conflicts that can trigger a return to use, both partners then agree not to discuss past or possible future substance use, instead reserving these discussions for the therapy sessions. For clients taking recovery-related medication (e.g., disulfiram or naltrexone), the SO witnesses the ingestion of the medication and verbally thanks or praises the client for doing so. The SO then records completion of the trust discussion on a calendar that is on the back of the recovery contract. Any other daily or weekly recovery contract components (e.g., attending AA, Al-Anon, urine drug screens) are also recorded on the calendar. Following the first week, in which the couple has tried out the contract, they then agree to a specific length of time during which the contract will be in effect and agree to call the counselor immediately if the trust discussion does not take place for 2 days in a row. If this occurs, do whatever you can to see the couple as soon as possible to discuss possible problems and renew the trust contract in session.

Once the contract is in place, review the recovery progress record/calendar at the beginning of each session to determine whether each person has done his or her part, and praise all efforts and progress. The couple can also complete the trust discussion (and medication taking, if applicable) in each session to highlight its importance and to let you observe and offer suggestions for areas of improvement. From week to week, the contract will evolve as certain components are added and removed. Additional or replacement weekly activities to support recovery can be chosen by the couple in order to personalize the contract so it meets their needs. Examples are group or individual counseling, exercise, reading from the AA Big Book, spiritual practices, or pastoral counseling.

In addition to the recovery contract, there are more generic behavioral counseling methods not specific to BCT that can be used as appropriate to promote abstinence (e.g., Meyers & Smith, 1995; Miller, 2004). For example, you may decide to spend time reviewing substance use or urges or teaching substance use refusal skills. If the person does resume substance use, intervene before it persists for an extended period of time. One approach is to have a plan in place so that the client or SO calls you if substance use recurs or seems imminent. Another area you might focus on would be a discussion of triggers for use and ways to avoid or cope with these cues. A *functional analysis* might be used to figure out ways to get a similar benefit without using (Chapter 11). For example, if the person is struggling with wanting to use a substance to cope with the stress of working long hours, what else could the person do to cope with that stress without using a substance?

Substance use can be particularly difficult to avoid when exposure to substances is pervasive and frequent. How could exposure to alcohol and other drugs be decreased? Particularly early in recovery, avoidance of high-risk situations is helpful. Of course, the safest plan is for the person to avoid all contact with situations where alcohol and drugs are available, but this may not be feasible. Will alcohol be kept in the home? Will it be served to guests? Will the SO also abstain in solidarity with the client? (It's very hard, for example, for one partner to quit smoking while the other continues to smoke.) Will the couple attend functions that include alcohol or other drugs? Some couples are able to use partial avoidance, while others may need total avoidance and major life readjustments to avoid people and places that might trigger a return to use, at least early in the recovery process.

It is also useful to help couples find alternative ways of coping with significant life stressors and identify supportive community resources (see Chapter 8). Some issues you may be able to address directly while others might require referral to another source of help. Start with problems that may show quick progress, and defer more complex problems until initial encouraging gains in abstinence and relationship skills have been made.

You may also discover and need to address partner behaviors that encourage substance use. Avoid placing blame and shame. Partners often do such things inadvertently or with the best of intentions, perhaps to avoid conflict or protect the family from negative economic or social consequences. Help the couple to identify any such responses that have occurred in the past or may still be occurring. Then brainstorm alternatives with the couple so that they have a different way of responding.

Offer lots of encouragement, praise, and social reinforcement for positive changes, even small ones. Acknowledge periods of abstinence, notice and comment on positive coping responses, praise small steps in learning.

Also encourage the couple to share in mutually enjoyable activities when the client has not been using (Noel & McCrady, 1993).

Increasing Positive Relationship

The second common goal of BCT is to improve the couple's relationship. The relationship-focused interventions are directed toward increasing enjoyable couple and family activities to enhance positive feelings, goodwill, and commitment to the relationship.

INCREASING POSITIVE BEHAVIORS

John Gottman, who has spent four decades studying happy and unhappy couples, has described methods for strengthening relationships. One simple but important method is to increase positive communications and actions. Over time, relationships can drift toward negativity, focusing on partners' shortcomings and pet peeves. Early in a relationship the partners tend to exchange many positive comments and actions. As these positives decline over time, the partners can come to feel taken for granted and unappreciated. Increasing positive activities is a way to reverse this somewhat natural negative drift in relationships. The ratio of positive to negative comments made by partners is a fairly good indicator of relationship happiness. Increasing positives involves consciously and conscientiously practicing caring behaviors on a daily basis. The reciprocal role for each partner is to notice and appreciate the partner's caring actions. Together, these changes can greatly improve relationship satisfaction (Gottman, 1994).

A common recommended step is for each partner to make a list of personal "P's and D's" (pleasing and displeasing actions). Each person generates a list of positive things that he or she could say or do that would be likely to please the other, as well as things known to be displeasing to the partner. Usually the partners do not show these lists to each other. Instead, each person keeps records of his or her own P's and D's toward the partner and brings these back for the counselor to review. A goal is to have the P's substantially outnumber the D's. Sometimes each person is asked to secretly choose one "caring day" in the week in which to particularly increase P's for the partner.

Each partner is also asked to notice and appreciate the other's P's. A helpful instruction here is to "catch your partner doing something nice" each day. When the couple returns for a session, you can ask each one to take turns describing something nice that the partner did in the preceding week, perhaps using an appreciative "I" message ("I appreciated when you ... "; "I felt good when you ... "; "I liked it when you ... ").

This method sounds fairly straightforward, but there is a lot of clinical know-how to making it work well. A variety of books provide excellent and more detailed practice guidelines for counselors (O'Farrell & Fals-Stewart, 2006) and for couples (Gottman, Gottman, & Declaire, 2007; Gottman & Silver, 2000)

SHARING POSITIVE ACTIVITIES

It is common for distressed couples to stop doing enjoyable things together. As one partner spends more time acquiring, using, and recovering from drugs, the couple spends less time together and becomes more distant from each other. The nonusing person may understandably begin avoiding social events with the partner for fear of embarrassing consequences. This can lead to parallel lives, a sign that the partners are withdrawing from their relationship. Reversing this negative drift requires increasing positive couple or family activities that do not involve alcohol/drug use. Couples who share more positive activities have better recovery rates after treatment (Moos, Finney, & Cronkite, 1990).

So how can you help to reunite a couple? Help them plan and share in activities that they enjoy together each week. This begins by having them identify activities they would like to do. If the couple is having trouble thinking of some activities they may enjoy, it may be helpful to provide them with a menu of local recreational activities. Remember that offering your own solutions for clients will often be met with "yes, but ... " reasons why that activity won't work. Instead, start with an open question of "What things might you enjoy doing together?" or have them brainstorm activities at home and bring the list to the next session to discuss. A goal is for the couple to have some enjoyable time alone together, while also having some quality time with their family and friends.

Strengthening Communication Skills

A third common goal in working with couples, beyond supporting sobriety and increasing relationship positivity, is to strengthen communication skills (McCrady & Epstein, 2009a, 2009b). Couples with a painful history of addiction often become angry and defensive with each other, with communications dominated by hostility and withdrawal. Strengthening communication skills involves both improving positivity and clarity of expression and fostering good listening. The speaker and the listener have important complementary roles. The speaker should clearly state what he or she wants, thinks, and feels. The listener should seek to understand the message without jumping to conclusions.

Effective listening helps each person feel understood, prevents quick escalation of negative exchanges by slowing down the conversation, and helps make the message intended by the speaker equal to the message received by the listener (Miller & Rollnick, 2002; O'Farrell & Fals-

Stewart, 2006). Good listening includes restating in one's own words the message that was heard, and seeking clarification by asking open questions (see Chapter 10). The first goal is to be sure to *understand* what the partner is saying before responding. Also helpful are small acknowledging responses (e.g., "I know that bothers you") without jumping immediately to disagreement or refutation. This enhances the partner's feelings of being understood and valued (Gottman, 1994).

On the expressive side, the use of "I" messages is a common tool. Starting a statement with "I" focuses on one's own feelings, without blaming the other person (as is more likely to happen when the statement begins with "You"). One helpful formula originally suggested by Thomas Gordon (1970) is: "I feel _____ (emotion) when you _____ (behavior) because _____ (specific reason)." The speaker takes responsibility for his or her own feelings and reactions (rather than saying, "You make me feel … "), and the specifics leave more room for problem solving instead of blaming.

During sessions, it is important to practice, and not only discuss communication skills such as active listening and "I" messages. A good place to start when practicing listening and expressing skills is to discuss a neutral or positive topic. Don't start with the most contentious issues! The usual cycle is to first demonstrate the skill to be learned, then have the couple practice in session, and then assign a similar activity for home practice. Plan home assignments in such a way that they minimize the risk of negative escalation.

Negotiating Changes, Conflicts, and Problems

A fourth common goal in BCT is to manage and reduce negative interactions. Although increasing communication skills and shared positive activities usually will reduce negativity, it can also be useful to develop specific skills for requesting changes, resolving conflicts, and solving problems in the relationship.

REQUESTING CHANGES

Generalized, global, personal "You" messages (such as "You're lazy," or "You never care") tend only to create negative feelings, whereas being specific is more likely to result in a concrete change. Specific complaints and requests for change can be very healthy in a relationship (Gottman, 1994; Gottman & Silver, 2000). Such requests are most constructive (and likely to result in change) when they ask for specific behavior, and are stated positively. A positive request is to do *more* of something. If the request could be accomplished by general anesthesia—by doing nothing (e.g., "Stop being so messy")—try reframing it in the positive (e.g., "Please hang up your towel instead of leaving it on the floor"). Such messages are also *requests* and open for negotiation and compromise (e.g., "Would you be willing to ...?).

Once a couple has tried out changing the P's and D's on their own list and more positive communication skills are in place, you can ask each partner to make a list of requested changes for each other. These are essentially P's and D's from the partner's perspective. The usual approach here is not a quid pro quo where a couple agree to make certain changes if and only if the partner also makes specific changes. The problem with quid pro quo is that the whole thing can break down quickly into disagreements about whether each person is keeping his or her part of the deal. Rather, each partner unilaterally begins to make the requested changes that are acceptable. Again, the more specific and positive these requests are, the more likely they are to be successful. You can review each partner's request list and suggest modifications before the lists are shared.

CONFLICT RESOLUTION

Conflict happens naturally in every relationship. It emerges when people have different thoughts, beliefs, or preferences. What matters in a relationship is how such conflicts are resolved. The skills here involve active negotiation, rather than trying to resolve conflict through avoidance or dominance. Again, effective communication skills provide a good foundation. It can be helpful to set a specific appointment and a set amount of time (perhaps 20 minutes) to discuss a specific problem. Have the couple practice this first in your presence, with your feedback and coaching. The skills discussed above—such as making specific requests, using "I" messages, and active listening—are applicable here. Setting a specific amount of time averts the concern that the discussion will go on endlessly or escalate. It can also be useful to allow time-outs if certain signs of escalation emerge. Let them succeed with such a negotiation in your office before you make it a home assignment.

PROBLEM SOLVING

Some problems may not involve heated conflicts or desires for change, but can still cause a lot of stress when they remain unresolved (e.g., financial problems, extended family problems, legal problems). If partners disagree on desirable solutions or don't know what to do, they may avoid dealing with the problem, and so it drags on. Such unresolved problems can build up in a relationship. Here it can be useful to teach some generic problem-solving skills. The usual steps are:

1. To specifically describe the problem and desired outcome(s).
2. To brainstorm—generate as many different possible solutions as possible, without rejecting or criticizing any of them.
3. To discuss and compare the various options. What would be the likely outcomes of each possible solution?
4. To agree on a solution or at least one next step.
5. To try out the chosen solution.
6. To evaluate how the chosen solution is going and make changes as needed.

Continuing a Recovery Plan

Of course your sessions don't go on forever. Plan in advance when and how to begin stepping back to let the couple proceed on their own using their skills. You might fade sessions for a while—scheduling them farther apart. Discuss termination in advance and invite the couple to discuss remaining concerns and their plans to continue strengthening their relationship. What will each partner do specifically to support sobriety and a strong relationship? You can discuss possible high-risk situations for returning to use, and an action plan to prevent that from happening (see Chapter 19). Leave the door open for them to call back or return, and consider scheduling a follow-up appointment to check on progress.

FAMILY-INVOLVED TREATMENT FOR ADOLESCENTS

> Involving the parents or caregivers yields substantially better outcomes than treating an adolescent individually.

Involving the family in treatment is perhaps even more important for adolescents than adults. Involving the parents or caregivers yields substantially better outcomes than treating an adolescent individually (Kaminer, 2001) . The family of the adolescent can either significantly help or hinder the adolescent's engagement in treatment, and family factors such as home environment, family substance use, housing issues, and co-occurring disorders tend to have more of a profound impact on an adolescent's ability to recover from addiction (Henggeler, Melton, Brondino, & Scherer, 1997; Lawrence & Sovik-Johnston, 2010). Family-involved approaches seem to have more enduring treatment effects (Liddle, Dakof, Turner, Henderson, & Greenbaum, 2008).

Several effective family-based therapies have been developed, and represent the most thoroughly researched treatment methods for adolescent substance use. These include multisystemic therapy (MST; Henggeler, Melton, & Smith, 1992; Randall, Henggeler, Cunningham, Rowland, & Swenson, 2001), the adolescent community reinforcement approach

(A-CRA; Godley, Smith, Meyers, & Godley, 2009), brief strategic family therapy (BSFT; Robbins, Szapocznik, & Horigian, 2009; Szapocznik & Williams, 2000), multidimensional family therapy (MDFT: Liddle, Rodriguez, Dakof, Kanzki, & Marvel, 2005), and functional family therapy (FFT; Slesnick & Prestopnik, 2009; Waldron & Turner, 2008), all of which show encouraging efficacy with adolescents.

Though they have different names, these models have many similarities, and the common thread is a cognitive-behavioral family therapy approach (Kaminer, 2001). Another commonality is the integration of other services and addressing the multiple risk factors in a particular adolescent's life. In addition to reducing substance use, these approaches also have reduced long-term rates of rearrest and out-of-home placement for violent and chronic juvenile offenders (Henggeler, Schoenwald, Letourneau, & Edwards, 2002), reduced behavioral problems and engaged difficult families (Santisteban et al., 2003; Szapocznik, Hervis, & Schwartz, 2003), engaged runaway youth (Slesnick, Meyers, Mead, & Segelken, 2000; Slesnick & Prestopnik, 2009), and increased positive peer relations and improved relationship and communication between parent and adolescent (Liddle, Rowe, Dakof, Henderson, & Greenbaum, 2009). These approaches also seem to work well across cultures, particularly in those that emphasize family relationships (Santisteban et al., 2003). We highlight here three integrated family-based treatment models with support for efficacy. A fourth, CRA, was described in Chapter 11, and has also been successful with adolescents.

Multisystemic Therapy

MST is a family- and community-based treatment approach originally developed to address the full spectrum of mental health needs of adolescents involved in the juvenile justice system, with the goal of reducing the frequency of out-of-home placements and incarcerations. MST is a time-limited (typically 4–6 months), very intensive therapeutic program. The MST approach is unique in that MST therapists are full-time providers with small caseloads of approximately three families and are available to those families 24 hours a day, 7 days per week. To increase the family's access to treatment, services are provided in the family's home, in a treatment agency, or wherever the family feels most comfortable. This flexible arrangement allows the provider to have multiple contacts with the family during the week, sometimes even meeting daily.

A key feature of MST is its capacity to address the multiple challenges facing children with mental health problems and their families. MST interventions are focused on the present and are behaviorally oriented, targeting specific and well-defined problems such a reducing criminal activity, delinquency, risky sexual behavior, and drug use. Although substance abuse has always been one of the behaviors addressed, MST has more recently been adapted to include the adolescent CRA with contingency management so that providers are better able to treat adolescent substance use (Godley et al., 2009; Randall et al., 2001). Urine screens, functional analyses to identify triggers and consequences of drug use, and skills training in drug refusal skills are incorporated in this approach as a way to better target substance use.

In addition to addressing risk factors such as substance use, this approach also focuses on developing protective factors to maintain therapeutic change, such as enhancing the adolescent's educational and vocational skills and developing prosocial peer relationships. Through decreasing risk factors and increasing protective factors, interventions provide safety for the family, prevent violence, offer the family easier access to needed services, and increase the likelihood that the family will stay in treatment. The parental skills training also offers parents or caregivers the capacity to manage future difficulties and maintain change. MST has particularly received attention for its success in reducing long-term rates of rearrest and out-of-home placement for violent and chronic juvenile offenders (Henggeler, Schoenwald, Rowland, & Cunningham, 2002). Training and practice of MST are carefully regulated for quality control.

Brief Strategic Family Therapy

BSFT (Robbins et al., 2009) is a manualized brief intervention (approximately 8 to 24 sessions) used to treat co-occurring adolescent behavioral problems such as aggressive and violent and oppositional behavior, associating with antisocial peers, and drug use. BSFT is problem-focused and emphasizes modifying maladaptive patterns of family interactions and ineffective communication patterns that are presumed to be directly related to the adolescent's symptoms. For instance, if an adolescent's parents are fighting, the adolescent may act out so that the parents turn their attention toward the adolescent rather than continuing to fight. In addition to these maladaptive interactions within the family, the communication between family members may also become ineffective and full of anger and animosity.

The BSFT counselor attempts to develop alliances with each family member and the family as a whole, understand family strengths and problem relationships that affect the adolescent's behavior or the ability of parental figures to correct the behavior, implement effective communication strategies to reduce the negative tone of the family members' communication with one another, and develop behavioral strategies to correct problematic family relations. Specific change strategies (such as building conflict resolution skills and providing parenting guidance and coaching) are implemented, and effective family behaviors and communication are reinforced through the use of home assignments to practice new behaviors.

Multidimensional Family Therapy

MDFT (Liddle et al., 2005) is an outpatient family-based drug abuse treatment for adolescents with substance use disorders. The underlying assumption of the MDFT approach is that adolescent drug use results from a network of developmental and environmental influences within the individual, the family, the community, and peers. The multidimensional approach therefore targets multiple pathways as a way to reduce substance use and increase prosocial behaviors. The MDFT treatment format includes individual and family sessions. Sessions are held in the clinic, home, school, or by phone with the format and components modified to suit the individual needs of the adolescent.

Similar to the other approaches we have discussed, targeted outcomes of MDFT include reducing the impact of negative risk factors as well as promoting protective processes in as many areas of the adolescent's life as possible. During individual sessions, the therapist and the adolescent work on important developmental tasks such as decision-making skills, ways to more effectively communicate thoughts or feelings, and problem-solving skills to better deal with life stressors. Objectives for the adolescent include shifting from a drug-using to a normative lifestyle as well as improved functioning in developmental domains such as positive peer relations, healthy identity formation, bonding with school, and autonomy within the parent–adolescent relationship. Parallel to the adolescent's individual therapy, the MDFT therapist also works with the parents. The parents are taught how to be more effective in their parenting approach and to differentiate between controlling and influencing their child. Objectives for parental change include improved relationship and communication between parent and adolescent and increased knowledge about parenting practices such as limit setting.

KEY POINTS

🖈 Outcomes can be significantly improved by including an SO in treatment.

🖈 There is no scientific evidence that family members of people with addiction have unique or greater personal pathology relative to the general population, though of course they do often suffer distress and negative consequences.

🖈 Behavioral couple therapy focuses on skills for supporting sobriety, communication, resolving conflicts, and building a more positive relationship.

🔖 Family involvement is particularly important in treating substance use problems of adolescents.

🔖 Effective family-involved methods include multisystemic, brief strategic, and multidimensional family therapy.

REFLECTION QUESTIONS

❓ Various views are discussed in this chapter regarding how families are involved in addiction. Which one(s) of these best reflect your own current conception?

❓ How comfortable are you with including SOs when treating addiction? What are the biggest obstacles to doing so?

❓ What experience, if any, have you had with addiction in your own family, and how do you think this may influence your own work with individuals and families?

CHAPTER 14

Mutual Help Groups

F ew areas of health are so richly supplied with peer support networks as the world of recovery from addiction. Alcoholics Anonymous (AA) alone is arguably the world's largest mutual help network for any health topic, with over two million members and 100,000 regular meetings worldwide, half of them within the United States (Alcoholics Anonymous World Services, 2008). These networks provide important resources to support recovery, with which any professional working in addiction treatment should be well acquainted.

The term "mutual help" describes these networks because they consist exclusively or primarily of people who are themselves in or seeking recovery, and they exist for the sole purpose of helping those with addictions. "Mutual help" is more accurate than "self-help" because of the importance of reciprocal support in these networks, rather than trying to go it alone. Also, within the largest of these networks, the 12-step fellowships, strong emphasis is placed on seeking help from outside oneself, as discussed below and in Chapter 21.

Mutual help groups are not "treatment" or "therapy" per se. They fall outside the context of people seeking help from an expert professional. Rather they represent either an *alternative* or an *adjunct* to formal addiction treatment. Many

> Mutual help groups are not "treatment" or "therapy."

people do seek support from mutual help networks without ever entering professional treatment. It is furthermore the case that within the United States, a large minority if not a majority of those in treatment have been or will be at least exposed to one or more mutual help groups. In many areas, mutual help groups are available free of charge 7 days a week, with growing presence on the Internet. This alone warrants familiarity with mutual help resources in your area.

Strong preconceptions about mutual help groups have been fairly common among addiction professionals. Some have described AA in superlative terms, for example, as "medicine's crowning glory" (Martin, 1980) and "the only continuing and successful group dealing with alcoholism.... In comparison with other therapies, its success rate is nearly miraculous" (Madsen, 1974, pp. 156, 195). Others have viewed mutual help groups skeptically if not cynically, believing them to be ineffective or even harmful. In our view, neither extreme view is warranted. The large scientific literature on mutual help groups, particularly AA, described later in this chapter provides ample reason for professionals to be interested in and knowledgeable about these groups as an important resource for promoting and supporting recovery.

THE SPECTRUM OF MUTUAL HELP GROUPS

There is a wide array of mutual help groups covering a range of addictive behaviors including alcohol and other drug use, gambling, overeating, and compulsive sexual behavior. They also vary widely in conceptions of the causes of and remedies for addiction. What all of these varied groups share is the central idea of afflicted people helping each other to recover.

One way to conceptualize these groups is according to certain dimensions along which they differ (Humphreys, 1993; Nowinski, 1999). Here are a few:

• One obvious distinction is the addictive behavior on which they focus. Some are designed primarily or exclusively for people with a particular form of addiction—for example, gambling, alcohol problems, or cocaine dependence. Others span a range of addictions.

• Mutual help groups differ to the extent that they use trained leaders. Some groups, such as SMART and Women for Sobriety, use trained volunteer leaders to convey program content, whereas 12-step programs prohibit the use of trained or paid facilitators.

• Most groups are for people with addiction themselves. Others such as Al-Anon and Alateen are for family members and SOs affected by a loved one's addiction.

• Mutual help groups differ to the extent that they rely on spiritual beliefs and practices as useful in overcoming addictions. Twelve-step programs are explicitly spiritual in nature, whereas other programs such as the

Secular Organizations for Sobriety (SOS) were developed specifically for people who are uncomfortable with or skeptical of spiritual approaches.

• Groups differ in the extent to which they promote long-term connection among members. SMART meetings, for example, are not intended to be long-term support groups and are more like classes. Participants are not expected to continue in them once the core curriculum has been covered. In contrast, 12-step programs encourage lifelong membership, sometimes with the belief that a member who is not attending regularly is at risk to return to substance use.

• Mutual help groups also differ in their emphasis on ego deflation versus self-enhancement. The 12-step programs value humility, surrendering self-control, accepting one's powerlessness, and admitting and addressing character flaws. Other groups such as Women for Sobriety emphasize empowerment, self-confidence, and personal competence. There is an interesting theological parallel here. Traditional Protestant religion in which the 12-step programs are rooted emphasizes sin, confession, repentance, humility, and salvation through grace rather than one's own merit. Feminist theology has explored whether this emphasis on ego deflation is more appropriate for males, whereas women, who have historically been more powerless and self-denying, may be more in need of empowerment (Ruether, 1998).

• Finally, mutual help groups differ in their emphasis on abstinence. Most such groups, including all 12-step groups, regard total and lifelong abstinence as the only acceptable goal for change. Moderation Management (MM) was developed for less dependent problem drinkers who want to reduce their alcohol use.

12-STEP GROUPS

By far, the largest and most popular mutual help groups for addictions are those based on the 12 steps of AA. Within the United States, nearly one in every 10 people will attend an AA meeting during the course of their lifetimes (Room & Greenfield, 1993). By the time Americans with alcohol problems enter professional treatment, a majority of them have already attended AA (Tonigan, Connors, & Miller, 1996). Beyond AA itself, there are dozens of other mutual help groups patterned after AA and based on the 12 steps including Narcotics Anonymous, Cocaine Anonymous, and Gamblers Anonymous.

In understanding the 12-step groups, a distinction must be made between the 12-step *program* and *fellowship*. The program encompasses the written beliefs and practices of the organization, usually referred to as the 12 steps and the 12 traditions. The 12 steps (see Chapter 21) are meant to be worked on sequentially and involve spiritual processes such as asking God for help, practicing prayer and meditation, making amends, and performing service to others. The 12-step program explicitly involves inviting and relying on a spiritual higher power to provide the strength and wisdom needed to sustain sobriety. Although the understanding of God or a higher power is left to the individual and is intentionally flexible so as to avoid unnecessarily alienating potential members, it is clear that the founders of AA intended a personal relationship with a transcendent presence (Kurtz, 1991). The 12-step program is meant to be practiced not only in regard to addiction, but "in all our affairs" as a more general approach for living.

In addition to the formal program just described, 12-step organizations also offer a more informal fellowship, which can be described as the pattern of interactions among members that involves sharing of joys and hardships, helping out when others are in need, and enjoying social events together. Members are encouraged to have a sponsor, a mentor who has longer experience with sobriety and the program, to help them in progressing through the steps and to provide encouragement and support, particularly at times of risk for return to substance use. People at meetings often exchange phone numbers and other contact information to extend mutual support beyond the meetings themselves. In addition to meetings, AA and other 12-step programs operate 24-hour telephone coverage through local service centers in many areas. In larger cities, meetings are typically available 7 days a week, morning, afternoon, and evening, and are always free of charge. Members traveling to other cities, states, or nations can usually find a 12-step meeting nearby where they are warmly welcomed.

Twelve-step meetings typically last about 1 hour and may be either open or closed. Open meetings can be attended by anyone, but closed meetings are restricted to members—that is, anyone with a desire to stop their own addictive behavior. The format of the meeting may be one in which the formal program is reviewed (step meeting), or might be devoted to hearing the experiences of one person's struggle with an addiction (speaker meeting), or could involve discussion of particular problems likely to be encountered in recovering from addictions (discussion meeting). Finally, some 12-step groups are geared toward particular demographic groups such as women, adolescents, medical professionals, gays and lesbians, atheists and agnostics.

Some Common Myths about 12-Step Groups

There are some common misconceptions about AA and other 12-step groups that warrant consideration here. Certainly the way the 12-step program is practiced varies across groups and individual members. This sometimes gives rise to anecdotes that can be incorrectly generalized to stereotypes about the 12-step program or fellowship.

1. *AA believes only in a traditional disease model and discourages people from receiving any other kind of treatment. This position will contradict what I am doing in treatment and confuse my clients.* In fact, AA has no official position with regard to the etiology of alcohol problems, and by policy it does not get involved in controversies. Twelve-step literature describes a broad range of possible factors contributing to addiction including biological, psychological, social, and spiritual factors. Occasional points of philosophical disagreement in AA meetings can be addressed by urging clients to learn all they can with an open mind and choose what helps them, consistent with the AA advice to "take what works and leave the rest." In a 10-year follow-up of Project MATCH (Tonigan, 2003), clients who were most likely to be attending 12-step meetings were not those who had been given 12-step facilitation, but rather those in cognitive-behavioral and motivational enhancement conditions. Whatever advice we or others may give to people, they actively seek what seems appropriate to them.

2. *People are pressured to discontinue their medications if they attend 12-step meetings.* Although injunctions against psychoactive medications are sometimes expressed by individual members in 12-step meetings (Rychtarik, Connors, Dermen, & Stasiewicz, 2000), such a prohibition is not supported by the core 12-step literature. Tonigan (2003) found that despite what they might hear in meetings, 12-step attendees as a whole were *less* likely to endorse abstinence from medications for emotional problems than were clients in other forms of treatment. Thus, attending 12-step meetings is not incompatible with taking prescribed psychiatric medications, nor is there evidence that attendance has any detrimental effect on clients' attitudes toward doing so (Tonigan & Kelly, 2004).

3. *The 12-step program only works for religious clients. It won't help nonreligious people, even if they can be persuaded to attend.* Actually, people's religious beliefs do not predict whether they benefit from 12-step programs (Connors, Tonigan, & Miller, 2001). The "Big Book" of AA directly addresses atheists (Alcoholics Anonymous, 1976), and although agnostics and atheists are less inclined to attend AA, they are no less likely to benefit when they do (Tonigan, Miller, & Schermer, 2002). Clients who benefit from 12-step programs do tend to show changes in their spiritual beliefs and practices over time (Robinson, Cranford, Webb, & Brower, 2007).

4. *Clients who participate in 12-step programs are told that only someone who is in recovery can be an effective therapist for them.* Again, individual members may offer this opinion, but official AA literature does not support this view. While the unique perspectives of other recovering people are among the benefits of attending 12-step meetings, many studies confirm that personal recovery status makes one neither more nor less effective as a therapist, even when delivering 12-step facilitation therapy (Project MATCH Research Group, 1998d).

5. *Pressuring my clients to go to 12-step meetings can't hurt, even if they don't want to go.* Pressuring people into 12-step programs is unwise, particularly if clients express strong resistance or philosophical objection (Humphreys, 1993; Peteet, 1993; Tonigan et al., 2002). Coercing clients to attend 12-step meetings despite objections to religious content may even violate codes of professional ethics. AA has always been meant to be a voluntary association, and the few clinical trials of coerced AA attendance have shown no differential benefit (Brandsma, Maultsby, & Welsh, 1980; Ditman, Crawford, Forgy, Moskowitz, & MacAndrew, 1967; Walsh et al., 1991). We concur with Glaser's (1993) admonition to clinicians treating alcohol dependence that clients should be encouraged to try AA but no one should be required to do so. As discussed later in this chapter, a variety of other groups are available, and it is also the case that mutual help groups are not for everyone.

6. *There is no scientific evidence that AA actually helps people.* To the contrary, there is a very large research literature on AA that generally shows a positive association between attendance and better outcomes. Less is known scientifically about other 12-step programs besides AA. We turn now to a brief consideration of this research.

Research on 12-Step Groups

Many studies have examined the relationship between sobriety and 12-step group attendance. These studies are necessarily correlational, evaluating the extent to which these two factors—attendance and outcome—covary, without establishing whether one causes the other. The usual finding across this body of research is a modest inverse relationship: attending more 12-step meetings is associated with lower levels of addictive behavior in the same or subsequent periods of time. The largest number of studies pertains to AA and drinking outcomes. Across several decades of research, in both older (Emrick, Tonigan, Montgomery, & Little, 1993) and more recent studies, very frequent AA attendance predicts higher rates of abstinence in the first year (Fortney, Booth, Zhang, Humphrey, & Wiseman, 1998; Johnson & Herringer, 1993; Tonigan, 2001), 3 years after treatment (Chi, Kaskutas,

Sterling, Campbell, & Weisner, 2009; Kelly, Stout, Zywiak, & Schneider, 2006), and 5 years or longer after treatment (Gossop, Stewart, & Marsden, 2007; Moos & Moos, 2006). Taking these relational analyses one step farther, longitudinal studies have found that AA attendance predicts subsequent abstinence, whereas abstinence does not predict subsequent AA attendance (McCrady, Epstein, & Kahler, 2004; McKellar, Stewart, & Humphreys, 2003). This sequence is consistent with a positive influence of AA participation on treatment outcome. AA attendance also predicts long-term sobriety apart from treatment (Moos & Moos, 2005; Timko, Moos, Finney, & Lesar, 2000). Furthermore, participation in AA predicts changes in spirituality, which in turn accounts in part for the impact of AA on outcome (Kelly, Stout, Magill, Tonigan, & Pagano, 2011). Finally, clients who do receive formal treatment on the whole tend to have better outcomes when they also attend AA (Dawson et al., 2006; McCrady et al., 2004; Timko et al., 2000). In sum, there is ample reason to encourage people in treatment for alcohol dependence to also try AA. Studies are fewer regarding 12-step attendance and subsequent illicit drug use or gambling, but findings are generally similar to those for alcohol (Christo & Franey, 1995; Gossop et al., 2007; McKay, Alterman, McLellan, & Snider, 1994; Toumbourou, Hamilton, U'Ren, Stevens-Jones, & Storey, 2002).

It is not simply the number of meetings attended that predicts benefit from 12-step programs. A broader concept is *involvement* in the 12-step program and fellowship. An analysis of multiple studies of AA found that reaching out to others for help, having a sponsor, and working through the first four steps of AA were significant positive predictors of benefit (Tonigan & Rice, 2010). One study found that AA attendance per se did not predict posttreatment abstinence, whereas AA involvement did (Montgomery, Miller, & Tonigan, 1995). Attendance is modestly correlated with other 12-step practices such as prayer and reading core literature (Morgenstern, Kahler, Frey, & Lavouvie, 1996; Toumbourou et al., 2002).

> It is not simply the number of meetings attended that predicts benefit from 12-step programs.

Are there particular kinds of clients who are more likely to benefit from a 12-step group? One clear finding is that AA is especially beneficial for people whose social networks do not support abstinence (Longabaugh et al., 1998; Toumbourou et al., 2002). In essence, it provides something that such clients need but are lacking: an instant social support network that is rooting for their sobriety.

In sum, there is good reason to encourage substance-dependent clients, whether religious or not, to sample 12-step meetings. As stated earlier, we do not think that anyone should be required or coerced to attend, but there is good reason to expect that such mutual help groups may improve clients' chances for stable sobriety.

FACILITATING MUTUAL HELP GROUP ATTENDANCE

It makes a difference whether and how you encourage clients to sample mutual-help groups. Here are a few things to keep in mind in this regard.

1. People are most likely to try out mutual help groups while they are still in treatment, if they are not already involved in one. Said another way, if you don't encourage clients to sample mutual help groups while they are in treatment, they are not very likely to do so afterward (Tonigan et al., 2003). The period of active treatment is a window of opportunity to encourage mutual help involvement.

> If you don't encourage clients to sample mutual help groups while they are in treatment, they are not very likely to do so afterward.

2. Mutual help groups vary widely, so that it makes sense to sample several rather than just one. Even within AA, there are large differences in the social environment from one group to another (Montgomery, Miller, & Tonigan, 1993). You can't know what AA is like just by going to one meeting, any more than you know what churches are like by attending one service, or colleges by attending one class. There is a natural process over time of finding a "home group," the place where one feels most comfortable, supported, and at home.

3. Similarly, don't just try once to encourage mutual help involvement and then give up. One practice guideline is a "three strikes" approach, in which clients who initially decline a referral to a mutual help group are asked if they would be willing to revisit the issue further along in treatment (Miller, 2004). As the name implies, the counselor is advised to try three times to refer to a mutual help group. This should be done, of course, in a way that does not engender client resistance (see Chapter 16).

4. If you want people to try out a mutual help group, do more than just provide information. The largest treatment effect ever reported in the alcohol literature involved procedures for encouraging clients to attend AA (Sisson & Mallams, 1981). Half of all clients in this study (randomly assigned) were advised to attend AA and given a list of the local meeting places and times. The other half were given the following systematic encouragement procedure. The counselor had prearranged help from volunteers who were themselves AA members. While the client was still in the office, the counselor (with the client's permission) telephoned one of these volunteers and then gave the phone to the client. The volunteer introduced himself, offered to accompany the client to a first meeting and provide transportation, and arranged a meeting time. In the advice group, no one actually attended an AA meeting. In the systematic encouragement group, everyone got to a first meeting.

What should you tell people to expect when attending 12-step meetings? First and foremost, explain that people often do benefit from attending, even if they don't agree with every aspect of the program. For example, as mentioned earlier, atheists and agnostics who go to AA show just as much benefit as theists do. Explain the strong emphasis in AA on personal choice, to "take what works and leave the rest," and that the only requirement for membership is a sincere desire to abstain. The program does not encourage hostile confrontation or "cross-talk" (uninvited advice or arguments), and participants are not required to speak or disclose personal information.

Even for those who try AA, many do not stay with it in the long run. In the Project MATCH study, for example, 95% of those in 12-step facilitation did attend AA during treatment, but 41% of these were no longer doing so at 9 months (Tonigan et al., 2003). Very similar findings were reported in another study with 2,778 men treated in 12-step-oriented programs (Kelly & Moos, 2003), of whom 91% attended at least one meeting. Of these attenders, 40% were no longer attending after 1 year. Longitudinal research, however, shows that dropping out of AA (not regularly attending) is not the same as disaffiliation. Some prior AA attenders nevertheless still describe themselves as AA members and report that they continue to live the 12-step program. This suggests that some people may internalize the 12-step program and continue to practice it, even though not regularly attending meetings.

Clients with concomitant addiction and major mental disorders offer a special challenge (see Chapter 18). For some, groups may be particularly intimidating or rejecting because of their psychological problems. In many areas there are mutual help or professionally facilitated support groups especially for people with dual diagnoses (e.g., "double trouble" 12-step groups). Approach referral to such groups with cautious optimism, and of course use your clinical judgment.

12-STEP TREATMENTS

What you do during treatment makes a difference in whether people will attend and affiliate with a mutual help group. Some professionals and programs describe themselves as 12-step-oriented, which can have a variety of meanings. Many encourage clients to become involved in the fellowship and practice the 12-step program. The design for Project MATCH included developing and formally testing a 12-session outpatient 12-step facilitation (TSF) treatment approach to parallel what was then the most commonly reported American program philosophy. TSF is delivered by a professional counselor and is designed to help clients find, attend, and become comfortable and involved in AA meetings. It reviews core 12-step beliefs and literature, discusses etiquette for meetings, helps clients know what to expect at AA, and encourages them to sample a variety of meetings. The therapist's primary goal is to help the client become engaged and involved in AA as a long-term recovery program (Nowinski & Baker, 1998; Nowinski et al., 1992).

It is fair to say that none of the nine principal investigators in Project MATCH was an ardent promoter of TSF. All had previously worked with behavior therapies. The study was very carefully executed, and all three treatments were delivered by therapists who were trained and believed in the approach they were delivering. TSF was designed and supervised by professionals who were highly knowledgeable and enthusiastic about a 12-step approach (Nowinski & Baker, 1998; Nowinski et al., 1992). A total of 1,726 clients were randomly assigned to receive TSF, CBT, or MET. As discussed in Chapter 7, all three treatments yielded excellent and similar results on the two primary outcome measures, with no significant differences between them (Project MATCH Research Group, 1997a, 1998b).

> In the percentage of clients who were totally abstinent, the 12-step treatment maintained a significant advantage.

On an outcome measure of most interest to AA, however—the percentage of clients who were totally abstinent—the 12-step treatment maintained a significant advantage of about 10 percentage points throughout the course of follow-up. Thus this methodologically strong clinical trial indicates that TSF was at least as effective as the two state-of-the-art treatments with which it was compared.

Further evidence emerged from a large naturalistic study examining outcomes for 3,698 men treated for alcohol problems at 15 U.S. Veterans Administration hospitals (Ouimette, Finney, & Moos, 1997). The programs in which they had been treated were classified as 12-step, cognitive-behavioral, or mixed (both) in orientation (five of each type). As in Project MATCH, overall outcomes were very good, with significant improvement on all 11 measures. At 1-year follow-up, 25% of those treated in 12-step programs were abstinent, compared with 18% in cognitive-behavioral programs and 20% in mixed programs, a statistically significant difference. Those receiving 12-step treatment also showed significantly lower health care utilization in the year after discharge (Humphreys & Moos, 2001).

Similar findings were reported in a clinical trial comparing group therapies for cocaine abuse based on a cognitive-behavioral or a 12-step approach (Wells, Peterson, Gainey, Hawkins, & Catalano, 1994). Clients were assigned in order of admission to one group until it was filled, then the next clients were assigned to the other condition. Both groups showed substantial improvement, with no between-group differences in outcome at 6 or 12 months on cocaine, marijuana, or alcohol use. In a Ukrainian randomized trial, adding 12-step oriented outpatient treatment to detoxification (vs. no additional treatment) substantially reduced posttreatment drinking (Vlasova et al., 2011).

Treatments delivered in these studies involved far more than simple referral to attend AA. Such referral without systematic encouragement in some form is unlikely to be sufficient to help clients attend and benefit from mutual-help groups.

BOX 14,1. Personal Reflection: Learning about AA

In the 1970s when I entered the field of addiction treatment, there was a polemical battle raging. In one corner were the "traditionalists" who generally endorsed a disease model of the etiology of alcoholism, regarded lifelong abstinence as the only acceptable treatment goal, and lauded AA as the golden road to recovery. In the opposite corner were the "revisionists" who typically regarded drinking as behavior subject to the same rules of learning as any other response, touted "controlled drinking" as a treatment goal option, and demeaned AA as outdated, unscientific mumbo-jumbo (Maltzman, 2008). We seldom met in the same venue. Each camp had its own professional meetings at which to despise and denounce the other. I was professionally born and raised in the behavioral camp and dismissed AA without investigation. One traditionalist averred in print that concerned colleagues ought to do "an intervention" to shake people like me out of our denial.

It didn't happen, but over time I did have the good fortune to meet and work with bright and compassionate colleagues who introduced me to the world of Bill W. I am grateful to my friend Ernie Kurtz for his patient conversations with me. When we collaborated to publish an article about AA (Miller & Kurtz, 1994), *both* of us had colleagues asking us incredulously, "What on earth are you doing working with *him*?" I went to AA meetings, felt the heart in them, and began reading in earnest not only the AA literature but also the voluminous research about AA. With Barbara McCrady I organized a scientific conference on AA research (McCrady & Miller, 1993), and we visited the home office of AA in New York together. For two decades I also had the privilege of collaborating with my friend and colleague Dr. Scott Tonigan to do and foster AA research.

Bill W. (W. W., 1949) welcomed collaboration with clinical professionals and encouraged AA members to participate in research (Alcoholics Anonymous General Service Office, 2002). The more I read his gentle writings about how to work with others, the more it sounds to me like motivational interviewing, and so different from the in-your-face confrontational methods that have sometimes been practiced and promulgated in the name of "12-step" treatment. I will never have an insider's understanding of alcoholism or AA, but I have come to a heartfelt appreciation of the breadth and depth of AA, and its untiring ministry to those who continue to suffer. In this sense, I became a friend of Bill W.

—W. R. M.

RELIGIOUS MUTUAL HELP GROUPS

Because 12-step programs are described as "spiritual but not religious" and are nondenominational, avoiding dogmatic faith statements, members of religious faith communities sometimes prefer recovery programs that are specifically consistent with their own religious beliefs. Both Overcomers Outreach (OO; *overcomersoutreach.org*) and Alcoholics Victorious (AV; *www.alcoholicsvictorious.org/av-faq.html*) are mutual support groups that bridge 12-step philosophy and biblical teachings. OO meetings are held in churches and may focus on many problems including use of pornography, gambling, depression, and substance use. Meetings are open, and current religious faith is not a requirement to attend, although meetings are explicitly focused on encouraging devotion to Jesus Christ as the higher power and biblical teachings as a means of overcoming addiction. AV meetings are more specifically focused on alcohol/drug problems. Similarly, the Calix Society (*www.calixsociety.org*) was founded in 1947 to provide Catholics with a faith-consistent mutual support group to augment the 12-step program. Meetings are typically facilitated by priests who assist members in using the 12 steps in a manner that is consonant with Catholic teachings (Nowinski, 1999). Searching the Web readily yields resources adapting the 12 steps to many other faiths including Buddhism, Judaism, Mormonism, and Islam. We are aware of no scientific studies of the effectiveness of these religiously based mutual help groups.

SECULAR MUTUAL HELP GROUPS

In contrast, some people find 12-step programs to be *too* "religious" (e.g., Copeland, 1997). All of the organizations described in this section were developed in part as a secular alternative to the 12-step programs for people who for whatever reason find that a 12-step approach doesn't fit or work for them. Some of these groups are more widely available than others. All of them maintain a website, some of which include online chat rooms. What all of them have in common, as of this writing, is the absence of scientific evidence of efficacy (Humphreys et al., 2004). We describe them in alphabetical order.

Moderation Management

Moderation management (MM) is the only alcohol mutual help organization that targets nondependent problem drinkers and considers moderation as an option (Kishline, 1994). It was developed specifically for people who do not have lifelong abstinence as a personal goal, but who want to reduce their drinking to a problem-free level. The program begins with 30 days of abstinence, a procedure originally tested by Sanchez-Craig (1980, 1996; Sanchez-Craig, Davila, & Cooper, 1996) to break habitual drinking patterns in preparation for moderation. The guidelines essentially follow behavioral methods for self-management of drinking (Hester, 2003; Hester & Delaney, 1997). MM provides services both in face-to-face and online formats.

The introduction of MM triggered impassioned controversy in the 1990s (Humphreys, 2003), renewing long-standing debates over abstinence and moderation goals (Fingarette, 1988; Heather & Robertson, 1984) and more recently harm reduction (Klaw, Horst, & Humphreys, 2006; Miller, 2008a). Media attention was fueled when in 2000 the founder of MM, Audrey Kishline, opted for abstinence, resigned from MM, joined AA and 2 months later drove while intoxicated, causing a tragic car crash in Washington that killed two people and resulted in her imprisonment. Pundits variously blamed either AA or MM for what Ms. Kishline acknowledged to be her personal responsibility (Kishline & Maloy, 2007).

Research to date indicates that MM does indeed tend to engage low-dependence problem drinkers, particularly women and youth, who are disinclined to seek treatment or accept a lifelong abstinence goal (Humphreys, 2003; Humphreys & Klaw, 2001), although this may be shifting over time (Kosok, 2006). This low-dependence group is precisely the subpopulation who are more likely to sustain moderation than abstinence (see Chapter 23). In this sense, MM appears to attract a relatively underserved population most of whom have never been treated for alcohol problems, though most had previously attended AA (Humphreys & Klaw, 2001).

Very little is known about the outcomes of people who participate in MM. Most professionals would discourage more severely dependent drinkers from trying MM. The MM website (*www.moderation.org*) is more permissive in this regard, leaving the choice to the individual (where, of course, it does reside), but does indicate that moderation is more feasible for people with less severe problems. Indeed, a series of studies of moderation-oriented treatment identified a level of dependence above which no one had succeeded in maintaining problem-free moderation* (Miller, Leckman, Delaney, & Tinkcom, 1992; Miller & Muñoz, 2005). Those with less severe problems and dependence were most likely to establish stable moderation. Many who tried moderation and found it difficult tended ultimately to abstain and said that the experience of trying moderation had helped convince them of the necessity of abstention (Miller, Leckman, et al., 1992). *Alcoholics Anonymous* (Alcoholics Anonymous, 1976) describes failure at

---

*In these studies, moderation was defined as averaging less than three standard drinks per day, with blood alcohol peaks below .08%, with no evidence of problems or dependence symptoms related to current drinking, by consensus of two interviewers (a psychologist and a psychiatrist) who evaluated each person independently.

moderation as one way in which people realize their alcoholism, and clearly recognizes the difference from problem drinkers who can moderate their drinking (Humphreys, 2003). Interestingly, in studies of treatment with a moderation goal, abstinence outcomes were not limited to those who tried moderation and failed. More-dependent people who ultimately abstained often simply had found moderation not worth the white-knuckle effort that it required of them!

Secular Organizations for Sobriety

As of 2004, Secular Organizations for Sobriety (SOS) was estimated to be the largest non-12-step mutual help group in the United States, albeit with still less than 1% of the membership of AA (Humphreys et al., 2004). SOS was founded in 1986 by James Christopher to provide a secular humanist alternative to the spiritual focus of the 12-step program. The practice of SOS groups is similar to 12-step groups in the focus on mutual support and pragmatic, healthy interpersonal interactions, but the SOS program specifically separates the concept of sobriety from spirituality. Distinctly secular-humanist, SOS encourages mutual support for members as well as the use of science-based methods for achieving abstinence. The objectives of SOS (Connors & Dermen, 1996) focus on peer support for abstinence and providing a safe atmosphere for individuals to share experiences related to sobriety while avoiding religious practices. Information about SOS meetings and philosophy can be found at *www.cfiwest.org/sos/brochures/overview.htm*.

Self-Management and Recovery Training

Self-management and recovery training (SMART) is a secular nonprofit organization that offers both face-to-face and online meetings teaching rational-emotive (Ellis & Velten, 1992) and cognitive-behavioral coping skills, as well as a web chat room format (*www.smartrecovery.org*). SMART-trained volunteer facilitators lead the meetings, focusing on practical coping skills such as problem solving, refuting irrational beliefs, and responding to urges as methods for achieving and maintaining abstinence. Meetings are free of charge, although as in 12-step meetings a freewill collection may be taken. Meetings are open to the public unless specifically announced as closed meetings, and walk-ins are welcome.

SMART incorporates a range of evidence-based behavioral treatment and self-management strategies (Horvath, 2000). A comparison of participants in SMART groups with AA participants found, not surprisingly, that the former were less spiritually oriented and perceived greater personal control over their alcohol use.

The historic roots of SMART lie in an organization known as Rational Recovery (RR), founded in 1986 by a social worker named Jack Trimpey. During its first decade, RR groups met with both educational and mutual help purposes. In 1999, however, Trimpey ordered the disbanding of all RR group meetings, summarily denouncing mutual help groups, spiritual approaches, and professional treatment as routes to recovery. A court battle led to a parting of ways, with SMART breaking off from RR (which remains aa for-profit organization offering classes and online services; Trimpey, Velten, & Dain, 1993). A caution regarding RR is that, given its program philosophy (*www.rational.org*), RR participants are likely to be encouraged to shun both professional treatment and mutual help groups. This is not true of SMART, which publicly supports evidence-based treatment methods.

Evidence for the effectiveness of SMART is sparse, with no controlled studies to date. One study followed 433 individuals attending RR groups before the mutual help format of RR was disbanded, thus providing a plausible proxy for SMART groups (Galanter, Egelko, & Edwards, 1993). In general, longer and more consistent group attendance was associated with longer self-reported abstinence from alcohol but not cocaine. A small pilot study assessed 20 participants in an RR group before and after the class. Significant reduction in substance use was reported, and questionnaire scores indicated increased openness to admitting substance use problems (Schmidt, Carns, & Chandler, 2001).

Women for Sobriety

Much has been written about the particular needs of women who attempt to recover from addictions (Beckman & Amarno, 1986; Finkelstein & Mora, 2009; Kaskutas, 1994; Lisansky, 1999), especially when treatment involves mixed-gender groups. Women in mixed groups may feel more stigmatized than men about their drinking and the reasons for it, especially if there are feelings of inadequacy in fulfilling gender roles (Wilsnack, 1973) or a history of sexual abuse (Beckman, 1993; Simpson & Miller, 2002). Women for Sobriety (WFS) is intended to be an alternative recovery program for women, which addresses addiction as a coping mechanism that women may turn to in response to problems in their relationships. The active elements of WFS involve building self-esteem; eliminating negative thinking and guilt; and encouraging competence, self-actualization, and personal responsibility for recovery. Women are regarded as having a special need for cultivating self-acceptance that cannot be accomplished readily in mixed-gender groups, including AA. Founded by Jean Kirkpatrick (1999), WFS is an abstinence-based, nonspiritual program with meetings facilitated by trained volunteer moderators.

In a survey of WFS programs, Kaskustas (1994, 1996) found that women who affiliate with WFS do so for reasons other than simply achieving or sustaining abstinence. For example, of 600 respondents, 60% of women stated that they would be able to remain abstinent without attending WFS, indicating that women are finding some benefit to meetings above and beyond the need for sobriety (Kaskutas, 1994). The main reasons women gave for attending WFS in this survey focused on gaining support from other women, the positive and self-enhancing focus of the program philosophy, the unique benefits of an all-woman milieu (including cross-generational sharing and strong female role models), and the safety of the environment (including an absence of religious themes). Some WFS participants stated that they did not attend AA because they felt they didn't fit in, found AA too negative and male-oriented, and did not like discussion of God or spiritual themes. However, consistent with the WFS philosophy that AA and WFS programs can be complementary, nearly a third of the women in this survey reported attending *both* AA and WFS meetings. Despite the apparent contradiction in program philosophy along the ego deflation versus self-enhancement continuum, these women reported that AA offered an appealing program, as well as the opportunity to enjoy friends and fellowship, avoid drinking, and take advantage of the wide availability of AA meetings. Of those attending both, only 21% gave coercion as a reason for attending AA.

In summary, if a WFS group is available in your area, consider WFS as a mutual help group referral for female clients, especially those who might be uncomfortable in mixed-gender groups or who do not wish to discuss spiritual themes as part of their recovery. Locations of groups and more information about WFS can be found at *www.womenforsobriety.org*.

PRACTICAL CONSIDERATIONS FOR CLINICIANS

As indicated earlier, the best window of opportunity for getting a client engaged in a mutual help group is *during* treatment. This is the time to be proactive in encouraging people who are unfamiliar with or disengaged from mutual help groups to try them out (again).

You can be more clear and credible if you are yourself familiar and comfortable with the resources available. A first step is to find out what mutual help groups are in your service area or online. Most such groups welcome professional visitors who want to learn and make referrals, unless they are explicitly closed (some 12-step) or specialized meetings (e.g., women only in WFS). Have a cancellation? Try out chat rooms on mutual help websites to which you might refer clients. Find out where and when face-to-face groups meet in your area and keep a schedule or website links handy. Some groups also have literature or fliers that you can keep in your office to distribute. If you are in a larger city, the local AA service office can often informally advise you by phone about meetings that could be a good match for a particular kind of client.

> COUNSELOR: I have a client I'd like to get to an AA group. She's a middle-aged professional, divorced, kind of shy, no prior AA, and pretty skittish about religion, so a church might not be the best meeting place for her to start. Have any suggestions?
>
> AA PHONE VOLUNTEER: Why don't you suggest the noon brown-bag discussion meeting tomorrow over at the university? They're really friendly, there are some professional women who've got years of solid sobriety, and they're great with newcomers. There's also a step meeting that's good for newcomers, every Tuesday and Thursday night at 7:00 at the Serenity Club downtown. Do you know where that is?

In accord with the systematic encouragement procedures described earlier in this chapter, it's great if you can find some longer term participants who would be willing to talk with newcomers and accompany them to a meeting. In general, a same-gender match is advisable.

Also prepare your client in advance to not generalize from first impressions. It is common for people to shop around among meetings, which can be very different from each other, before finding a group that suits them. Groups differ not only in content and format, but also in their interpersonal atmosphere on dimensions such as warmth, cohesiveness, expressiveness, and aggression (Montgomery et al., 1993; Tonigan, Ashcroft, & Miller, 1995).

If you are in recovery yourself, should you share this information with a client? In the addiction treatment field it is quite common to do so, but professionals do vary in their preferences on whether, when, and how to do this. Conventional wisdom is that it's unwise to refer your client(s) to your own home group, although of course you can't prohibit them from attending if they happen in. If that should occur, it is best to offer a friendly greeting but not call the person by name or reveal that you have a professional relationship. Then discuss the situation at your next session—privately if it is a group session.

KEY POINTS

📌 Involvement in the 12-step program of AA is consistently correlated with abstinence from alcohol. Less is known about other mutual help groups.

- People are most likely to try mutual help groups if encouraged to do so during treatment.

- TSF therapy (which involves far more than encouraging people to attend) has been found to be at least as effective as other evidence-based treatment methods.

- A variety of both religious and secular mutual help groups have been developed.

- Groups vary widely in structure, content, and social climate, so that clients are well advised to investigate several before deciding whether and which to attend.

REFLECTION QUESTIONS

What do you know about mutual help groups that are available in your community or the Internet? Which have you visited and what was your experience?

Of the common myths about 12-step groups discussed in this chapter, which (if any) have you found to be most prevalent among your professional colleagues?

What (if anything) surprised you about the research findings discussed in this chapter?

CHAPTER 15

Pharmacological Adjuncts

As effective medications have been developed, pharmacotherapy has played an increasing role in the treatment of addictions. Medications can be used to manage the negative effects of withdrawal, reduce cravings and urges to drink or use drugs, and/or impede the reinforcing effects of alcohol or other drugs. They help individuals to become less preoccupied with drug use and drug seeking and to decrease impulsive drinking and drug use, which in turn increases the likelihood of maintaining a longer period of abstinence.

This chapter examines the current state and recent advances in medication development for addiction problems. We emphasize in particular how medications can be used as part of addiction treatment to address various symptoms and problems. Behavioral and pharmacological treatments can be combined in productive ways, and we examine the evidence for the efficacy of various types of medication.

MEDICATIONS FOR WITHDRAWAL AND MAINTENANCE

People with severe physical dependence may need medications to reduce the aversive effects of stopping or reducing their use of alcohol and other drugs. As is true more generally in addiction treatment, medication to manage withdrawal is only a first step, one part of the stabilization process (see Chapter 7), and should be accompanied by behavioral interventions to enhance motivation and skills to avoid a return to substance use (Barber & O'Brien, 1999).

Medications that attenuate withdrawal tend to be longer acting *agonists*, those that have similar effects to the primary problem drug. For this reason, they can be used not only for detoxification, but as substitution drugs. Thus these medications can be used as a replacement drug for immediate detoxification (Chapter 6), for gradual tapering over time, or for long-term maintenance (Chapter 19).

Nicotine Substitution

Tobacco use and nicotine dependence are disproportionately high among people with other substance use disorders. Historically, addiction treatment programs often tolerated cigarette smoking, but social trends toward smoke-free environments have increased pressure to ban smoking in most treatment programs as well. Concerns that smoke-free facilities (or efforts to treat nicotine dependence more generally) might compromise the efficacy of treatment proved to be unwarranted. To the contrary, smoking cessation can facilitate abstinence from alcohol and other drugs (Bobo, McIlvain, Lando, Walker, & Leed-Kelly, 1998). Successful abstinence from alcohol or other drugs, however, does not address nicotine dependence; tobacco use needs to be addressed specifically and is obviously relevant to clients' long-term health and survival. Among smokers who are in recovery from other substance use disorders, tobacco is the most common cause of premature death and disability.

> Smoking cessation can facilitate abstinence from alcohol and other drugs.

Most effective approaches for smoking cessation involve some form of nicotine substitution such as nicotine patches or chewing gum (Lancaster, Stead, Silagy, Sowden, & Group, 2000). Here the drug that is being "substituted" is the same one that is the primary addictive substance in cigarettes: nicotine. Substitution strategies are used because of the low success rate of total cold-turkey withdrawal from nicotine. Typically clients are switched to an alternate source of nicotine, and dosage is then gradually tapered over time to minimize withdrawal symptoms. Some clients, however, continue to use a nicotine substitution source such as chewing gum, at least periodically, to deal with experienced nicotine cravings. More effective programs combine nicotine substitution and tapering with behavioral interventions. The website *www.treatobacco.net* provides information for health professionals about evidence-based methods to help clients quit smoking.

An alternative strategy to nicotine substitution is a partial nicotine agonist intended to provide some of the dopamine release that is afforded by nicotine, while also blocking nicotine receptors so that nicotine itself has less positive impact. This partial agonist strategy is similar to that of buprenorphine for opioid dependence (described on pages 234 and 244). The partial nicotine agonist varenicline (trade name Chantix), while not without side effects, appears promising in early research as an aid in smoking cessation for people in recovery (Hays, Croghan, Schroeder, Ebbert, & Hurt, 2011). Dopamine agonists are also being tested as aids in abstaining from other stimulants such as methamphetamine and cocaine (Pérez-Maña, Castells, Vidal, Casas, & Capella, 2011).

Opiate Withdrawal and Maintenance Medications

Methadone Maintenance

Oral methadone is a well-known and effective replacement therapy for opiate dependence. It does prevent opiate withdrawal symptoms, but is more often used as a long-term maintenance medication than in short-term detoxification. Methadone relieves the aversive effects of opiate withdrawal (e.g., anxiety, agitation, insomnia, abdominal cramping, and diarrhea) and reduces motivation for opiate use. In addition to preventing opiate withdrawal, methadone also substantially reduces the euphoria or highs associated with opiate use (Batki, Kauffman, Marion, Parrino, & Woody, 2005).

When beginning this medication, clients are typically required to attend a methadone clinic daily to receive their dosage. This provides daily contact and the opportunity for additional evaluation, case management, and treatment services. Urine screening for illicit drug use is commonly required. When clients attend clinic reliably, are stabilized on methadone, and free from other drug use, they may be offered take-home methadone for up to 30 days, provided they continue to refrain from other drug use or criminal activity. The convenience of take-home doses serves as an incentive for continued adherence to program requirements and can alleviate problems with transportation, employment, and child care.

Buprenorphine

The development of buprenorphine (trade name Subutex) and the combination of buprenorphine plus naxolone (tradename Suboxone) provided an effective alternative to methadone for alleviating opiate withdrawal and weaning clients from opiate use. Buprenorphine offers several practical advantages over methadone. Its action is longer lasting, which means that the dosing schedule is less frequent (three times a week instead of every day; O'Malley & Kosten, 2006). Self-administration of the medication can be easily observed because buprenorphine is absorbed sublingually (under the tongue). Buprenorphine is generally considered to have a less euphoric effect as compared to methadone and therefore is less likely to be sold on the open market. In short, buprenorphine is fast becoming the treatment of choice in withdrawing clients from opiate use, whereas methadone continues to be used for long-term opiate replacement therapy.

Buprenorphine is administered in three phases: (1) induction (2) stabilization, and (3) maintenance (Batki et al., 2005). The induction phase focuses on stopping opiate use by reducing aversive effects of withdrawal such as nausea, headaches, diarrhea, and cravings. The stabilization phase focuses on eliminating withdrawal symptoms and managing any side effects. In this phase, clients are tested regularly for illicit drugs. In the maintenance phase, other treatment can be provided to address psychosocial aspects and prevent a return to illicit drug use (see Chapter 19). Buprenorphine dosage can then either be maintained or tapered down. Because withdrawal from buprenorphine is typically easier than from methadone, buprenorphine is preferable when the client's goal is to be drug-free rather than being maintained on a replacement medication.

Alcohol Withdrawal Medications

Pharmacologically assisted detoxification is unnecessary for most people with alcohol use disorders. A minority of clients in a typical treatment population have sufficiently severe alcohol dependence to require pharmacological management for safe withdrawal, and even this can in most cases be done in a medically supervised outpatient setting (see Chapter 6). The majority of alcohol clients can be successfully detoxified with mainly supportive (i.e., nonpharmacological) care. Nevertheless, severe alcohol withdrawal is a serious medical condition, with potential consequences including seizures, delirium, and death (Kosten & O'Connor, 2003).

Effective medications are available to suppress seizures and delirium as well as the discomfort of alcohol withdrawal, and their use in detoxification may also improve ultimate treatment outcome (O'Malley & Kosten, 2006). There is no evidence that allowing clients to suffer during withdrawal benefits their recovery, and of course there is a medical risk in doing so. Medications such as benzodiazepine, chlordizaepoxide, and lorazepam are effective in treating alcohol withdrawal. Other medications such as beta-adrenergic blocking drugs, anti-convulsants, and antipsychotics can also be used to alleviate withdrawal symptoms and complications.

> There is no evidence that allowing clients to suffer during withdrawal benefits their recovery.

How can you know whether medical/pharmacological management of alcohol withdrawal is likely to be needed for a particular client? The Revised Clinical Institute Withdrawal Assessment for Alcohol scale (CIWA-Ar; Sullivan et al., 1989) is the most widely used instrument for this purpose, assessing the severity of alcohol withdrawal symptoms such as tremors, disorientation, and seizures. It is useful both in predicting severity of withdrawal and in titrating medications during detoxification, that is, adjusting treatment to the individual client (Swift, 2003).

Remember that detoxification is only a preparation for treatment. Used alone, it rarely changes substance use problems, leading to the familiar and expensive revolving door of people returning for dozens, even hundreds of episodes of detoxification. Detoxification provides an opportunity and responsibility to engage the person in treatment beyond stabilization (see Chapters 6 and 7).

MEDICATIONS TO ATTENUATE SUBSTANCE USE

Medications can be used to reduce cravings for and reward from substance use, thus helping clients to achieve and sustain recovery. Establishing an initial period of abstinence is an important part of stabilization, interrupting prior use patterns and enabling clients to benefit from psychosocial treatment. The medications described here have been tested with various clinical populations and have demonstrated efficacy in suppressing the use of alcohol or other drugs.

Naltrexone

Naltrexone (U.S. trade name Revia) selectively blocks opiate receptors. If given to a person using heroin, it immediately triggers withdrawal, and thus is used to reverse opiate overdose. While maintained on naltrexone, a person experiences no high from injecting heroin. It would seem, therefore, an ideal drug to treat heroin dependence, but the problem is that the vast majority of heroin users simply refuse to take it. Treatment with naltrexone has also been difficult to initiate because clients should be drug-free for 2 weeks prior to starting them on naltrexone, and many clients resume drug use while waiting to receive the medication. It blocks the effects of heroin, but provides none of the benefits of agonist (replacement) therapy like methadone or buprenorphine. For most clients naltrexone does not sufficiently reduce opiate cravings, and it can be discontinued at any time without withdrawal effects. All of these factors work against heroin-dependent clients continuing to take the medication (O'Malley & Kosten, 2006).

Naltrexone does, however, appear to be a useful aid in treating alcohol dependence, presumably by blocking the rewarding aspects of drinking that are mediated through opiate receptors. Clinical trials have shown significant albeit modest benefits, and side effects are typically mild (the most frequent being temporary nausea). Naltrexone appears to reduce the frequency and intensity of drinking, as would be expected if it reduces the rewarding effects of alcohol, and to help people return to abstinence more quickly after drinking (Garbutt, 2009; Garbutt, West, Carey, Lohr, & Crews, 1999; Kranzler & Van Kirk, 2001). In a large rigorously designed multisite clinical trial known as the COMBINE study (Anton et al., 2006), naltrexone was significantly more effective than placebo when given within the context of medical management, a low-intensity primary care approach (Pettinati et al., 2004, 2005); benefits were still present 1 year after medication had been discontinued. It is worth noting that people who were admitted to these studies generally did not have severe psychiatric disorders or other serious drug use problems beyond alcohol dependence and were required to complete a brief period of abstinence. Retention rates have also been low in some of these trials (Garbutt et al., 1999; Oslin et al., 2008). In short, individuals benefitting from naltrexone in these studies may represent a more stable, manageable population than typically seen in alcohol treatment settings (Anton et al., 2006). In a Veterans Administration study with patients having more severe and chronic alcohol dependence, no benefit from naltrexone was found (Krystal et al., 2001).

More recently, an injectable form of naltrexone (trade name Vivitrol) has been offered for clients with alcohol dependence. Administered once monthly, the injectable form offers an advantage in increasing medication adherence. Initial findings have been promising. In a multisite efficacy trial of injectable naltrexone, individuals who received the active medication had significantly fewer days of heavy drinking at follow-up (3.1 vs. 6 days) than their counterparts in the placebo group (Garbutt et al., 2005). Prescription and monitoring of this medication seems to be feasible and effective in primary care settings (Lee et al., 2010). Within the context of psychosocial treatment, it has also been used to reduce drinking during high-risk periods such as holidays (Lapham, Forman, Alexander, Illeperuma, & Bohn, 2009).

Disulfiram

Disulfiram (trade name Antabuse) has long been used in treating alcohol problems. It works by selectively blocking the metabolism of acetaldehyde, a by-product produced as the body breaks down ethyl alcohol. The resulting buildup of acetaldehyde produces highly unpleasant and potentially dangerous symptoms such as nausea, vomiting, racing heart, dropping blood pressure, and shortness of breath (Ait-Daoud & Johnson, 2003; Burnett & Reading, 1970). The strategy assumes that clients, knowing that they will have such an aversive reaction if they drink, will refrain from using alcohol. Disulfiram is not intended to be an "aversion therapy" because ideally the person would never experience the disulfiram–ethanol interaction. (During the 20th century, patients were sometimes given disulfiram and then alcohol while hospitalized as a "challenge" to let them experience the unpleasant interaction, but this is no longer done.) The person must be abstinent for at least 12 hours before taking the initial dose and not have medical or psychiatric contraindications. The intended use of disulfiram is to help the person achieve an initial period of abstinence by taking the medication daily (Barber & O'Brien, 1999; Strain, 2009), which in turn can facilitate psychosocial treatment during Phase 3 rehabilitation (see Chapter 7).

Clinical trials of disulfiram for alcohol dependence have produced mixed results (Brewer, 1992; Miller & Wilbourne, 2002). What seems clear is that clients who faithfully *take* disulfiram fare better than those who do not (Fuller & Gordis, 2004; Garbutt et al., 1999). Medication adherence is the principal problem. Studies suggest that men who are older, more socially stable, have more severe alcohol problems, and attend Alcoholics Anonymous may be more likely to adhere to and do well on disulfiram (Swift, 2003).

Additional measures can be taken to increase disulfiram adherence. Pharmacist-supervised daily administration can be used, with the obvious inconvenience that the person must come to the pharmacy daily. An effective alternative is to engage a supportive significant other (SSO) monitor in a daily disulfiram ritual with the client. The SSO's role is not to nag or enforce, but rather to witness and lovingly encourage daily dosage (Azrin, 1976; Azrin et al., 1982; Meyers & Miller, 2001; Meyers & Smith, 1995). SSO-monitored disulfiram has been found to significantly increase abstinence when added to psychosocial treatment (Brewer, 1992; Meyers & Miller, 2001). People who do not have such a SSO or who have had several unsuccessful treatment experiences may benefit from daily disulfiram supervised by clinical staff to establish an initial period of abstinence (Fuller & Gordis, 2004; Swift, 2003).

Another potential use of disulfiram (in Canada, trade name Temposil) is as a protective drug taken as needed. In this situation, the client does not take the medication daily but carries a supply and pops a tablet if feeling in danger of drinking. Clients report that this strategy helps them to "make the decision once rather than a hundred times" in a day.

Disulfiram has also been used successfully as an aid in treating cocaine dependence, and acceptance of the medication may be better when cocaine rather than alcohol is the drug of choice (Carroll et al., 1998). One obvious mechanism is that drinking is a common antecedent to resumed cocaine use, so that suppressing alcohol use may improve cocaine abstinence. Disulfiram may also have a direct pharmacological effect on cocaine use and craving. In a randomized trial (Carroll et al., 2004), clients receiving behavioral or interpersonal psychotherapy showed significantly greater reduction in cocaine use when they were also given disulfiram than when receiving placebo. In this study, the impact of disulfiram on cocaine use was not attributable to changes in alcohol use. Another clinical trial found that it was necessary for disulfiram dosage to be no less than 250 mg for the drug to suppress cocaine use in methadone-maintenance patients (Oliveto et al., 2010).

Acamprosate

Acamprosate (trade name Campral) which affects various neurotransmitters (particularly glutamate and GABA), has also been approved in the United States and other nations for the treatment of alcohol dependence. The results of clinical trials, however, have been quite mixed. Early studies conducted in Europe found that acamprosate (vs. placebo) significantly increased the proportion of already-abstinent clients who remained continuously abstinent (Lhuintre et al., 1990; Mason & Ownby, 2000; Sass, Soyka, Mann, & Zieglgansberger, 1996; Whitworth et al., 1996). These European findings were not replicated in three large randomized trials. In an industry-sponsored multisite U.S. study, no advantage was found for acamprosate relative to placebo (Mason, Goodman, Chabac, & Lehert, 2006). Similarly, acamprosate showed no greater benefit than placebo for alcohol-dependent clients in the largest study, the federally supported multisite COMBINE trial (Anton et al., 2006) and in a 20-site randomized trial in the United Kingdom (Chick, Howlett, Morgan, Ritson, & Investigators, 2000).

It is unclear what might account for the differences between the U.S. and European studies. The European participants typically had undergone a longer period of abstinence stabilization prior to entering the studies. It is possible that the benefits of acamprosate may appear only in Phase 4 maintenance after a sustained period of abstinence has been achieved. This would be consistent with the claim that acamprosate attenuates the negative effects of protracted withdrawal. Also, no attempt was made to standardize and assess the behavioral treatments that were provided in the earlier European trials, so little is known about how the various behavioral platforms in these studies impacted response to the medication. In the COMBINE trial, the psychosocial treatment (essentially a cognitive-behavioral community reinforcement approach; see Chapter 11) was manual-guided and monitored (Miller, 2004), and acamprosate yielded no additional benefit beyond either placebo or psychotherapy. In any event, given the lack of effect in three large multisite trials, the efficacy of acamprosate seems doubtful. A preliminary trial of acamprosate for cocaine dependence also found no benefit (Kampman et al., 2011).

Topiramate

Advances in neuroscience research have suggested that neurotransmitters (such as GABA and serotonin) and receptor subtypes linked with the development of alcohol and drug problems may parallel those for other common psychological disorders such as depression and obsessive–compulsive behaviors (Schuckit et al., 1999). Consequently, medications found to be effective in treating other disorders have also been tested in addiction treatment.

One such medication is the anticonvulsant topiramate (trade name Topamax) that is already approved for treating epileptic seizures. Topiramate's mechanisms of action were hypothesized to be relevant for treating alcohol and cocaine misuse. A clinical advantage is that topiramate (unlike naltrexone and disulfiram) can be started without an initial period of abstinence. Following on promising initial studies (Johnson et al., 2003), a 17-site clinical trial for alcohol dependence (Johnson et al., 2007) found that topiramate was more effective than placebo across a number of consumption measures including drinks per drinking day, percent of heavy drinking days, and percent of abstinent days. The medication was also found to reduce cravings on various obsessive–compulsive drinking scales that are highly correlated with self-reports of drinking. Topiramate was also found in a single-site randomized trial to be more effective than placebo in producing clinically meaningful improvement with cocaine-dependent clients (Kampman et al., 2004).

Medication Development

The development and testing of new medications for addiction treatment is currently a very active area of research. While it seems unlikely that any medication will be found to cure drug problems by itself, new discoveries will continue to emerge from research, providing promising adjuncts for treatment.

It is also worth saying that many other medications have been tested and found ineffective. An astonishing array of pharmacotherapies have been evaluated in clinical trials for alcohol dependence including antidepressants, anxiolytics, lithium, hallucinogens, and even antibiotics, with little success (Miller & Wilbourne, 2002; Miller, Wilbourne, et al., 2003).

ADAPTING MEDICATIONS TO CLIENTS' TREATMENT NEEDS

Combining Medications for Addiction Treatment

There may be advantages in combining different medications in the treatment of alcohol and other drug problems. Medications have different purposes and mechanisms of action. Some are geared to achieving abstinence whereas others are designed to diminish a drug's reward value if use resumes. For example, disulfiram and naltrexone might be used in combination during stabilization. Disulfiram could help a client achieve enough days of continuous abstinence to start naltrexone. Once abstinence is achieved, disulfiram could be continued or discontinued as naltrexone is initiated (Fuller & Gordis, 2004).

It is also possible, of course, for different medications to be used to address concomitant disorders. Pharmacotherapies described in this chapter might be used to attenuate substance use while those discussed in Chapter 18 treat a concomitant psychological disorder.

Combining Medication and Behavioral Treatment

As mentioned earlier, when medications are prescribed in addiction treatment, they are not typically used alone, but in combination with some form of behavioral treatment. There are several good reasons for doing so. One of the main limitations of pharmacotherapies is that adherence is important, but often poor. Behavioral treatment can have as one of its goals to increase medication adherence (Miller, 2004; Pettinati et al., 2004), which should improve the efficacy of pharmacotherapy. Similarly, medication can help to establish an initial period of abstinence, improving retention and adherence in psychotherapy. In both pharmacological and behavioral treatment, retention and adherence are associated with better treatment outcome, and thus these treatments may combine in a synergistic way. Clients frequently need reliable exposure to a medication regime in order to achieve a period of sustained abstinence. A stable period of abstinence in turn allows clients a greater opportunity to benefit from the motivational and coping strategies used in behavioral treatments to achieve lasting change. Medications and behavioral treatments also may focus simultaneously on different aspects of addiction (e.g., cravings and lifestyle changes), thereby complementing each other.

BOX 15.1. Personal Reflection: Pharmacotherapy as a Motivator for Change

In my own experiences in conducting pharmacotherapy trials, I have found that offering an addiction medication helps to recruit and engage into treatment a group of people who have been reluctant to participate in more traditional substance use programs such as those focusing on a 12-step approach or "talk" therapy. A construction worker who was working in the area where our clinic was located happened to see our announcement of a program combining medication and behavioral treatment for people with alcohol problems. He applied and was accepted, regularly attended sessions during his lunch hour, and did very well in the program. In a termination interview, he mentioned that having a pill available is what had motivated him to attend. Before coming to our program, he had never participated in treatment despite having a serious drinking problem. Programs that involved only talking didn't appeal to him. He thought that just talking was a waste of time and that people in talk therapy were using a "crutch" to deal with their addiction problems.

For this man, having a medication available helped to reduce the stigma associated with help seeking. It helped him view his drinking behavior more as a medical concern than a moral deficiency. It also increased his optimism about change, which is an important element in changing addictive behaviors.

—A. Z.

Research on Combined Treatments

There is accumulating evidence that combining behavioral and pharmacotherapies for addiction can be useful (Chick, Anton, et al., 2000; Pettinati et al., 2000; Volpicelli, Pettinati, McLellan, & O'Brien, 2001; Zweben & Zuckoff, 2002). Pharmacotherapy trials have successfully incorporated behavioral components to facilitate medication adherence and improve treatment outcomes (Carroll, 1997b), and indeed it is rare to find a pharmacotherapy study for alcohol/drug problems that did not also provide psychosocial intervention. (Nicotine replacement therapy, however, appears to be effective regardless of the additional support provided; Lancaster et al., 2000). Forms of behavioral treatment that have been combined with pharmacotherapies include: (1) contingency management with disulfiram for cocaine-dependent clients (Carroll et al., 1998), (2) the community reinforcement approach (Chapter 11) with disulfiram for alcohol-dependent clients (Azrin, 1976; Azrin et al., 1982; Meyers & Miller, 2001), (3) motivational and behavioral therapy with naltrexone for alcohol-dependent clients (Anton et al., 2006), (4) motivational interviewing and compliance enhancement therapy with a selective serotonin reuptake inhibitor (Heffner et al., 2010), and (5) motivational (Saunders et al., 1995), behavioral family therapy (Dattilio, 2009), or individual counseling with case management and social services for methadone maintenance clients (McLellan et al., 1998, 1999; Morgenstern, Hogue, Dauber, Dasaro, & McKay, 2009).

One series of trials, for example (O'Malley et al., 2003), provided open-label naltrexone to clients who also received either supportive therapy (analogous to primary care) or CBT over a 10-week period. Patients who responded positively (e.g., no more than 2 days of heavy drinking and adherent to the medication regime 60% of the time) to either of the behavioral treatments were followed for an additional 24 weeks and given either naltrexone or placebo under double-blind conditions. Results showed that responders who had received CBT maintained their treatment gains throughout the 6-month period whether or not the medication was withdrawn. In contrast, responders who had received supportive therapy maintained their initial gains only if they were continued on naltrexone in the follow-up period. A reasonable conclusion is that the CBT treatment provided benefits beyond those from medication alone.

Implementing Pharmacological Interventions in Treatment Settings

Pharmacotherapies obviously require the involvement of a licensed medical provider who can prescribe and monitor medication—something that many addiction treatment agencies have lacked historically. If you already work in a setting with such medical consultation available, collaborate as a team. If not, it is worth considering how such collaboration might be arranged with health professionals in your area. This makes a broader range of therapies available to your clients, and facilitates the integration of treatment. Similarly, if you work in a medical setting (e.g., primary care) without staff who have expertise in health behavior, consider how psychological/behavioral consultation might be integrated (Blount, 1998; Dunn & Ries, 1997; Ernst et al., 2007; Willenbring & Olson, 1999).

What are the issues that need to be considered in offering effective medications along with behavioral interventions? How does one choose a pharmacotherapy, ensure the safety of clients, and facilitate medication adherence? This section offers some guidelines for including pharmacological adjuncts in addiction treatment.

Medical Evaluation

Obviously a medical examination and evaluation are important in choosing the appropriate medication and ensuring its safety. This includes consideration of any preexisting health conditions such as liver or kidney disease, hypertension, or heart disease. It is also important to review all other medications (both prescription and nonprescription) to consider potential drug interactions. Prior experience with specific medications (e.g., their effectiveness, and any adverse reactions) can be informative. Behavioral factors such as psychological symptoms, past experience with taking medications (i.e., adherence to the medication regime), and overall motivation for change are also relevant considerations.

Therapeutic Relationship

Medications are prescribed and monitored within the context of a therapeutic relationship. A strong working alliance can help in explaining important information about the medication, clarifying misunderstandings, preventing misuse of medication, and improving adherence to the prescribed regime for taking it.

Formulating a Plan for Medication Use

Because medication is usually only part of treatment, it is important to consider how it fits within the larger treatment plan. It can be important for nonmedical members of the treatment team to understand the purpose and plan regarding medications, and to help encourage adherence. When two or more medications are used concomitantly or sequentially, develop a specific plan for when and how each one is to be taken. It is wise to check in early and periodically to monitor adherence and discuss any adverse reactions or other problems.

As discussed earlier, some medications are used intermittently as needed. In this case, the plan should specify the circumstances under which it should be used (e.g., to forestall a return to drinking or drug use), as well as the appropriate dose and method for taking it.

Developing a Medication Adherence Plan

A variety of factors can affect whether medications as taken as prescribed and intended. These include the person's

Overall motivation for change.
Knowing the purpose and importance of the medication.
Understanding how it is to be taken.
Unpleasant side effects.
Ability to afford and obtain the medication.
Lifestyle factors that interfere with reliable adherence.

Before prescribing and starting a pharmacotherapy, review and address potential obstacles to adherence. When and how will the person take the medication? What reminders might be used? How will the person respond to side effects? Can a family member help with adherence? If the person is ambivalent about the goals of treatment (and therefore about taking the medication), strategies from Chapter 10 may be helpful.

Combining Behavioral Treatment and Pharmacotherapy

Medications normally are but one part of a larger addiction treatment plan. Pharmacotherapy may be helpful in establishing abstinence and diminishing urges or cravings, but the sudden absence of substance use raises other issues that medication does not address (see Chapter 11). How will the person spend the time that was previously devoted to getting, using, and recovering from the effects of alcohol or other drugs? With whom will he or she share time and activities, particularly when a change of friends is needed? How will the person cope with feelings and situations that previously triggered use? How can relationships be repaired that have been damaged by addictive behavior? What will be the new sources of fun, pleasure, and meaning in life? Medications are not designed to solve these problems, and ignoring them is a recipe for failure. The treatment methods described in Chapters 8–14 can be combined with pharmacotherapy for an integrated approach. Family involvement in treatment can reengage spouses or relatives who have been distanced, strengthen family relationships, and support the client's own motivation and efforts to change (see Chapters 11 and 13). Engagement with a mutual help group (Chapter 14) can also support change.

TREATMENT IN HEALTH CARE SETTINGS

With this said, we also recognize the potential and advantages of treating addictions within the context of regular health care and social services. Specialist addiction treatment programs simply cannot meet the needs of the full spectrum of alcohol/drug problems that are so prevalent in society. Substance use disorders should be screened for and addressed wherever people receive general health and social services (Hilton et al., 2001; Miller & Weisner, 2002; Weisner et al., 2001), where people with addictions are typically seen first, earlier in the development of problems. Many are reluctant or refuse to seek specialist care, but are willing to talk to their primary provider about substance use.

The development of effective pharmacotherapies has made it more feasible to address addictions within the primary health care setting. Most health professionals involved in primary care have neither the time nor the training to provide comprehensive treatment for addictions, but they *can* screen, evaluate, prescribe, and monitor (Saitz, 2005; Saitz, Horton, Larson, Winter, & Samet, 2005; Samet, Friedmann, & Saitz, 2002). This is the *normal* role of a primary care practitioner in treating chronic illness. Chronic conditions are often first diagnosed in primary practice. If a patient with asthma, diabetes, cancer, or heart disease is then treated by a specialist, ongoing care and monitoring are still provided as part of primary care. For this reason, it is important to foster closer relationships and collaboration of addiction treatment professionals with ongoing health care systems.

Clearly, people with addictions can benefit from pharmacotherapy delivered within primary health care (Saitz, 2005). In the studies described earlier in this chapter, clients who benefited from topiramate and naltrexone received only supportive therapy, such as could be provided within primary care, while receiving the medication. Those taking topiramate were not required to be abstinent prior to receiving the drug, and all clients were drinking at enrollment (Johnson et al., 2007). These findings suggest that addiction treatment can be done, or at least started, in nonspecialized medical settings. The need for this grows when funding for specialty treatment of addiction problems is curtailed. Most people with addiction problems never receive treatment within a specialty program. It has been estimated that only 12% of addiction treatment programs use alcohol pharmacotherapies, for reasons including lack of medical staff, cost, and ideology (Abraham, 2010). Combining medications and primary care supportive therapy can improve access to effective addiction treatment to large number of individuals with addiction problems seen in medical settings.

Looking ahead, it will be useful to integrate broader behavioral health treatment services with the pharmacotherapy and supportive treatment that can be delivered in primary health care. Although pharmacotherapy is often better than no treatment, many people can benefit from the additional treatment that addiction professionals are trained and able to provide. Such care can be provided on-site at primary care clinics when behavioral health specialists work in those settings. Close collaboration makes it feasible for a person to be diagnosed and receive initial treatment in primary care, then be referred for specialist treatment, and return for ongoing monitoring and case management (Samet et al., 2002). Integrating care can be accomplished in a cost-effective manner through cooperation between a medical professional and a case manager. The former provides medication-assisted treatment including ambulatory detoxification, and the case manager facilitates medication adherence while keeping medical staff informed of any change in symptoms or side effects that may warrant a dosage change or further medical evaluation. The case manager also coordinates care with other professionals who are providing services during active treatment. With appropriate training the case manager can help to educate clients and their families as well as referral sources about the importance of medications in addiction treatment.

In the future, much more needs to be known about how best to integrate these services for people with addictions. More specifically, it will be helpful to learn more about how to (1) determine what behavioral treatment modalities are more effective with what pharmacological agents; (2) sequence medications and behavioral interventions to address different symptoms and problems that may stem from alcohol/drug misuse; and (3) adapt or modify the combined approach to help nonresponders who appear not to be benefiting from treatment. Important questions also remain regarding the long-term cost-effectiveness of a combined approach particularly in generalist practice settings. More treatment is not necessarily better treatment, and sometimes combinations of treatments are no more effective than an evidence-based pharmacotherapy or behavioral treatment alone (Anton et al., 2006). Further experience with stepped care will clarify what treatment is enough for whom, and how best to help those who do not respond to initial treatment (Sobell & Sobell, 2000).

KEY POINTS

🖈 Effective medications are available to reduce or prevent withdrawal symptoms and help patients safely through detoxification.

🖈 Substitution drugs (such as buprenorphine and nicotine) can also be used for longer term maintenance.

🖈 Pharmacotherapies are also available to help reduce urges to drink or use drugs, facilitate initial abstinence and treatment participation, enhance motivation, and maintain change.

🖈 Pharmacotherapies should be seen as complementary to and not a replacement for psychosocial interventions.

🖈 Pharmacotherapy also can improve access to effective treatment for many untreated individuals with addiction problems who are currently seen in health care settings.

REFLECTION QUESTIONS

💬 What attitudes have you encountered with regard to the use of pharmacotherapies in addiction treatment? What is your own current attitude?

💬 If you are not a prescribing professional yourself, what are the various ways in which clients you serve can access pharmacotherapies?

💬 What could you do to help clients who are on pharmacotherapy take their medication reliably as prescribed?

PART IV

Issues That Arise
in Addiction Treatment

B eyond the evidence-based treatments for addiction described in Part III, there are practical clinical issues that commonly arise when treating addictions. Perhaps none of these issues is more widely discussed than how to deal with client resistance in treatment. In Chapter 16 we describe an evidence-based way of thinking about resistance and effective strategies for reducing it. A related issue is how to encourage clients to stick with whatever treatment is chosen and to take the needed steps in order to recover. These issues of treatment retention and adherence are the subject of Chapter 17.

Practitioners who treat addictions are likely to encounter the entire DSM spectrum of disorders, and therein lies yet another challenge (Chapter 18). What is the best way to address co-occurring disorders? Is it better to treat one first and then the other or to work on them simultaneously? Chapter 18 also discusses the use of therapeutic psychotropic medications to treat disorders that commonly accompany substance use disorders.

It is common knowledge that addictions are chronic conditions, and that the real challenge is not in getting sober, but in staying that way. In Chapter 19 we take up this issue of how to help your clients maintain the gains they have made and how best to deal with recurrences.

Systems of managed care often encourage or require practitioners to provide treatment in groups, rather than in individual client sessions. Chapter 20 describes various aspects of and approaches to group treatment and the evidence base for its effectiveness.

Particularly in the Americas, spirituality has been strongly emphasized in understanding and addressing addictions (Chapter 21). There are few other classes of disorders for which spiritual factors have been so frequently stressed as crucial. What is the evidence for spiritual/religious factors in the development and resolution of alcohol/drug problems, and how can practitioners, regardless of their own personal beliefs, address the spiritual side of addictions?

Professional ethics are a vital concern in all forms of health and social services. In addiction treatment, there are special protections and particular ethical concerns of which professionals need to be aware. Chapter 22 outlines major ethical issues of the addiction field.

Why is there a concluding chapter (23) on prevention in a book about treatment? These may seem like different endeavors. Prevention specialists and treatment practitioners often speak different languages, work from differing assumptions, and have separate professional meetings and journals. Yet both are pursuing the same fundamental goal: the reduction of suffering related to the use of licit and illicit drugs. What is called "treatment" lies along a continuum of prevention, where approaches vary in how early and with whom one intervenes. We believe treatment professionals should be knowledgeable about and supportive of the efforts of prevention specialists, and vice versa.

CHAPTER 16

Responding to Resistance

Warren Farrell once quipped that when a client disagrees with a therapist, it is called denial; when the client subsequently comes to agree with the therapist, it is called insight.

The concept of resistance entered into addiction counseling through the door of psychodynamic psychotherapy. From this perspective, the expert psychotherapist gently seeks to make conscious what are unconscious motivations (Khantzian, Halliday, & McAuliffe, 1990; Prochaska & Norcross, 2009). Timing is everything. If the psychotherapist moves too fast (e.g., a premature interpretation), the client resists. Through psychoanalysis, a whole catalog of ego defense mechanisms such as denial, projection, and rationalization entered everyday discourse (Vaillant, 1993).

As discussed in Chapter 2, during the mid-20th century it was widely believed that addiction was inherently linked to immature character defenses, particularly denial. This view of clients being "in denial" furthermore casts clients "as unable to read and know themselves, and therefore unable to speak authoritatively" about themselves (Carr, 2011, p. 235). These pathological aspects of personality were regarded as "just part of the disease." There never was scientific evidence that people with addictions have unique personality characteristics or manifest unusually high levels of particular defense mechanisms (Vaillant, 1995). In fact, it is widely recognized that addiction afflicts a very broad range of humanity, and that is certainly our own experience. People with addictions are just as varied and unique as snowflakes.

How, then, did so many professionals come to believe that all "alcoholics" or "addicts" were the same—resistive, denying, lying? Vernon Johnson (1973, p. 44) wrote that "the alcoholic evades or denies outright any need for help whenever he is approached. It must be remembered that he is not in touch with reality." A front page story in the *Wall Street Journal* (Greenberger, 1983) quoted as an example of good practice a medical director shouting at an executive who was alcohol-impaired: "Shut up and listen.... Alcoholics are liars, so we don't want to hear what you have to say."

Some claim mistakenly that this confrontational view came from AA. The writings of AA cofounder Bill W. are quite at variance with such an authoritarian approach. Commenting on how one should work with others, he wrote (Alcoholics Anonymous, 1976, p. 95):

> Let him steer the conversation in any direction he likes.... You will be most successful with alcoholics if you do not exhibit any passion for crusade or reform. Never talk down to an alcoholic.... He must decide for himself whether he wants to go on. He should not be pushed or prodded.... If he thinks he can do the job in some other way or prefers some other spiritual approach, encourage him to follow his own conscience.

> The American detour into a denial-busting confrontational style for addiction treatment was, from our perspective, an aberrant wrong turn justifying treatment practices that would be blatantly unprofessional and unethical in any other area of health care.

The American detour into a denial-busting confrontational style for addiction treatment was, from our perspective, an aberrant wrong turn justifying treatment practices that would be blatantly unprofessional and unethical in any other area of health care, and clinical trials of such approaches have yielded uniformly negative results (Miller, Wilbourne, et al., 2003; White & Miller, 2007).

What is particularly seductive about this belief in denial and confrontation is that it is a self-fulfilling prophecy (Miller & Rollnick, 1991). Defensiveness is a *normal* human reaction to confrontation, labeling, judgment, and being told what to do. Counsel in this way, and people are likely to minimize their problems, disagree with you, deny a diagnostic label, reject your advice, and not come back (thereby confirming the stereotype). Client resistance is strongly influenced by the counselor: You can turn it up or down just like a volume control, by altering your counseling style (Glynn & Moyers, 2010; Patterson & Forgatch, 1985).

> Denial is not a client problem. It is a counseling skill issue.

In other words, denial is not a client problem. It is a counseling skill issue, and a serious one at that. Counsel in a way that evokes a lot of resistance, and your clients are unlikely to change their addictive behavior; provide a therapeutic atmosphere that minimizes resistance, and change happens (Miller et al., 1993). If you find yourself arguing for change while your client argues against it, you're in the wrong chair.

So if resistance is a response to what the counselor is doing, then it is in essence *a signal not to do more of whatever you just did*. Try something different to reduce resistance. This is precisely the opposite of what was once taught: if you meet resistance, dig in and turn up the volume on confrontation (which is, by the way, something that a classical psychoanalyst would never do). Resistance is not a challenge to try to win the argument, but an immediate in-session feedback from your client to try something different. This is quite consistent with a psychodynamic understanding of resistance—that it signals therapists that they are moving too fast.

RESISTANCE VERSUS SUSTAIN TALK

We find it helpful to differentiate true resistance from what we in motivational interviewing (MI) call *sustain talk* (Rollnick et al., 2008). Sustain talk is the opposite of change talk (see Chapter 10); it is a stated reason not to change. A neuroimaging study supported meaningful differences between change talk and sustain talk: spontaneous sustain talk (favoring continued substance use) was associated with activation of appetitive reinforcement channels, whereas change talk was not (Feldstein Ewing, Filbey, Sabbineni, & Hutchinson, 2011).

If clients are ambivalent about their addictive behavior, as most are, then they have within themselves both sides of the conflict: the arguments to quit or cut down (change talk) and the arguments to maintain the status quo (sustain talk). It is perfectly normal for clients to express both sustain talk and change talk when they are ambivalent. They are simply airing the arguments that are going on within them. It is even quite common to hear sustain talk intermixed with change talk. Here's an example, with change talk in *italic font* and sustain talk in **bold font**.

> *"I know I ought to cut down on pot, maybe quit. It hangs around in the body for a long time, and if I get drug tested I'm busted.* **But the drug testing makes me mad—who are they to tell me what I can and can't do? It's like they're my parents, all over again. So I just keep on smoking,** *and the weeks go by and I don't do anything to get my life moving, and I don't care. I'm at a dead end.* **I mean, I really like how pot makes me feel, and I enjoy kicking back and not caring or thinking about my life and just listening to music,** *but how long am I going to keep on like this?*

The transitions from change talk to sustain talk in client speech are often marked by a "but." Both arguments are there inside the client. It matters which one you call forth. If you take up the "good" arguments for change yourself, then the client is likely to respond with sustain talk defending the status quo, and literally talk him- or herself out of changing. It certainly is tempting to argue against sustain talk when you hear it, but doing so only tends to evoke more arguments from the client against change!

Anyhow, sustain talk is perfectly normal. It is a client statement *about the behavior* that you are discussing. Ideally over the course of a session you gradually hear more change talk and less sustain talk—a pattern that presages change (Amrhein et al., 2003). The ratio of change talk to sustain talk that a client expresses is directly related to the probability of behavior change (Moyers et al., 2007), but hearing sustain talk is not in itself reason for concern. It happens normally whenever people are ambivalent.

Resistance, in contrast, is not about the behavior but *about your relationship*, or even about you. It is client behavior that tells you there is some dissonance in your working relationship at the moment. If a client statement contains the word "you," it is probably resistance rather than sustain talk. Here are some examples of resistance responses that are inversely associated with behavior change (Chamberlain, Patterson, Reid, Kavanagh, & Forgatch, 1984; Miller et al., 1993):

- Arguing: "I'm not quitting (sustain talk) and you can't make me (resistance)."
- Discounting: "How can you understand me? Did you ever do heroin?"
- Ignoring: (Not paying attention, changing the subject) "Whatever."
- Interrupting: (Talking over you at the same time you're speaking, breaking in)
- Hostility: "To hell with you! You don't care about me."

Such responses indicate at least temporary tension in your working alliance that needs some repair.

Either way—sustain talk or resistance—there are certain ways to respond (and not respond) to a client. Fortunately, the ways of responding to either one are the same.

ROLLING WITH RESISTANCE AND SUSTAIN TALK

At the entrance to and the exit from the security area of the Albuquerque airport there are revolving doors that begin to turn automatically whenever a motion sensor detects someone approaching. Emblazoned on the glass doors in big red letters are the words: DO NOT PUSH. DOORS WILL LOCK. And sure enough, when someone fails to heed the warning and tries to push the door to make it go faster, the whole thing locks up and the impatient or unobservant traveler is slowed down. The traveler who moves *with* the door instead of getting ahead of it is the one who moves through the fastest.

This is the general lesson in responding to resistance and sustain talk. A directive, authoritarian style of counseling is a particularly poor match for clients who are more angry or resistive (Beutler, Harwood, Michelson, Song, & Hollman, 2011; Waldron, Kern-Jones, Turner, Peterson, & Ozechowski, 2007; Waldron, Miller, & Tonigan, 2001). Don't push against it. Don't oppose, argue with, or try to refute it. Doing so only strengthens it. Move with it rather than against it.

Reflective Responses

One effective way to respond to resistance or sustain talk is to reflect it (see Chapter 4), which directly acknowledges what the client said and affirms that you heard it.

> CLIENT: I don't think I have a drinking problem.
>
> COUNSELOR: Alcohol really isn't a problem in your life.

This may feel like an uncomfortable "siding with" the client's perspective, and the urge is there to say, "How can you sit there and tell me it's not a problem for you?," in order to correct what seems like an irrational misperception. However, those two counselor responses are likely to yield quite different responses from the client. Consider this exchange from early in a first session with a man referred by his physician to talk about his drinking.

> THERAPIST: Your doctor asked me to talk with you about your substance use. Tell me what you're struggling with.
>
> CLIENT: Well, I think my biggest problem really is cigarettes.
>
> THERAPIST: Smoking is really what concerns you most.
>
> CLIENT: And alcohol to some extent [change talk], but really that was more of a problem for me a year or two ago [sustain talk]. I've cut down quite a bit.
>
> THERAPIST: So you've put that one behind you [reflection].
>
> CLIENT: Well, not completely. I mean I probably still drink too much [change talk], but it's just that I can't drink like I used to [change talk].
>
> THERAPIST: You're drinking less now because you can't keep up like you used to [reflection].
>
> CLIENT: That's right. I really can't. It takes too much of a toll on me [change talk].

THERAPIST: Tell me a little more about that. In what ways has alcohol been affecting you?

What's going on here? The client offers some sustain talk, hears it reflected back, and then responds with the other side of his ambivalence. Reflection of an ambivalent person's sustain talk has a way of bringing back the other side.

But why not just go ahead and defend the good side yourself? Why not say, instead of reflecting, "Well, *I* think alcohol is still a serious problem for you!"? The client's likely response would be to continue to defend the status quo (no problem), and it is what *the client* says about change that predicts outcome. You want clients talking themselves into, not out of, change.

> You want clients talking themselves into, not out of, change.

The above are examples of simple reflection. They don't add much to what the client has said. It's not just parroting, but basically the reflections say in different words what the client has already told you. There are two other kinds of reflection that can be helpful in responding to resistance and sustain talk (Miller & Rollnick, 2002).

The first of these is an *amplified reflection*. You reflect back what the client has said but turn up the volume a bit, increasing the intensity of the statement.

CLIENT: I really don't have a problem with drugs.

THERAPIST: Using drugs hasn't ever caused any problems for you.

The amplification is a step up in the sustain talk. It hasn't *ever* caused *any* problems for you. Now, it's possible that the client could say, "That's right," but if there's ambivalence there, it's much more likely that the client will offer a bit of the other side: "Well, I wouldn't say it hasn't caused *any* problems. My girlfriend doesn't like it, and sometimes I blow off working when I should study.... " By upping the intensity of the sustain talk or resistance, you make it more likely that the client will explore the other side. Note that it is important for there to be no hint of sarcasm in your reflection. If you say, "So *YOU* think that you don't have *ANY* drug problem!" you're not reflecting, but rather confronting through your voice tone.

Another useful response is a *double-sided reflection*. Here you are voicing both sides of the client's own ambivalence (which means you need to have been listening long enough to hear both sides). You include both the sustain talk and the change talk in the same reflection. Two tips about this are that it is usually best to put the sustain talk first and to join the two parts with "and" rather than "but" (unless you're trying to deemphasize the first part, which is what "but" does).

THERAPIST: What have you noticed about your drinking?

CLIENT: Well, sometimes I don't feel too good in the morning when I wake up [change talk].

THERAPIST: With a hangover [reflection].

CLIENT: Yes, but I don't think I'm an alcoholic or anything [sustain talk].

THERAPIST: That label just doesn't fit you, and at the same time you have some concerns about how drinking is affecting you [double-sided reflection].

The same reflective style works well in responding to resistance:

CLIENT: How can you understand me? Have you ever been a drug addict [discounting]?

THERAPIST: It's pretty hard for you to imagine how I might be able to understand and help you [reflection].

CLIENT: Yeah, whatever. You don't really care about me. You're just here to get a paycheck [discounting].

THERAPIST: You'd like to work with somebody who really cares about you [reflection].

CLIENT: Yeah. Well, I guess I'm just mad about having to be here.

THERAPIST: I hear that loud and clear. It's no fun having to come here [reflection].

Emphasizing Personal Choice

Sometimes a conversation about substance use can feel like a power struggle to the client. When people feel like a freedom may be taken away from them, they naturally resist and want to assert their freedom—a phenomenon called *reactance* (Brehm & Brehm, 1981). If you push against reactance by telling people that they "must," "have to," "don't have a choice," "can't," and so forth, the result is usually more reactance.

A simple (and truthful) way to respond to this is to acknowledge that the person *does* have a say, a choice. One thing that we can never take away from people is their ability to choose how they will be. We don't get to make those decisions for somebody else. By emphasizing this fact we are simply telling the truth. Again, it's said without any hint of irony or sarcasm.

> One thing that we can never take away from people is their ability to choose how they will be. We don't get to make those decisions for somebody else.

CLIENT: Well I'm not quitting drinking, and that's final!

THERAPIST: Right you are. Nobody else can decide that for you. It's your choice.

CLIENT: I just don't want to feel like I can't have something.

THERAPIST: Of course! You're the one who chooses how to think about it. If you say, "I can't have it" you feel trapped, and then naturally you want it. Or you can say, "I could take a drink, but I choose not to, just for today." Then you don't feel so trapped. It's up to you.

Shifting Focus

Sometimes it helps to take the spotlight off of the hot-button issue and focus on where you can collaborate.

CLIENT: Are you saying that I'm an alcoholic?

THERAPIST: No, I'm not really invested in labels. That's not the issue. What I'd like to talk about is what's happening in your life and what, if anything, you might like to change.

Addiction treatment is not a contest about who's going to win. With adults, and particularly with adolescents, if you square off to win the argument, it is the client who ultimately pays the price. The pro-change motivations are already there inside the client. Let your client have the good lines!

> If you square off to win the argument, it is the client who ultimately pays the price.

LISTENING FOR WISDOM

Finally, remember that when clients appear to be resistive, they are usually trying to tell you something. A familiar theme in effective sales is "The customer is always right," and the parallel is worth considering: that your client is always right. At one level, this could mean coming alongside and joining with your clients even when you think they are wrong, in hopes of steering them aright. We mean something deeper than this—that clients have real wisdom about what will work for them, and of course they also retain the autonomy to choose whether and what they will change. What feels like resistance may be a message:

"You're not listening to me."

"What we're talking about is not the most important thing for me right now."

BOX 16.1. Personal Reflection: A Lesson Learned

He came to the clinic complaining of an odd obsession, and perhaps because of my interest in addictions he was referred to me. Raul was a professional artist who used a form of meditation to quiet his mind and tap into the deep creative river within him. For several months, however, whenever he had entered this meditative state he encountered an intrusive image: the face of a man who was a stranger to him. The face was always the same, not particularly threatening, but just there "in the upper left-hand corner" of the blank canvas behind his eyelids. He found it terribly distressing and distracting, and it was seriously interfering with his creative productivity. "I think it might help if you hypnotized me," he said. I had training in clinical hypnosis but was also aware of the literature at the time on treating obsessions, so I explained to him that there was no good scientific evidence that hypnosis would help him. For 2 months or so I tried a variety of behavioral strategies—systematic desensitization, prolonged exposure, functional analysis to identify evoking cues or reinforcing consequences—all to no avail. Finally in desperation I hypnotized him with a classic trance induction and a posthypnotic suggestion that the obsession would be gone. He called me 4 days later. "Doc! It's amazing! He's completely gone! Thanks—I don't need to come in any more." And I never saw him again.

—W. R. M.

"I don't have much hope that I can change."
"There is something else that concerns me more."
"You're pushing too hard."

Listen hard for what your client is trying to tell you. Ask: "It seems like I'm not hearing something that is really important to you, and I'd like to understand. Tell me what's bothering you right now." Then listen.

KEY POINTS

- Client sustain talk is the opposite of change talk, and is a normal part of ambivalence, whereas resistance is a signal of dissonance in your working relationship.

- Arguing with sustain talk or resistance typically strengthens it and decreases the likelihood of change. Don't push back, even if it feels like the right thing to do.

- Resistance is strongly influenced by counseling style; it takes two to resist. Change is promoted by counseling in a way that diminishes (rather than evokes) defensiveness.

🖈 Reflective listening is a good tool for rolling with resistance, and can include amplified and double-sided reflections.

🖈 People get to make the choices about whether and how they will change. Recognizing and emphasizing this fact can diminish resistance.

REFLECTION QUESTIONS

Q Where did the idea that "If you can just make people feel *bad* enough, then they will change" come from?

Q How have you understood the causes of client "resistance"?

Q What counseling approach(es) would follow logically from the way in which you have thought about "resistance"?

CHAPTER 17

Enhancing Adherence

No matter what particular treatment people are receiving, there is one fairly good predictor of outcome, and that is their level of personal involvement and adherence. In general, taking active steps toward change is a good predictor that the change will actually happen. This does not mean that the *kind* of treatment a person receives is irrelevant. As we have maintained throughout this book, some treatments do generally work better than others; the amount of evidence for (and against) efficacy varies widely across specific treatment methods (Miller & Wilbourne, 2002). It also matters *who* delivers treatment and *how* (Chapter 4), but in addition to these factors, the client's own involvement in and effort toward change is a strong predictor of outcome (Bohart & Tallman, 1999).

> The client's own involvement in and effort toward change is a strong predictor of outcome.

This chapter is about how to increase client *adherence* to treatment and other change efforts such as attending mutual help groups (Chapter 14). There is much that you can do to increase adherence in order to improve outcomes. We begin with a definition of adherence, a brief consideration of why adherence matters, and a discussion of reasons why people decide not to continue in treatment. We then turn to practical things that programs and individual providers can do to prevent attrition and facilitate engagement in treatment.

DEFINING ADHERENCE

The term "adherence" refers to how fully and well a client participates or engages in a particular treatment or change effort. One common indicator of adherence is simple: attendance. In general, the more treatment sessions people attend or the longer they stay in treatment, the better the outcome. Treatment noncompletion, tardiness, sessions missed and cancelled are associated with less positive outcomes.

Another meaning of adherence is the extent to which people engage in prescribed tasks such as home assignments, rehearsal of new skills, choosing a sponsor, attending AA meetings, bringing an SO to the sessions, and sticking to a medication regime (taking the prescribed dosage at the appropriate times). Even when clients are prescribed a placebo medication (as in a randomized clinical trial), the extent to which they faithfully take their "doses" predicts successful outcome (Zweben et al., 2008). Usually such adherence is closely linked with good attendance, but not always. People may show up faithfully for their sessions but not actively participate or take the steps needed to change. This is more often the case when individuals are coerced into treatment (Carroll, 1997a).

For purposes of this chapter, we will use a broad definition of adherence to describe both attendance (e.g., length of stay in a program and number and frequency of sessions completed) and in-session task assignments (e.g., taking medication as prescribed, bringing an SO to the sessions, attending NA/AA meetings, or self-monitoring of drug and alcohol use). Both kinds of adherence are steps toward recovery.

WHY IS ADHERENCE IMPORTANT?

Adherence has been particularly troublesome in the treatment of substance use disorders. A high proportion (averaging 44–60%) of those who enter addiction treatment leave within the first month (Carroll, 1997a; Greenfield et al., 2007). In some settings, the modal (most common) number of treatment sessions completed is one. If people do not return, they are unlikely to benefit from treatment. Increased adherence (including attendance) is associated with improvements in individual and social coping resources (e.g., managing negative mood states, building or rebuilding supportive relationships, reducing cravings or urges to drink, and enhancing motivation) as well as a reduction or cessation of drug and alcohol use and problems. Poor adherence may be particularly problematic for people with serious concomitant medical and psychiatric problems (Weiss, 2004). For example, people with alcohol/drug problems and HIV-AIDS are seriously at risk if they do not adhere to the combined medication and behavioral treatment regime (Parsons, Rosof, Punzalan, & DiMaria, 2005).

There are some circumstances, however, where leaving treatment "early" can be viewed as a positive step. Clients might be well advised to leave a program and go elsewhere if the program does not adequately address their needs. Individuals with co-occurring addiction and psychiatric or psychological problems, for example, tend to fare better in settings that address both areas than in an alcohol/drug-specific programs (Mueser, Drake, Turner, & McGovern, 2006; see Chapter 18).

The therapeutic "working alliance" is also a good predictor of treatment outcome, and when the client–counselor match is not good, it is probably best for the person to move on (Zweben & Zuckoff, 2002). When there is a fixed number of prescribed sessions, it also happens that some clients drop out "early" precisely because they have already successfully achieved their change goals. Nonetheless, the preponderance of evidence indicates that people with addiction problems do better if they attend treatment and adhere to a change plan.

REASONS FOR NONADHERENCE

Clients' reasons for seeking and staying in treatment may be different from their reasons for adhering (or not adhering) to various components of the treatment offered. To illustrate, people may attend sessions regularly to avoid legal consequences stemming from a court-ordered referral, without being ready to adopt particular recommended changes such as AA attendance. Individuals may be open to seeking help as a consequence of job loss or pressure from a spouse, but object to certain program components like taking medication or providing urine and blood specimens.

Moreover, people's readiness to engage in treatment has much to do with how they perceive their drinking or drug use. Problems with retention and adherence may reflect a mismatch between the counseling approach and the client's level of readiness. Some individuals are uncertain about whether their drug or alcohol problem is

> Problems with retention and adherence may reflect a mismatch between the counseling approach and the client's level of readiness.

serious enough to warrant formal treatment. They may compare themselves with their heavy-drinking or drug-using peer group and not perceive a problem. Others attribute their recognized problems such as job loss to external factors like having a "mean supervisor" rather than to their own behavior. For some, the immediate benefits of the drug use (such as getting high) may outweigh whatever costs there are. Finally, some may think that they lack the individual and social resources (e.g., child care, social support for abstinence, and transportation) to engage in treatment or undertake a lifestyle free of drugs and alcohol.

In addition, there are various individual and contextual factors that may impact on clients' readiness to participate in treatment. There is still social stigma attached to alcohol/drug problems, and people may be fearful of being labeled as a "junkie" or "alcoholic" by family members or peers. Sometimes the barrier is as simple (and vital) as lacking bilingual counselors who speak their primary or only language. Some may be reluctant to participate because of concerns about confidentiality—for example, that information on substance use might be conveyed to their employer, causing them to lose their jobs.

Moreover, clients' lives may be too disorganized and stressful to accept and fulfill the requisite demands of treatment. Such clients may be overwhelmed by everyday hardships resulting from unstable living situations, violence, or poverty. Some may lack the needed supports from family and friends to engage in treatment. Some have had negative interactions with prior providers or programs or rejected a particular treatment approach previously offered or imposed. All together, these factors serve as powerful *demotivators* for change (O'Toole et al., 2006; Zweben & Zuckoff, 2002).

Our message, then, is that there are *many* different reasons for encountering adherence problems in addiction treatment, and it is important to understand the reasons for an individual's reluctance. It is not good practice to blame and dismiss clients as "unmotivated," "difficult," "in denial," or "resistant." Rather it is important to understand the unique circumstances confronting each client that may interfere with entering, participating, and remaining in treatment. We suggest here a variety of strategies that programs and clinicians have used to understand and address barriers to adherence.

> It is not good practice to blame and dismiss clients as "unmotivated," "difficult," "in denial," or "resistant."

WHAT PROGRAMS CAN DO TO ENHANCE RETENTION AND ADHERENCE

Creating a Client-Friendly Environment

It seems an obvious point, but one that is overlooked in a surprising number of programs. When people arrive for treatment, they should feel welcomed and comfortable. Make your program and setting a place that people *want* to come to! Some practical points are friendly and courteous reception staff, an attractive and safe waiting area, a cup of coffee (AA has known this for a long time), and prompt appointment times. Clients should not feel like you're grudgingly doing them a favor to let them in, but rather that you are glad to see them. Each individual should be treated with warmth and respect.

Matching Treatment to Clients' Needs (and Not Vice Versa)

In Greek mythology, Procrustes was an unscrupulous innkeeper on the road from Athens to Eleusis. He had one iron bed in which he invited all comers to sleep. If they were too short, he stretched them to be the same size as the bed, and if they were too tall he amputated accordingly. Needless to say, few guests survived. Programs in which "one size fits all" are thus termed "Procrustean." Imagine a shoe store that carried only one kind of shoe, and in only one size. Few would want to shop there.

Another program aspect to improve retention and adherence, then, is to give people a real voice and choice in the design of their own treatment. It means adjusting treatment plans to fit the individual, and not the other way around (see Chapter 7). This means, first of all, offering a menu of options, services, hours, and formats from which people can choose (McLellan, 2006). Clients who have a choice among options are more likely to stay and to adhere to what they have chosen.

Selecting Appropriate Staff

Client retention and adherence can also be promoted by hiring and staffing policies. One of the fastest ways to change the climate of a treatment program is to be the person who selects new staff. Remember that one of the stronger determinants of retention is the counselor to whom a client is assigned. How are individual staff members doing at retaining clients? When hiring, pay attention

> One of the fastest ways to change the climate of a treatment program is to be the person who selects new staff.

to specific skills such as accurate empathy (Chapter 4) that promote client retention and change (Miller et al., 2005).

In contrast, counselors who practice a more authoritarian, confrontational, coercive interaction style tend to evoke resistance and defensiveness, threatening clients' sense of personal autonomy and freedom (Dillard & Shen, 2005; Longshore & Teruya, 2006; Miller et al., 1993). Because dropout from treatment often happens early, the communication style of those whom clients first encounter in a program can be particularly influential.

WHAT PROVIDERS CAN DO: A MENU OF STRATEGIES

Motivational Interviewing

As an overarching approach MI (see Chapter 10) has much to offer in promoting treatment retention and adherence. A single conversation with an empathic counselor can substantially promote motivation and change, even when this is not the dominant program style (Bien, Miller, & Boroughs,

1993; Brown & Miller, 1993) The nonauthoritarian, collaborative style of MI affirms client motivations and intentions to change and helps facilitate a therapeutic alliance, itself an important factor in predicting better adherence rates (DeWeert-Van Oene, Schippers, De Jong, & Schrijvers, 2001).

Supporting Client Autonomy

When people come for an initial consultation, they are beginning a choice, a decision-making process about whether to engage in treatment. MI emphasizes respect and support for clients' choice and autonomy, factors that help promote retention and adherence. You can express this directly with statements such as "It's really up to you," "It's your choice," and "No one can decide this for you." Reminding people of their freedom of choice makes it more possible for them to consider alternatives, even unpleasant ones. In contrast, telling people that they have no choice, "have to," or "must" tends to evoke resistance and *reactance*—the need to reassert personal freedom (Chapter 16).

Related to this theme, MI posits that retention is improved when you help clients to focus on personal, individualized reasons for seeking treatment while also accepting external motivators such as family, legal, and employment pressures (O'Toole et al., 2006; Wild et al., 2006). People are more receptive to treatment when they have their own reasons for change and perceive that they have a voice in the change process

Negotiating a Trial Period

Where there is reluctance, one approach is to suggest trying out a goal or treatment on a "trial basis." A trial period allows a client to take steps in the right direction without making an initial commitment. This is a strategy commonly used in sales (e.g., free samples, test drive) as well as in AA ("One day at a time"). The method of sobriety sampling (described in Chapter 11) is an example of this approach—just "trying out" sobriety to see how it feels. This lets clients commit to a specified try-out period and retain the option to revisit the matter later. This kind of approach can also provide the client with an opportunity to gain confidence about reaching the initial goal and gives you time to foster a therapeutic alliance, both of which are factors that can increase a client's receptiveness to treatment (DeWeert-Van Oene et al., 2001).

Assessing and Addressing Barriers to Adherence

Attention to adherence begins, ideally, with the very first contact. An assessment can be a simple conversation or a more structured interview, the purpose of which is to explore practical barriers as well as motivators for treatment engagement (Zweben & Zuckoff, 2002). A primary focus here is to understand what services the client needs and wants (see Chapter 7). Also consider clients' practical barriers to participation such as a need for transportation, child care arrangements, flexible appointments, and housing assistance. Case management services may be needed to stabilize their living situations in order to engage them in treatment (see Chapter 8). People with co-occurring disorders (Chapter 18) may require stabilization via psychotropic medication to facilitate their engagement. Those whose social networks revolve around substance use may need help in building a social support system for sobriety to persist in treatment (Liddle, 2004).

Consider whether what you (or your program) have to offer is consistent with the person's needs, hopes, and expectations for treatment. A clash of expectations often leads to adherence problems. Some individuals initially want to cut down on their drinking and are alienated by a program that only supports lifelong abstinence. Some may be willing to take medication but don't want behavioral therapy, whereas for others the reverse is true. Some folks are uncomfortable with groups, and others prefer them. It matters what's on the treatment menu and how much flexibility you have in individualizing treatment plans.

> It matters what's on the treatment menu and how much flexibility you have in individualizing treatment plans.

Conducting a Role Induction Interview

Another method to stave off potential adherence problems is a role induction interview. Role induction is an effective method to reduce misunderstanding and misperceptions of treatment and obtain a mutual agreement about the treatment situation (Zweben & Li, 1981). It entails informing about and clarifying issues related to the content, length, and frequency of sessions; explaining the roles/responsibilities of clients and counselors; and discussing potential obstacles that may interfere with the completion of treatment. This can include handouts and pamphlets giving details such as appointment times, contact person, fees, insurance coverage, and emergency coverage. It is also possible to provide this orientation via videotape or former clients. Ascertain how the individual's own perceptions and expectations square with the information being presented. Such an approach helps to clarify misperceptions on the part of clients which in turn enables you to establish a viable treatment contract. When multiple treatment options are available (rather than a single program for all clients), this orientation can describe the menu of options.

Again, it is important to take a nonjudgmental, collaborative stance with clients to forge a therapeutic alliance. Encourage clients to express differences between what you have described and what they want and expect from treatment. This helps to reduce client distrust and enables you

BOX 17.1. Personal Reflection: Is Double-Booking a Good Way to Deal with Adherence Problems?

When I teach students about treatment adherence, I often begin the discussion explaining how I became interested in adherence issues. "Noncompliance" was once considered the norm in addiction treatment settings. Having clients who arrive late for treatment sessions or don't show up, cancel appointments without rebooking, and abruptly terminate treatment was just expected, and it was thought that we could do little to change the problem. People with addictions were seen as an unmotivated, difficult, "hard-to-reach" group who were unable or unwilling to effectively engage in treatment. Practitioners would therefore schedule two or more clients for the same time period, with the expectation that at best one might show up for the scheduled appointment.

Such was the case when I became the chief social worker in a large multidisciplinary addiction treatment center. Our staff attributed high dropout rates to "the addictive personality": manipulative, deceitful, and untrustworthy people who were in denial about their problem. The normative view was that clients would tell you what you wanted to hear about change, but what they really wanted was to drink and use drugs. Attending treatment was just a ruse to satisfy an angry spouse or employer. Some practitioners also expected very little from clients because of their "counterdependency" problems, or being incapable of handling a close relationship. (It is a great pleasure now to have incredulous audiences ask me, "No one ever *really* believed that, did they?").

As a program administrator, I decided to address the adherence problem. Working with two recently hired staff members, we read the literature on motivation and decision making and became convinced that we could change the status quo. True, many clients were pressured to enter treatment by family members, employers, and friends. Many were uncertain about whether their drinking or drug use was serious enough to warrant formal treatment. We thought that staff may have been mistakenly attributing this to pernicious personality traits, rather than to understandable ambivalence, and guessed that disagreements with staff about the seriousness of clients' problems may partially explain why so many were dropping out. (Of course, it also didn't help that clients would show up for appointments and not be seen because of double-booking.)

Suppose that instead of arguing about severity, we conducted a comprehensive evaluation? We started by adopting a set of reliable and valid assessment measures such as the time line followback (see Chapter 5). After this careful evaluation, we offered clients objective feedback based on their own responses. We hoped that doing so in a supportive, consultative (rather than confrontive) manner would help clients to take an honest look at their alcohol/drug use, increasing their awareness and motivation for change. We taped our sessions, reviewing them together and discussing how we could improve our practice with clients. Over time this led to a variety of methods for enhancing adherence, which I termed "facilitative strategies" (Zweben et al., 1988), some of which became part of the motivational enhancement therapy (see Chapter 10) developed and tested in multisite trials (Longabaugh, Zweben, et al., 2005; Miller, Zweben, et al., 1992; Project MATCH Research Group, 1993).

—A. Z.

to establish a mutuality of expectations about what will be happening in treatment, thereby reducing the likelihood of premature dropout. Having common expectations improves retention.

Preventing and Responding to Missed Appointments

"No shows" or missed appointments are common in addiction treatment, and there are several beneficial ways to prevent or respond to this situation (Carroll, 1997a). One way is to provide clients with a calendar listing scheduled appointment dates. Ask clients to keep the schedule in a familiar place as a reminder. As with medical or dental appointments, you can also ask support staff to call clients a day or two before the scheduled visit to remind them about the forthcoming session.

If a client misses a session without canceling, it is important to follow up with a call to determine what happened and facilitate continued engagement. It is best if you, rather than support staff, do this. The basic components of the call are to (1) express your regard and concern for the client, (2) briefly explore with empathy and acceptance the reasons for the missed appointment, and (3) state your desire to see the person again and reschedule. Consider following up this telephone contact with a handwritten, personalized note summarizing what you said.

In the next session spend some time exploring further the reasons for not attending. Ask whether not attending might reflect a change in motivation, resumption of alcohol/drug use, emergence of new problems, or some specific concern about treatment. Be careful not to sound judgmental or moralizing about the missed session. Normalize client concerns (e.g., "Many people feel uncomfortable at first discussing personal problems with someone who is not a family member"). At the same time, affirm the clients' willingness to discuss obstacles that interfere with attendance.

Before the session ends, explore potential or future difficulties that may arise in attending sessions. Negotiate a plan for dealing with these. End the session by expressing your regard for the client and optimism for change.

Detecting "Early Warning Signs"

A sizeable proportion of clients do not stick with their original treatment plan. Willingness to take certain steps (e.g., taking medication, attending mutual help meetings, avoiding high-risk situations) may increase or decrease. Significant life changes can disrupt original plans, and failing to detect and address these adherence difficulties can lead to resumption of drinking or drug use, which in turn may lead to abrupt withdrawal from treatment.

An early signal of emerging adherence problems can be missed or cancelled visits or arriving late for sessions. Another warning sign can be increased defensiveness or evasiveness, which can be manifested in persistently talking about irrelevant issues ("chatting"). Attending to such signs may prevent premature dropout. Case monitoring (Chapter 8) can be helpful here. Ask whether these possible warning signs may be connected to other problems or concerns the client is having. Discussing these matters openly and directly may reduce future nonadherence, facilitating trust and change (Stout et al., 1999). Case management can also help stabilize the clients' living situation so that they can attend treatment. In some cases it may be helpful to involve family members or supportive others to facilitate the client's participation in treatment.

A particularly good approach for detecting early warning signs is to ask clients to provide ongoing feedback after each visit. The Outcome Questionaire and the briefer Outcome Rating Scale are simple client feedback tools with well-established reliability and predictive validity (Bringhurst, Watson, Miller, & Duncan, 2006; Lambert et al., 1996). Comparing clients' ratings from session to session can alert you to a perceived lack of progress, and obtaining such regular feedback has been shown to improve both retention and outcome (Lambert et al., 2001; Miller, Duncan, Brown, Sorrell, & Chalk, 2006; Miller, Duncan, Sorrell, & Brown, 2005). Client feedback scales can be obtained free of charge from *www.talkingcure.com*, and by registering at *www.scottdmiller.com/?q=node/6*.

Involving Concerned Significant Others

The community reinforcement and family training (CRAFT) approach described in Chapter 13 is another way to encourage adherence. Concerned significant others (CSOs) can have quite a positive effect on treatment engagement and retention when taught how best to make use of their influence (Meyers & Smith, 1995; Meyers & Wolfe, 2004; Smith & Meyers, 2004). The value of CSOs is not limited to initial treatment engagement. It can also be very helpful to include CSOs in treatment sessions (see Chapter 13). Involved CSOs can facilitate client retention and adherence and thereby improve outcomes (Burke, Vassilev, Kantchelov, & Zweben, 2002; Soyez, DeLeon, Broekaert, & Rosseel, 2006; Zweben, 1991). The CSO can support client motivation by offering constructive feedback and encouragement, recognizing and reinforcing positive changes, and directly participating in adherence plans (see Chapter 11). Involving family members can also reveal important other problems that need to be addressed either in treatment (e.g., Chapter 13) or by intensive case management (Chapter 8).

Using Incentives

As discussed in Chapter 10, the use of monetary incentives or vouchers has proven to be a useful tool in achieving and maintaining treatment adherence. Providing cash or vouchers that are exchangeable for food and other items (e.g., bus tokens, gas coupons, and other goods or services) can significantly increase treatment retention, adherence, and outcomes (Hamilton et al., 2007). Incentives have been used successfully to promote negative urine specimens or taking daily doses of disulfuram (Garcia-Rodriguez et al., 2009; Higgins et al., 1994; Petry, Martin, Cooney, & Kranzler, 2000; Petry et al., 2005). Monetary incentives have been effectively used in treating opiate- (Bickel et al., 1997), marijuana- (Budney, Higgins, Radonovich, & Novy, 2000), and stimulant-dependent clients (Carey & Carey, 1990; Higgins et al., 1994; Killeen, Carter, Copersino, Petry, & Stitzer, 2007).

We recognize that providing concrete incentives can clash with a particular agency's philosophy of serving clients. Such an approach may be seen as "bribing" or "manipulating" clients, or as too costly. It is fairly clear, however, that positive reinforcement in the form of motivational incentives can be quite effective in increasing treatment retention and adherence (Petry et al., 2005; Stitzer et al., 2007), which in turn improve client outcomes. Newer incentive strategies, such as draws from a fishbowl for prizes, appear to be equally effective and considerably less expensive, and can be fun to implement (Hamilton et al., 2007). We therefore encourage you to consider how such incentives might enhance retention and adherence in your own setting.

KEY POINTS

🔱 Regardless of the treatment approach being used, client adherence is a good predictor of change. Taking steps matters.

🔱 Client adherence is highly responsive to counseling style and program milieu.

🔱 Adherence problems often reflect a clash of client goals and preferences with program characteristics and counselor style.

🔱 Clients who have a choice among options are more likely to stay and participate actively in treatment.

🔱 It is important to detect and respond to early warning signs of adherence problems.

REFLECTION QUESTIONS

Q There can be large differences among providers in what percentage of
   their clients drop out versus remain in treatment. What do you think
   accounts for these differences?

Q From the *client's* perspective, what considerations are most likely to
   influence the extent to which he or she adheres to treatment advice?

Q If you were assigned to train new counselors in how to improve
   retention and adherence among their clients, what would you teach
   them?

CHAPTER 18

Treating Co-Occurring Disorders

In the context of addiction treatment, the term "co-occurring disorders" (like "dual diagnosis" and "comorbidity") refers to the simultaneous presence of at least two different diagnosable conditions, one of which is a substance use disorder (e.g., alcohol dependence and depression). In treating addictions, you are sure to encounter a broad range of concomitant conditions since having a substance use disorder significantly increases the prevalence of other disorders (Mueser, 2004). In a typical addiction treatment population, roughly half will also have another significant mental disorder (Grant et al., 2004; Ouimette, Gima, Moos, & Finney, 1999; U.S. Department of Health and Human Services, 1999). Anxiety and mood disorders are particularly common. The prevalence of co-occurring mental health and substance use issues is so high in behavioral health services that co-occurring disorders are the norm rather than the exception (Mueser & Drake, 2007).

The same is true in mental health services. Substance use disorders are the second most common DSM diagnosis in the general population (after depression), and the most frequent co-occurring disorder among people with a serious mental illness, a category that includes bipolar disorder, schizophrenia, and severe depression. In both epidemiological surveys and studies of clinical populations, about half of individuals diagnosed with schizophrenia also develop a co-occurring substance use disorder at some point in their lifetime (Cantor-Graae, Nordström, & McNeil, 2001; Margolese, Malchy, Negrete, Tempier, & Gill, 2004; Regier et al., 1990; Swartz et al., 2006), and this concurrence rate may be increasing (Kessler & Merikangas, 2004). The good news is that effective treatment for substance use can improve the course of the co-occurring mental disorder (Smelson et al., 2008).

Which comes first? Is the substance use a cause or a result of the mental disorder, or do both result from some third factor? All of these are possibilities. The two disorders may be independent of each other, or one may be secondary to another and subside after the primary disorder is treated. Some clinicians try to determine which emerged first in time, although this can be challenging and still does not resolve the question of independence.

A point of clear agreement, however, is that the combination of two disorders is generally more serious than either disorder alone (Kessler, 1995). When substance use and mental disorder co-occur, the course of each problem area is worsened (Swann, 2010). Co-occurring disorders each tend to be more severe and have a greater effect on clients' quality of life than does a single diagnosis (Burns & Teesson, 2002; Kessler, 1995). Among those with severe mental illness, substance use problems are associated with more frequent psychosocial consequences such as legal, housing, financial, and health problems (McLellan, Luborsky, Woody, O'Brien, & Druley, 1983). The presence of a co-occurring substance use disorder may also affect symptomatology in people diagnosed with a severe mental illness (Talamo et al., 2006). Treating those with co-occurring disorders is certainly more challenging than treating people with a single disorder.

WHY ARE CO-OCCURRING DISORDERS SO COMMON?

The Self-Medication Hypothesis

One of the most popular explanations for co-occurring disorders is the self-medication hypothesis: that people are using alcohol, tobacco, or other drugs in an attempt to manage their psychiatric symptoms. This explanation has a certain intuitive appeal in that these drugs are psychoactive, and indeed many people report that substance use offers them some symptom relief (e.g., "It helps me relax and forget my problems"). It would seem to follow logically that people with depressive symptoms would prefer stimulants, and those with anxiety symptoms would choose more anxiolytic substances. Research findings, however, do not support such clear associations between the person's symptoms and the types of substances used. Drugs of choice tend to be influenced more by peers, and use persists despite fluctuations in symptoms over time (Mueser et al., 2006). In addition, many people report continuing use despite their clear awareness that the drug actually makes their psychiatric symptoms worse. This is just a specific example of the more general puzzle of addictions: that people persist in use in the face of clear adverse consequences.

Although the self-medication hypothesis doesn't seem to be a satisfactory general explanation for comorbidity, it still may be correct in specific cases and is worth considering. Perhaps the more general question is what is motivating someone with a concomitant disorder to use particular substances. Even if drug use does not directly alleviate psychiatric symptoms, it may be motivated by fun or excitement, escape, or to facilitate social interactions. It is not necessary that the drug actually yields the desired effect, but only that the person believes it does so. Alcohol, for example, tends to produce both stimulant and depressant effects depending on dose and time since consumption (Holdstock & de Wit, 1998). Within this *biphasic* effect, drinkers may remember (and drink for) the earlier stimulant effects, with selective forgetting of the depressive rebound that occurs later and with higher doses. A list of perceived motivations for drinking is shown in Box 18.1. In any event, attempting to self-medicate psychiatric symptoms does not seem to account for the high rates of comorbidity.

> It is not necessary that the drug actually yields the desired effect, but only that the person believes it does so.

Supersensitivity to Alcohol and Other Drugs

Another hypothesis suggests that people with co-occurring disorders may have a biological *diathesis*, a vulnerability that increases their likelihood for developing a psychiatric disorder. Gene expression interacts with a person's environment, and if certain stressors are present, then the person will develop the disorder. In this case, the "stressor" is exposure to the effects of certain psychoactive drugs. It is further hypothesized that people with such psychiatric vulnerability may be particularly sensitive to the effects of certain drugs. In this case, even use at a level that might be considered low to moderate could trigger psychiatric problems (Mueser et al., 2006). The reasons for such vulnerability are not yet understood.

An anecdotal example is a person who experiences a first psychotic episode during or after taking a hallucinogenic drug. The vulnerability was there, but symptoms were triggered by the drug experience. This in turn may have a *kindling* effect such that experiencing a first episode places the person at increased risk for further or more severe episodes—something that appears to be true of major depression (Muñoz et al., 2009) and alcohol withdrawal-induced seizures (Becker, 1998; Becker & Hale, 1993). Seizures are also associated with increased risk for psychosis (Smith & Darlington, 1996). Given these factors, people with serious mental illness seem to reach a threshold for serious negative consequences of substance use at a much lower level than others (Mueser et al., 2006). The essential idea here is that substance use triggers expression of a genetic vulnerability.

BOX 18.1. Desired Effects of Drinking

Tracy L. Simpson, PhD, Judith A. Arroyo, PhD, William R. Miller, PhD, and Laura M. Little, PhD

Drinking alcohol can have many different effects. What results or effects have you wanted from drinking alcohol *during the past 3 months?* Read each effect/result of drinking on the left and indicate how much this was an effect of drinking you *wanted* during the past 3 months.

During the past 3 months, how often did you want this effect from drinking alcohol?	Never 0	Sometimes 1	Frequently 2	Always 3
1. to enjoy the taste	0	1	2	3
2. to feel more creative	0	1	2	3
3. to change my mood	0	1	2	3
4. to relieve pressure or tension	0	1	2	3
5. to be sociable	0	1	2	3
6. to get drunk or intoxicated	0	1	2	3
7. to feel more powerful	0	1	2	3
8. to feel more romantic	0	1	2	3
9. to feel less depressed	0	1	2	3
10. to feel less disappointed in myself	0	1	2	3
11. to be more mentally alert	0	1	2	3
12. to feel good	0	1	2	3
13. to be able to avoid thoughts or feelings associated with a bad experience	0	1	2	3
14. to feel more comfortable in social situations	0	1	2	3
15. to get over a hangover	0	1	2	3
16. to feel brave and capable of fighting	0	1	2	3
17. to be a better lover	0	1	2	3
18. to control my anger	0	1	2	3
19. to feel less angry with myself	0	1	2	3
20. to be able to think better	0	1	2	3
21. to celebrate	0	1	2	3
22. to control painful memories of a bad experience	0	1	2	3

(cont.)

From Miller (2004). This instrument is in the public domain and may be reproduced without further permission. For psychometrics, consult Doyle et al. (in press).

BOX 18.1. *(cont.)*

During the past 3 months, how often did you want this effect from drinking alcohol?	Never 0	Sometimes 1	Frequently 2	Always 3
23. to be able to meet people	0	1	2	3
24. to sleep	0	1	2	3
25. to be able to express anger	0	1	2	3
26. to feel more sexually excited	0	1	2	3
27. to feel less shame	0	1	2	3
28. to feel more satisfied with myself	0	1	2	3
29. to be able to work or concentrate better	0	1	2	3
30. to relax	0	1	2	3
31. to forget about problems	0	1	2	3
32. to have a good time	0	1	2	3
33. to stop the shakes or tremors	0	1	2	3
34. to be able to find the courage to do things that are risky	0	1	2	3
35. to enjoy sex more	0	1	2	3
36. to reduce fears	0	1	2	3
37. to feel less guilty	0	1	2	3

SCORING INFORMATION

Sum the scores for these four items in each scale:

	Scale	Items				Totals
A	Assertion	7	16	25	34	
D	Drug Effects	6	15	24	33	
M	Mental	2	11	20	29	
N	Negative Feelings	9	18	27	36	
P	Positive Feelings	3	12	21	30	
R	Relief	4	13	22	31	
S	Self-Esteem	10	19	28	37	
SE	Sexual Enhancement	8	17	26	35	
SF	Social Facilitation	5	14	23	32	
	Total Score					

Common Factors

A third hypothesis regarding comorbidity is that an underlying vulnerability independently increases the risk for both the addiction and the psychiatric disorder. This third factor might be familial, social, environmental, neurocognitive, or genetic and could likely vary from person to person, even for those who develop the same disorders. One example of a proposed common factor is neurocognitive impairment of self-regulation. Generalized self-regulatory deficits that are observable in the first decade of life predict a host of later problems and diagnoses including substance use disorders (Brown, 1998; Diaz & Fruhauf, 1991; Miller & Brown, 1991; Tarter et al., 2003). A common neurocognitive vulnerability may underlie risk for antisocial personality disorder, psychosis, and substance use disorders (Mueser et al., 2006).

A variety of other common vulnerability factors have been proposed. For instance, environmental stressors such as abuse and trauma (Simpson & Miller, 2002), poverty, or deprivation may predispose people to developing both psychiatric and substance use disorders. Another example would be emotional blunting. There is evidence that individuals with antisocial personality disorder may not experience negative consequences as intensely as people without antisocial personality disorder, and if so, the prospect of adverse consequences might not be as great a deterrent (Miranda, Meyerson, Myers, & Lovallo, 2003). This underlying emotional blunting may be the common factor that underlies childhood conduct disorder and adult antisocial personality disorder.

Evidence does not support genetic factors as an explanation for increased rates of co-occurring disorders. Apart from the genetic factors that have been studied fairly extensively, most of the proposed common factors have not been examined empirically.

In sum, various hypotheses have been proposed to explain co-occurring disorders, and the evidence thus far does not support any one of these as the whole story. Chances are that each contains some element of truth. The continuation of science in this area may yield new insights that inform treatment. In the meantime, much is already known about how to help people with concomitant disorders.

WHAT DISORDERS ARE OVERREPRESENTED?

One thing that we do know is that certain disorders are overrepresented in people with substance use disorders. Some of the most common co-occurring problems are mood disorders (major depression, bipolar disorder), anxiety disorders (posttraumatic stress disorder [PTSD], generalized anxiety disorder, panic disorder), thought disorders (schizophrenia and schizoaffective disorder), and personality disorders (borderline personality and antisocial personality). We briefly consider each of these diagnostic groups and key issues and concerns that they can raise in addiction treatment.

Mood Disorders

The most common concomitance is that of substance use with mood disorders, particularly among women (Lyne, O'Donoghue, Clancy, & O'Gara, 2011).

> The most common concomitance is substance use with mood disorders.

Approximately 25% of people with alcohol dependence and 50% of those with drug dependence have current co-occurring depression (Grant et al., 2005). About 60% of those with bipolar disorder also meet criteria for a substance use disorder (Regier et al., 1990).

A diagnostic complication is that the effects of intoxication and detoxification include mood disturbance. Dysphoria, for example, can result from alcohol or other depressant drug use, or from cessation of stimulants. Stimulant-induced episodes of mania can include paranoid symptoms that last from hours to days. Since nearly all psychoactive drugs have some effect on mood, it is unsurprising to find mood disturbances associated with alcohol/drug use and withdrawal.

It is a mistake, however, to assume that mood disturbances are merely secondary to substance use. Independent mood disorders are common in addiction treatment populations and may appear, persist, or worsen with abstinence. Drug use in turn can exacerbate the swings of affective disorders, specifically the highs of mania and the lows of depression. In almost all studies of completed or attempted suicide, alcohol or drug use and major depression are among the top associated conditions. Having both conditions simultaneously leads to one of the highest statistical risks for suicide. When you are working with someone who suffers from a mood disorder and addiction, it is important to assess and reassess danger to self or others since the use of psychoactive substances can lower inhibitions and result in impulsive action.

Anxiety Disorders

Like mood disorders, anxiety disorders are among the most common co-occurring conditions affecting people with substance use disorders. Anxiety disorders can be diagnosed in approximately 25% of alcohol-dependent individuals and about 40% of those who are drug-dependent (Grant et al., 2005). Psychoactive drugs can increase psychomotor stimulation and manifestations of anxiety including generalized anxiety and panic attacks. Anxiety symptoms that are merely alcohol- or drug-induced and withdrawal-related anxiety usually resolve within a few days or weeks.

Again, it is unwise to assume that anxiety symptoms are merely side effects of substance use. Independent anxiety disorders co-occur with addictions at a much elevated rate, as does a history of child abuse, trauma, and PTSD (Simpson & Miller, 2002). Substance use may be motivated by a desire to manage, avoid, or escape from the suffering related to anxiety disorders. Short-acting sedatives are used in this way, either with or without prescription. Benzodiazepines reduce symptoms of panic disorder with agoraphobia. The effects of such medications wear off quickly, however, and the rebound effects can increase anxiety. The same can occur with alcohol. This in turn can cause people to believe they need more frequent and higher doses. If medicating is the only means clients know for managing anxiety symptoms, they are vulnerable to resumed use when encountering even normal life stressors.

Thought Disorders

Among people with a lifetime diagnosis of schizophrenia or schizophreniform disorder, almost half have also met criteria for an alcohol/drug use disorder (Grant et al., 2005). Again there can be confusion as to whether psychotic symptoms represent a primary psychiatric disorder or are secondary to substance use or withdrawal. Symptoms of substance intoxication and withdrawal can strongly mimic symptoms of thought disorders, including hallucinations, paranoia, agitation, or delirium. These tend to resolve relatively quickly. Yet it is important to be alert for independent thought disorders that preceded substance use or persist well into abstinence. As discussed above, it is also possible for drug use to trigger the first episode of what becomes an independent disorder.

People with acute psychotic symptoms are most likely to be taken to mental health facilities, but may also present in addiction treatment systems. The first priority is typically to stabilize the crisis and determine whether the person needs emergency medical care, psychiatric hospitalization, or detoxification. Often, people with psychoses are experiencing social issues such as homelessness or housing instability, victimization, poor nutrition, and poverty, and immediate crises may need to be addressed. You should also assess the risk of danger to self or others, considering any current hallucinations or thought disorders.

A thorough assessment should follow as soon as feasible. Collateral information from family or significant others is especially important if the person's speech and thought patterns are disorganized and his or her ability to give a history is impaired. Find out if there is a history of significant medical disorders, loss of consciousness or head trauma, and psychiatric treatment.

Personality Disorders

People with Cluster B personality disorders (American Psychiatric Association, 2000) have the highest incidence of concomitant substance use disorders. Personality disorders are diagnosable in about half of all alcohol-dependent clients and in 7 of 10 drug-dependent clients (Grant et al., 2005). Likely because of the impulsivity of this population, the most common co-occurring personality disorder among substance using clients is antisocial personality disorder, found in about 20% of alcohol-dependent patients and 40% of drug-dependent clients, followed by borderline personality disorder (Grant et al., 2005).

Individuals with antisocial or borderline personality display impulsive behaviors, and when combined with substance use, this can be dangerous. Because of this increased impulsivity, there is also an increase in high-risk behaviors. Chaotic patterns of substance use are typical in this population and increase the likelihood of risks including infection from unprotected sex or contaminated needles.

Avoiding Misdiagnosis

Across these areas there is a common issue of sorting out the effects of drug use and withdrawal from those of co-occurring disorders (McKetin, Hickey, Devlin, & Lawrence, 2010). This process can involve considerable skill in differential diagnosis, and provisional diagnoses are appropriate earlier in the evaluation process, given the number of diagnoses that can be mimicked by drug effects (see Box 18.2). An early question is differentiating substance-induced conditions (resulting from intoxication or withdrawal) from concomitant disorders that exist independent of the substance use disorder. A diagnosis of a separate (not substance-induced) disorder is clearest when there was evidence of symptoms prior to the onset of substance use, if symptoms persist for a month or more after acute withdrawal, or the symptoms are in excess of what would be expected given the type and amount of substance used.

Waiting until the withdrawal process has fully subsided is one approach to differential diagnosis and gives perhaps the clearest indication of what additional conditions may require clinical attention. It is possible, of course, that persisting problems are severe enough during the first month to require a more rapid clinical decision and treatment, particularly if symptoms are worsening. After initial stabilization, it is usually easier to construct a time line of when substance use and psychiatric symptoms began. What was the person's quality of life during substance-free periods? Meeting diagnostic criteria for a disorder prior to the onset of substance use is strong evidence for an independent disorder. Remember, however, that onset during sub-

BOX 18.2. Drug Effects That Can Mimic Mental Disorders

	Some Possible Psychiatric Symptoms during:		
	Intoxication	**Acute Withdrawal**	**Protracted Withdrawal**
Alcohol	• Euphoria • Mood lability • Disinhibition • Slurred speech	• Agitation • Anxiety • Tremors • Insomnia • Hallucinations • Delirium	• Mood instability • Hostility • Fatigue • Low sexual interest • Sleep disturbance
Stimulants	• Euphoria • Impulsivity • Grandiosity • Paranoia • Rapid pressured speech	• Depression • Fatigue • Agitation • Sleep disturbances	• Anhedonia • Lethargy • Dysphoria • Anxiety
Hallucinogens	• Sensory dissociation • Visual hallucinations • Panic • Paranoia • Delusions	• Anxiety • Delirium	• Depression • Flashbacks
Cannabis	• Euphoria • Agitation • Lethargy • Grandiosity (high doses) • Perceptual distortions	• Irritability • Depression • Anxiety	• Irritability • Depression • Anxiety
Inhalants	• Euphoria • Slurred speech • Psychomotor retardation	• Insomnia • Agitation • Anxiety • Hallucinations	• Anxiety • Depression • Irritability
Sedatives	• Euphoria • Disinhibition • Mood lability • Slurred speech	• Mood instability • Depression • Anxiety • Insomnia • Hyperactivity	• Anxiety • Depression • Perceptual distortions • Depersonalization
Opioids	• Euphoria • Indifference • Apathy	• Agitation • Irritability • Anxiety • Depression • Anhedonia • Insomnia • Delirium	• Anxiety • Depression • Sleep disturbance

From Sacks and Ries (2005).

stance use does not rule out an independent disorder (e.g., the first episode of which may have been triggered by substance use).

APPROACHES TO TREATING CO-OCCURRING DISORDERS
Quadrant Model

The quadrant model offers a framework for conceptualizing subgroups of individuals with co-occurring disorders by understanding the severity of each disorder (McGovern, Clark, & Samnaliev, 2007). Four different subgroups correspond to combinations of high and low severity of psychiatric disorders and substance use. The theory behind the quadrant model is that those who differ in the severity of their addiction and psychiatric disorders have different treatment needs and may require different treatment settings.

		Psychiatric severity	
		Low	High
Substance use severity	Low	I	II
	High	III	IV

   • *Quadrant I.* These individuals display low severity of both substance use and psychiatric illness. It is typical for people in this quadrant to be treated in nonspecialist settings, with specialist (e.g., psychiatric, psychological, or addiction) consultation as needed.

   • *Quadrant II.* These individuals display low substance use severity and high psychiatric illness severity. Services for individuals who fall in this quadrant are typically provided in mental health settings. A collaborative or integrated model is preferred, in which substance use and mental health service providers work in tandem or where services are blended with a single team of providers.

   • *Quadrant III.* These individuals have high substance use and low psychiatric severity. Services for people in this quadrant have been offered primarily in addiction treatment settings. Similar to Quadrant II, a collaborative or integrated model is preferred, in which substance use and mental health service providers work in tandem or where services are blended with a single team of providers.

   • *Quadrant IV.* People in this quadrant have severe substance use and severe mental illness. They may be seen in mental health clinics or hospitals, correctional facilities, and emergency departments. They may also be bounced back and forth between mental health and addiction treatment facilities. It is for people in this quadrant that an integrated service model is most indicated.

Integrated Treatment Models

The problem of deciding where to send people from each quadrant stems from the fact that treatment for substance use disorders historically has been isolated from other health care systems. It has been relatively rare for specialist addiction treatment services even to be colocated with mental health or primary care systems. Thus referring agents, clients, and their families have had to choose which system to access. This has resulted in referrals back and forth, sequential treatment of one and then the other problem, or at best parallel treatment within different systems. Some people would enter treatment through mental health services, and when it was discovered that substance use was also part of the clinical picture, they might be referred to an addiction treatment program to resolve that problem first. Many such referrals were not completed because of client reluctance or practical barriers such as waiting lists.

The problem of isolated treatment for different disorders is also in part a function of professional specialization. For decades, substance use disorders in the United States were treated primarily by specialist counselors whose training and expertise were focused on addictions. Educational requirements (as well as salaries and status) were lower for addiction counselors than for professionals working in other health care settings, including mental health. As recently as the first decade of the 21st century, it was controversial in state laws whether even a bachelor's degree should be required for addiction counselors—a contention that would be unthinkable for the treatment of virtually any other life-threatening illness. Conversely, those trained in mainstream mental health professions such as psychology, psychiatry, and social work rarely received adequate preparation, training, or even encouragement to treat addictions, one of the most common disorders they would encounter throughout their careers (Miller & Brown, 1997). In most other developed nations, substance use disorders have been addressed by mainstream health care professionals. The professionalization of addiction treatment has been occurring in the United States as well, both with gradually increasing educational and training standards for addiction counselors and with greater inclusion of addiction training in medicine and mental health professions. "Behavioral health" has come to describe expertise and services in both addiction and mental health, and addiction specializations and journals have emerged within health professions including psychology, psychiatry, social work, and nursing.

Since the 1980s, integrated outpatient or day treatment programs have emerged for people with co-occurring severe disorders (Quadrants III or IV), which combine services within a single system of care. Integrated residential facilities have also been developed (Drake, Mueser, Brunette, & McHugo, 2004).

Integrated treatment models combining mental health and addiction services are optimal in addressing co-occurring disorders (Horsfall, Cleary, Hunt, & Walter, 2009; Weiss & Connery, 2011). Unlike parallel treatment, integrated treatment uses the same team of providers combining mental health and addiction treatments in the same setting to offer coordinated care. The uncertainty surrounding etiology and clinical presentation hints at the complexity of co-occurring disorders: they are so intertwined that it makes sense to deal with them simultaneously rather than try to isolate which symptoms should be treated by whom. By having the same treatment providers in one centralized location, treatment-related stress is minimized and engagement and retention is increased.

Integrated dual disorder treatment (IDDT) is designed for people with co-occurring disorders as a way to address both disorders simultaneously, in the same clinic, and by the same team of treatment providers. The multidisciplinary team meets regularly to discuss the person's progress and coordinate all aspects of recovery. Different services are offered at different stages of treatment. For example, for someone ambivalent about engaging in treatment, the focus is on providing practical help, outreach, and crisis intervention. As a way to build an alliance with clients, clinicians engage in assertive outreach in the community where a client lives. As clients progress through stages of IDDT they are given access to comprehensive services including case management, substance abuse and mental health counseling, medical services, supported employment, and family services. Continuous access to services is one feature that sets IDDT apart from other interventions. People are able to receive services throughout their lifespan, even when symptoms are mild or infrequent (essentially a primary care model). Staying connected with the care system is an important aim in itself; people are not discharged if they stop taking their medications or continue using substances. IDDT essentially mirrors a chronic disease management approach.

An integrated approach seems to work well across the board for concomitant substance use and psychiatric disorders with one potential exception: people with antisocial personality disorder (ASPD). A recent study (Frisman et al., 2009) suggested that people with ASPD benefit when assertive community treatment (ACT) is added to IDDT, showing greater reduction in alcohol use and incarceration than with IDDT alone. For people without ASPD, IDDT worked equally well with or without the addition of ACT.

So what is ACT (Horsfall, Cleary, & Hunt, 2010)? It is a more intensive treatment approach developed particularly for helping people with more severe disorders function in the community. A significant difference between ACT and other treatment models is that ACT takes treatment to the person rather than always asking the person to come in for treatment. The goal of ACT is to help people avoid crisis situations in the first place or, if that proves impossible, to intervene quickly at any time of the day or night to keep crises from turning into unnecessary hospitalizations. Another way ACT differs from IDDT is the inclusion of peer support specialists as part of the multidisciplinary team. These individuals have had personal successful experience with the recovery process and can offer a variety of recovery approaches from their own lived experience of receiving services.

Some Helpful Perspectives

Following are some points to consider particularly when working with people with co-occurring disorders. They are also useful perspectives in addiction treatment more generally, but can be especially helpful with concomitant disorders in all four quadrants.

1. Think of recovery as something positive beyond the disorders, just as peace is more than the absence of war and health more than the absence of illness. What are the person's broader goals and values (see Chapter 21)? What would "recovery" or a "good life" mean to this person? Some continuing symptoms are likely, and are not incompatible with a path of recovery.

> Think of recovery as something positive beyond the disorders.

2. Because of possible cognitive difficulties, give smaller bits of information and use some repetition, particularly by presenting the same thing in different ways or by giving specific examples. It can be helpful to use a behavioral approach in which you first demonstrate the behavior to be learned, then have the client practice during the session. This way you can offer suggestions and troubleshoot any difficulties the person is having with the new skill. Another suggestion is to break down goals into smaller concrete steps in the right direction. If a client is interested in attending a self-help meeting, for example, a goal of "go to one meeting this week" might be too big. Instead, break the goal down into smaller steps such as (1) find the list of self-help groups in town, (2) look at meeting times to find a time that would work with my schedule, (3) go to the meeting. Asking questions to ensure that the person is actively processing the information and frequently reviewing the material are other ways to help clients who may have cognitive difficulties.

3. Empower clients, within a broad perspective of helping them to self-manage their symptoms. Educating and involving the family, caregivers, and SOs is also important as a way to promote understanding of the symptoms and effects of mental illness, substance use, and the medications

used in treatment. Such involvement and support for the family can also reduce their stress. Organizations such as the National Alliance on Mental Ilness (NAMI) offer support and outreach to family members affected by mental illness.

4. Mutual help groups can be an important adjunct to treatment. Particularly explore groups that are specifically designed for people with concomitant disorders. Groups such as Double Trouble in Recovery (DTR) can provide greater acceptance, understanding, and support than may be encountered in addiction-focused groups. A significant benefit of DTR (as compared to traditional 12-step programs) is the increased understanding of the importance of managing psychiatric conditions through the use of pharmacotherapy. DTR groups tend to encourage clients to practice adherence to their medications. Participation in DTR groups can have both direct and indirect beneficial effects on several important components of recovery, including medication adherence, abstinence, and quality of life (Magura, 2008).

THE USE OF PSYCHIATRIC MEDICATIONS

Some counselors or mutual help groups have been skeptical about or even opposed to the use of psychiatric medications in addiction recovery. This issue is still somewhat controversial on the front lines of addiction treatment, though there is evidence that it is changing. The opposition to the use of psychiatric medications in addiction treatment arose in part from a confusion of therapeutic medications with drugs of abuse (since there is indeed some overlap), and in part from a sense that people ought to be able to recover on their own without relying on chemicals. The same argument was not made regarding insulin for people with diabetes, or for medications to reduce blood pressure and cholesterol, but ambivalence has been greater about psychoactive medications, even among clients themselves.

There is a large difference between an unprescribed drug used to get high and a medication taken as directed to manage a diagnosed disorder. Many psychiatric medications have little abuse potential or street value. Effective medications are available and are an important component of treatment for severe mental disorders including psychoses (such as schizophrenia), mood disorders (like major depression and bipolar disorder), and anxiety disorders (such as PTSD, panic disorder, and generalized anxiety disorder). It is, we believe, unethical to deny such effective treatment options to people suffering from mental disorders because they also have a concomitant (or history of) substance use disorder. Even if you are not the prescriber of such medication, it is important to have a working knowledge of the main classes of psychotropic medications, their uses, side effects, and possible interactions with illicit substances. An understanding of these medications will also help you know how to respond when a client expresses ambivalence about taking psychiatric medication. You may, for instance, work with a client who is upset after being criticized in a 12-step meeting for continuing to rely on chemicals such as antidepressants and who feels torn between the benefits of the medications but facing shame during recovery meetings. This is a situation where a working knowledge of the main classes of psychotropic medications and understanding the difference between drugs used to get high and those used to manage a psychiatric disorder is beneficial.

Antidepressants

Medications used to treat affective disorders like major depression are known as antidepressants. Some examples are fluoxetine (trade name Prozac), sertraline (trade name Zoloft), and amitriptyline (trade name Elavil). There are several major classes of antidepressant medications. For many years, tricyclics were the first-line agents used to treat depression and are still used in certain cases. Tricyclics (like amitriptyline, desipramine, and imipramine), however, can produce anticholinergic side effects such as dry mouth and abnormal heart rhythm, and can be extremely toxic with overdose. More recently, selective serotonin reuptake inhibitors (SSRIs) have been the preferred first choice to try in the treatment of depression. SSRIs (like fluoxetine and sertraline) have fewer side effects, improving patient acceptance and compliance with treatment. Serotonin–norepinephrine reuptake inhibitors (SNRIs) like venlafaxine (trade name Effexor) and selective dopamine reuptake inhibitors (SDRIs) like bupropion (trade name Wellbutrin) are also commonly prescribed with concomitant affective disorders and addiction. Some possible side effects of SSRIs, SNRIs, and SDRIs are nausea, headaches, insomnia, and sexual dysfunction. Because monoamine oxidase inhibitors (MAOIs; like those with trade names Marplan, Nardil, and Parnate) can produce lethal reactions when combined with certain drugs or foods, they are usually used only for patients who do not respond to other antidepressant medications.

There is little professional controversy about the use of antidepressants for patients with co-occurring depression and addiction. Most antidepressants are relatively safe and there is no real potential for abuse of these medications. There have been some reports of antidepressants like SSRIs causing suicidal ideation. For patients who are using substances and prone to impulsive actions, this is something to monitor, especially with adolescents. Alcohol should be avoided by those taking antidepressants. The MAOIs uniquely can cause fatal interactions with certain foods (including cheese and chocolate), beer, and many prescription and illicit drugs. In all cases, patients taking antidepressants should be medically monitored.

Anxiolytics

Anxiolytics are medications used to treat disorders in which the prevailing symptom is anxiety. There are many classes of anxiolytic medications including benzodiazepines, barbiturates, and other sedative hypnotics. Certain antidepressants have also been used effectively to treat anxiety disorders.

For people with a history of substance use disorders, there have been good reasons for caution in the long-term use of benzodiazepines like chlordiazepoxidl (trade name Librium) and diazepam (trade name Valium), particularly because of their similarity to alcohol (which makes them useful in alcohol withdrawal). Benzodiazepines can produce tolerance and dependence, particularly for people with a history of addiction, and like alcohol can harm an unborn child during pregnancy. Alcohol and benzodiazepines show cross-tolerance and inhibit each other's metabolism so that their combined effects can be multiplied rather than additive.

Why, then, would benzodiazepines be prescribed for people with a history of addiction? The reason is their efficacy in managing concomitant anxiety disorders that persist or worsen in abstinence. Benzodizepines are rarely a primary drug of abuse; their misuse tends to be in combination with other drugs, and as a prescribed medication they do not appear to increase the risk of return to prior problematic alcohol/drug use (Mueller, Goldenberg, Gordon, Keller, & Warshaw, 1996; Posternak & Mueller, 2001). Furthermore, there is little evidence that a history of addiction is a significant risk factor for future benzodiazepine addiction.

The picture for barbiturate sedatives is clearer. Their potential for misuse, tolerance, dependence, and overdose is very high. Once used to manage alcohol withdrawal and treat anxiety disorders and insomnia, barbiturates were largely replaced by benzodiazepines.

Because of concerns about safety and addiction, a variety of other medications have been used to treat concomitant anxiety disorders. Buspirone is a commonly prescribed anxiolytic with lower potential for misuse, tolerance, and dependence. SSRI antidepressants are also prescribed to manage anxiety disorders including social anxiety, obsessive–compulsive, and panic disorders.

Stimulants

Stimulants, particularly methyphenidate (trade name Ritalin) are effective in treating attention-deficit/hyperactivity disorder (ADHD), which is a common concomitant as well as a risk factor for substance use disorders. Because stimulants have street value and are subject to misuse, there has been concern that using them to treat ADHD in youth and adults could increase the risk of developing substance use disorders. A meta-analysis of six studies found precisely the opposite: Untreated ADHD was associated with twice the risk of later substance use disorders, compared with those receiving pharmacotherapy (Wilens, Faraone, Biederman, & Gunawardene, 2003). Initiation of methyphenidate treatment for ADHD at a younger age has also been found to reduce risk for developing antisocial personality disorder (Mannuzza et al., 2008). Thus it appears that years of *untreated* ADHD increase risk for problems in adolescence and adulthood.

Antipsychotics

Antipsychotics are medications used in the treatment of major mental and emotional disturbances such as psychoses. Typical antipsychotics such as haloperidol have good efficacy, but do increase risk for enduring extrapyramidal side effects (EPS) and tardive dyskinesia. EPS causes uncontrollable movements with tremors and gives patients a feeling of needing to move around. More recent "atypical" antipsychotics (such as those with the trade names Geodon, Seroquel, and Abilify) also have good efficacy with lower risk of EPS and tardive dyskinesia. These medications are also being used increasingly to treat bipolar disorder and depression. There is no risk of abuse with these medications and no known significant interactions with alcohol or illicit drugs. Like all medications, however, the atypicals can have significant side effects including metabolic abnormalities such as diabetes, weight gain, elevated cholesterol, and high blood pressure.

BOX 18.3. Personal Reflection: Demons in the Mirrors

He came to the mental health center agitated and frightened, with a long history of methamphetamine use. What particularly distressed him was that he had begun seeing demons in the mirrors of his home. He complained that they were hard to see and that he was exhausted from staying awake trying to monitor their whereabouts. After some discussion, I suggested that medication might be a way to help make the demons go away.

"Will the medicine make me sleepy?" he asked.

Assuming that restful sleep would be a welcome change for him, I replied, "Yes, it should also help you to sleep better."

He looked up at me, startled. "Well then, I'm not interested one bit in taking those pills. I need to be able to stay awake to protect myself from the demons. That's what I need the meth for—to stay alert."

To me, this nicely highlighted the dilemma of medication compliance in psychiatric clients. Sometimes symptom relief is what the client fears!

—A. A. F.

Mood Stabilizers

Mood stabilizers include lithium (trade name Lithobid), valproate (trade name Depakene), and carbamazepine (trade name Tegretol). These medications are typically used for mania and hypomania. Lithium is the oldest, and must be monitored carefully because of potential toxicity. Valproate and carbamazepine appear to be generally safer and at least as effective as lithium, but tend to have sedating effects, so patients taking these medications have to be careful with alcohol consumption. There is not a risk of abuse of these medications and no known interactions with illicit drugs.

MEDICATION NONADHERENCE

Low adherence to prescribed medication is a widespread challenge in medical practice that undermines treatment effectiveness (McDonald, Garg, & Haynes, 2002). Failure to take medications as prescribed is a frequent cause of recurrence of major mental disorders, and is also a problem in addiction treatment (as described in Chapter 15). Strict adherence is also vital in the treatment of infectious diseases that are more prevalent in addiction treatment populations, including TB, hepatitis, and HIV. People may dislike or fear side effects, believe that a medication is not working, or discontinue it when symptoms abate in the belief that it is no longer needed. As discussed earlier, some clients may believe (or be told) erroneously that any psychiatric medication will endanger their recovery from addiction. Poor adherence can also arise from disorganization, inattention, or apathy related to the concomitant disorders.

There is much you can do to support medication adherence in your clients, even if you are not a medical professional yourself (see Chapters 8, 9, 15, and 17). Certainly patients should be urged to stay in regular contact with their prescribing physician(s) to monitor progress and discuss any concerns. Involving supportive family members or SOs can improve medication adherence (see Chapter 11). Explore your clients' beliefs and concerns about medications they are taking, check in about and encourage adherence, and brainstorm ways to improve it. Direct communication and collaboration with the prescribing physician(s) are often appropriate.

A CLOSING NOTE OF OPTIMISM

Throughout this chapter we have been discussing the complexities of treating people with concomitant psychiatric and substance use disorders. This is indeed a professionally challenging area, but we want to close with the note that the prognosis for successful treatment is *good*. In a 10-year prospective study of clients with severe and persistent mental illnesses and substance use disorders treated concomitantly (Xie, Drake, McHugo, Xie, & Mohandas, 2010), 86% had at least one 6-month remission period. For those who achieved at least 6 months of abstinence, the average duration of continuous remission was 6 years. Remission from addiction was associated with better outcomes on employment, independent living, positive peer affiliations, and life satisfaction. As is the case with treatment in general (Miller, Walters, & Bennett, 2001), there were very large reductions in substance use and improvements in life functioning even among those who did not maintain perfect abstinence after treatment.

KEY POINTS

🔖 Substance use and other psychological disorders commonly co-occur. Each one increases risk for the other.

🔖 Simultaneous integrated treatment of addiction and a concomitant mental disorder is preferable. Treating one improves outcomes in treating the other.

🔖 The effects of intoxication and detoxification can mimic, trigger, or exacerbate other disorders.

🔖 Psychiatric medications can be both effective and appropriate in treating disorders that co-occur with addictions.

REFLECTION QUESTIONS

💬 How comfortable and prepared are you to treat clients in each of the four quadrants described in this chapter?

💬 Of the people you see in your daily work, what percentage would you estimate have a substance use disorder in addition to another psychological disorder?

💬 How would you define "recovery" for people with co-occurring disorders?

CHAPTER 19

Promoting Maintenance

THE COURSE OF RECOVERY

Like the development of substance dependence itself, recovery is typically a process that occurs over time. To be sure, there are fortunate individuals who have a sudden discrete, even mystical experience that ends their substance use once and for all (see Chapter 21). For most people, however, recovery and sobriety continue to emerge (Hibbert & Best, 2011). Members of AA describe themselves as still recovering, not recovered, and sobriety as involving far more than abstinence (Dodge, Krantz, & Kenny, 2010). The DSM-IV (American Psychiatric Association, 1994) added criteria for substance use disorders to be "in remission," defined as the absence of any symptoms of abuse or dependence for at least 1 month, and "partial remission" if one or more symptoms remained but the person did not meet full diagnostic criteria.

For illustration, consider a man we treated for alcohol dependence within a clinical trial. He came to treatment reluctantly, under pressure from his wife who had threatened to leave him and take the children if he did not seek help. He clearly met criteria for alcohol dependence. An initial assessment revealed some early neurocognitive and liver impairment. He decided on abstinence as his goal, particularly to keep his family together. Because he was participating in a clinical study, we obtained daily drinking data from 3 months before treatment through a 15-month follow-up. He had been averaging 96 standard drinks per week prior to treatment. He stopped drinking abruptly at the second week of treatment (with no apparent withdrawal symptoms!) and remained abstinent until week 16, near the end of treatment, when he drank on two consecutive days (2 and 5 standard drinks). He went back to abstinence again for 3 months, then had four drinking days in a row (total of 13 standard drinks), and again returned to abstinence. During the remaining 7 months of follow-up he had a total of five more drinking days, with the heaviest being 7 standard drinks, and at month 15 he had been abstinent for 4 months. In a clinical trial where outcomes were dichotomized as either abstinent or relapsed, his treatment had been a failure. On the study's binary "survival curve," he converted from abstinent to "relapsed" at week 16 even before treatment had ended, and remained there. Yet even a cursory examination of his data indicates that his drinking had changed dramatically (see Box 19.1). Compared to pretreatment levels, his drinking had decreased by 89% during treatment, and by 96% during follow-up. By DSM-IV criteria, he was in full remission throughout months 2–15, with no symptoms of abuse or dependence.

Such a clinical picture is normative in managing chronic diseases. If this were the blood glucose elevation chart of someone with Type 2 diabetes, it would be cause for celebration and the patient would be congratulated for excellent adherence. On the whole, with diabetes treatment and behavior change, glucose levels decline and symptoms abate. Spikes in blood sugar still occur, but they tend to be lower, farther apart, and shorter in duration than before diagnosis and disease management. A hypoglycemic crisis may put someone with Type 1 diabetes in the emergency room or hospital, but no one whispers that this person has "relapsed" or that treatment has failed, even though clearly the crisis was a direct result of the person's own choices. In treating asthma, a remarkably successful outcome of diagnosis and treatment would be for the person to *never* have another asthma

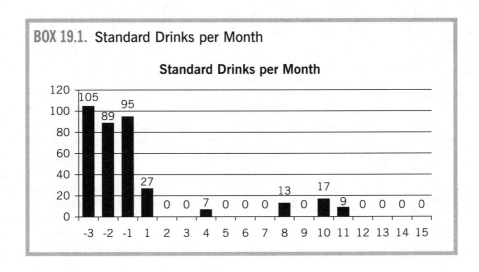

BOX 19.1. Standard Drinks per Month

attack, but a more typical outcome of asthma management is fewer, less severe attacks spaced farther apart in time, so that the person lives a longer life with better quality, and ultimately dies of some other cause.

McLellan has observed that addiction treatment has been held to a different standard for "success" in comparison with other chronic behavior-related diseases (McLellan et al., 2000; McLellan, McKay, Forman, Cacciola, & Kemp, 2010). If the onset of a treatment (such as a medication) for a chronic illness results in a significant reduction in symptoms and clinical indicators (like blood pressure or glucose), and the discontinuation of treatment subsequently results in a return to pretreatment levels, that is classic evidence that the treatment *works*. The same pattern with an addiction is often judged to constitute a treatment failure.

In fact, outcomes following a single episode of addiction treatment are rather good in comparison to those for many chronic diseases. Among 8,389 U.S. cases treated for alcohol use disorders (Miller, Walters, et al., 2001), 24% refrained totally from drinking throughout the year after treatment. For the remaining 76%, abstinent days increased by 128%, and total alcohol consumption decreased by 87% relative to pretreatment levels, a dramatic and certainly medically meaningful change. The 1-year mortality rate was 1.5%. (Mortality can be higher with illicit drugs. In an opiate substitution treatment program, the comparable annual mortality figure was 3% [Barnett, Trafton, & Humphreys, 2010].)

So what does all of this tell us?

1. After any single episode of stabilization or rehabilitation, most people will use again, most likely within the first few months after initial treatment.

> After any single episode of stabilization or rehabilitation, most people will use again.

2. Thus "treatment" is not over at the end of rehabilitation (Phase 3). The efficacy of inpatient substance abuse treatment, for example, depends heavily on whether people receive continuing outpatient care back home (once termed "aftercare"). In this sense, the initial phases of specialist treatment for stabilization and rehabilitation represent "forecare."

3. In Phase 4 (maintenance), treatment is likely to be less intensive and may resemble primary health care (and indeed may occur in that context): routine follow-up visits to review health status and adjust or intensify treatment as needed.

4. Finally, for goodness sake, don't discharge people from treatment for the same reason that you admitted them. Imagine if we "fired" patients from treatment for cancer, heart disease, diabetes, or asthma because their symptoms had recurred! If addiction is a chronic condition, then we should treat it like one.

BOX 19.2. Personal Reflection: What Is a Relapse?

It seemed like a fairly straightforward study. Three clinical sites were contracted to amass a large sample of clients, study the process of relapse to drinking after treatment, and examine factors that predict its occurrence (Lowman, Allen, & Miller, 1996). The study required us to define what would constitute a relapse. Would it be any consumption of alcohol at all after a period of abstinence? If so, how many days of preceding abstinence would be required before it could be considered a relapse? If a "slip" is differentiated from a "relapse," how many drinks or days would it take to qualify as a full-blown relapse? Should the volume of alcohol that qualifies as a relapse vary according to body weight or other factors (such as gender) that influence intoxication level? And all of this took into account only one drug: ethyl alcohol. What about using or substituting another drug? Is that a relapse? If a person has a drink, then abstains for 3 days, then has another drink, is that two relapses?

What became clear to us as we tried to superimpose these various filters on highly varied patterns of alcohol use is that the problem was in our binary assumption that there were only two possible states: abstinence and relapse (Miller, 1996b). What does it add to label such behavior as a "relapse"? Does it perhaps add something harmful? Clearly it adds a judgmental dimension, perhaps an implicit element of blame. It also communicates to clients (inaccurately) that there are only these two extreme states of being: perfect abstinence or relapse. Alan Marlatt described the "abstinence violation effect" (the belief that if one makes a single exception, one will then lose control) as a self-fulfilling prophecy. Having taken that first sip or puff or bite, the rule has been broken and there is now nothing to lose (Cummings et al., 1980; Marlatt & Donovan, 2005). Ironically, that belief—the abstinence or rule violation effect—is implicit within the term "relapse" itself.

Posttreatment drinking or drug use is common, even normative, and is highly variable in pattern and intensity. Some people take a drink, ask themselves "What am I doing this for?," and go right back on the wagon. Others revert quickly to full-blown alcohol dependence. In between are many degrees of variation. The course of recovery is rarely a single resolution that is never violated. More often it involves increasingly long spans of sobriety, interrupted by gradually shorter and less severe episodes of use. What, then, are we communicating to our clients if we tell them that they have "relapsed"? Does that really help them?

—W. R. M.

Understanding an illness as chronic does not absolve people of responsibility for their own health, of course. To the contrary, the management of chronic illness normally requires quite a lot from the patient. The course and outcomes of chronic disease are strongly related to the person's own health behavior: taking prescribed medications, managing diet and weight, keeping appointments. The same is true of health in general. Maintaining good health has much to do with lifestyle: diet, exercise, checkups, stress, and moderation.

PHASE 4: MAINTENANCE

Helping people to experience an initial period of weeks or months of sobriety is a necessary and important first step toward maintenance. Making the initial changes required to escape from substance use disorders is termed the *action stage* in the transtheoretical model of change (Prochaska, 1994). In Chapter 7 we described these initial

> In addiction, as with weight loss, after taking it off the challenge is keeping it off.

steps as palliative care (Phase 1), stabilization (Phase 2), and rehabilitation (Phase 3). That is not the end of treatment. Stopping smoking, drinking, or other drug use is often not all that difficult to achieve in itself. Even detoxification for severely dependent people, once an agonizing ordeal, is now a reasonably straightforward process. In addiction, as with weight loss, after taking it off the challenge is keeping it off.

Some people do just fine during maintenance (Phase 4) with no additional help. There is no reason to expect everyone to remain in active treatment for a certain period of time or to jump over a fixed number of hurdles. For some people, making the initial decision to quit and getting through the stabilization period (Phase 2) is sufficient. When asked how to have a successful addiction treatment program, the director of a prominent rehabilitation center once quipped, "Be the place where people go once they have finally decided to quit." For others, Phase 3 treatment is enough, but for many it is not. Maintenance (Phase 4) should be a normal part of addiction treatment services. Here are three general guidelines for helping people in the maintenance phase after initial stabilization or rehabilitation.

Keep the Door Open

Don't communicate that treatment is over, the process finished, or that clients are on their own from here on. Neither do we recommend telling people that they are likely to relapse, or scaring them into additional treatment. A reasonable middle ground is to keep the door open and the light on, inviting them back whenever they want additional consultation. A readily available visit or two may help the person stay in remission.

Use the Client's Wisdom

Most people are reasonably good judges of their stability, a fact that is particularly evident in research on self-efficacy. If you ask someone how likely he or she is to still be a nonsmoker (or sober, or drug-free) 3 months from now, his or her probability estimate is a reasonably good predictor of that specific outcome. Estimates lower than 80% provide some reason for concern and further exploration. In considering further visits, ask the person when he or she would like to check back.

Follow Up

A third guideline is to check back *routinely and proactively* on how people are doing. This is easiest in an ongoing health maintenance system, where the person returns for various kinds of care on a regular basis. During a health visit, it's easy enough to ask, "How's it going with _____?" In other contexts, it's a good idea to get in touch and check back on how they are doing. Because most people who return to drinking, smoking, or drug use do so within 3–6 months after rehabilitation, one option is to check back routinely at 2 months and perhaps again at 4 months. These need not be long contacts, but they keep the door open, and most people appreciate the continued concern and interest. We particularly noticed this in doing follow-up visits in our clinical studies. Even though people knew that we were seeing or calling them primarily to collect research follow-up data, they often perceived and appreciated it as continuing care. Scott and Dennis (2009) found in two randomized trials that adding quarterly "recovery management checkups" based on MI was effective in reengaging clients in treatment when needed and significantly increasing abstinence days during 2 years of follow-up.

MAINTENANCE STRATEGIES

> Sometimes the skills and strategies needed for successful maintenance are different from those that worked to get sober in the first place.

Sometimes the skills and strategies needed for successful maintenance are different from those that worked to get sober in the first place. Fortunately, many of the tools needed in Phase 4 have already been discussed in prior chapters. Here are some general maintenance strategies.

Use Mutual Help Groups

An excellent resource for maintenance is the mutual help groups that can be found in many communities (see Chapter 14). Encourage people to try out available groups as a source of ongoing support during the maintenance phase. How many meetings should a client attend? People who stick with AA after treatment tend to be those who attended at least two meetings a week during Phase 3 treatment (Tonigan et al., 2003). That is far fewer than the "90 meetings in 90 days" sometimes recommended or even mandated. Here again the client's own wisdom is a good resource, and ultimately people settle into their own patterns of involvement.

Maintenance Medications

Some medications are designed specifically to help people avoid their previously preferred drugs over the short or longer term (see Chapter 15). Disulfiram, methadone, buprenorphine, naltrexone, and nicotine gum are all examples. One general strategy is to transfer the patient from his or her previously preferred drug to the maintenance medication, a common approach in detoxification. Then the maintenance medication is gradually tapered over time. A second strategy is long-term maintenance on the medication. Agonist (substitute) medications are also generally addictive, but offer important advantages in terms of their pharmacological properties. Some medications, for example, have a longer half-life and avoid the rapid high followed by an abrupt crash. Also, unlike street drugs, the content and dose are known, decreasing risk of overdose. An antidipsotropic like disulfiram can be maintained at a protective dosage over time, or taken in anticipation of high-risk situations.

Case Management and Continuing Care

Besides mutual help groups, what kinds of services can be helpful in maintaining sobriety? We do not recommend any standardized set of services here. Instead we recommend a flexible menu of options from which clients can choose on the basis of their needs and preferences. In one public treatment system we literally presented such a menu to the people we served, empowering them to choose the options that met their needs. Helping clients to address the particular problems they face can aid maintenance of treatment gains (McLellan et al., 1997, 1998).

The perspective of case management (Chapter 8) is therefore also of value in Phase 4 maintenance. People with substance use disorders often have a broader range of social, legal, financial, health, and spiritual issues to deal with and can benefit from services far beyond those that directly address addiction. It can be useful to survey the range of services that clients may need and to develop a plan for accessing these in order of priority.

Self-Monitoring

Another strategy is to use self-monitoring as an early warning system. Keeping a daily record, particularly for the first few months of sobriety, can alert the client to emerging concerns before they turn into renewed substance use problems. Within the community reinforcement approach (CRA) (Chapter 11), for example, a general goal is for the person to be happy in sobriety, and simple daily mood monitoring on a 1–10 scale has been used to watch for slippage that could signal a drift toward renewed problems. You might instruct the client to call you if mood ratings fall below a certain point for 2 days in a row. Another obvious target for daily monitoring would be cravings or urges (see Chapters 6 and 12). For clients seeking to maintain moderate drinking, daily monitoring of alcohol use should be continued for a few months after Phase 3 treatment (see Chapters 12 and 23). This parallels the common method of keeping detailed food diaries as part of a weight loss program. The essential strategy here is to keep track of anything that could signal a drift toward prior patterns of substance use and to take steps early to head off problems.

Dealing with Old and New Problems

Some problems do abate with sobriety. Others continue or even worsen. Without alcohol or other drugs on board, the symptoms of PTSD may return with a vengeance, and mood disorders may become more apparent or severe. The financial, legal, family, social, employment, educational, and medical consequences of prior use can come home to roost during recovery. Conventional AA wisdom likens this to the inertia of a train wreck: after the locomotive has crashed and come to an abrupt stop, the boxcars continue to hit for some time thereafter.

A variety of Phase 3 strategies have been tested to help clients avoid a return to substance use during maintenance Phase 4 (Abbott et al., 2003; Marlatt & Donovan, 2005; Marlatt & Marques, 1977). Part of the challenge here is treating other disorders that have coexisted with addiction. As discussed in Chapter 18, this may be best done concomitantly with addiction treatment. However, some disorders are difficult to recognize or address while the person is still using. Addressing these in an effective and timely manner during Phase 4 can diminish the risk of resumed substance use.

Sometimes alcohol or other drugs were used as a way to cope with life problems that then persist into sobriety. In this case it can be important to help a client learn new coping strategies to replace substance use in these situations (Chapter 12). The "new roads" assessment presented in Chapter 7 is one way to anticipate and address these problems.

Responding to Resumed Use

Treatment services should seek not only to prevent recurrence of use and problems, but to detect it early and help the person get back on track. When people try to abstain from one or more drugs that they have been accustomed to using, perfect uninterrupted abstinence is the

> We are thus not surprised or even discouraged when clients return having resumed use after a period of abstinence.

exception rather than the rule on any given try. We are thus not surprised or even discouraged when clients return having resumed use after a period of abstinence. Imperfection is the normal human condition (Kurtz & Ketcham, 1992). A recurrence of substance use is not a reason to be excluded from AA, nor should it be cause to withdraw or withhold treatment.

It seems odd, then, that treatment professionals and programs have sometimes responded to resumed use in such a punitive manner. Renewed use has sometimes been seen as reason to reduce maintenance medication dose, revoke privileges, or even terminate treatment. As noted earlier, these would be strange professional responses to a recurrence of symptoms in someone with diabetes, heart disease, or chronic obstructive pulmonary disease. If anything, a resumption of prior problems would suggest a need to *increase* dosage (Maremmani, Balestri, Sbrana, & Tagliamonte, 2003) or provide intensified or different treatment. Further, don't assume that resumed use means that treatment (let alone the person) is failing. The course of recovery is seldom smooth, and a certain number of bumps are to be expected along the way. A message we like to give to clients is "I will work with you until we find what works for you."

It is also important to keep recurrent use in perspective. All that has happened is that the person violated a rule that he or she or you had (at least apparently) adopted as a goal. The client described earlier (Box 19.1) had been averaging nearly 100 standard drinks per week for several years—the equivalent of about two six-packs of beer per day. He committed to abstain from alcohol, and did so for 15 weeks. Then he came in looking sullen and defeated, his wife angry and dejected. "I relapsed," he said. On 2 days that week he had had two and five beers, respectively. Rather than joining his despondence, the therapist contrasted this with the amount he had previously been drinking in a period of 15 weeks (a ratio of roughly 200 to 1), emphasized that imperfection is normal, and explored what had happened.

So how is it best to respond when people deviate from their goal of abstinence or moderation? We suggest three simple questions:

"What's up?"
"What's new?"
"What's needed?"

What's Up?

First, make sure that you understand the client's goals. If abstinence is your goal but not your client's goal, then continued use is unsurprising. Clarify what your client wants, with motivational methods described in Chapter 10. Does the resumed use reflect a shift in the person's motivation and goals for change? It is normal for motivations to fluctuate over time. Try to distinguish here between motivational shifts that *preceded* the event, and responses (such as demoralization) to the event itself. Explore what the person wants, needs, and hopes for, and as appropriate renew commitment to change goals. Have the person's original motivations changed? If commitment to change seems shaky, it may be useful to explore the positive and negative consequences of continued use versus resumed abstinence. In the style of MI, you would particularly seek to hear from the person the advantages of resumed abstinence (or moderation, if that was the goal), and the risks and disadvantages of returning to prior use patterns. Beware the scenario where you champion a particular goal and the client argues against it.

Another important point in responding to resumed use is to help the person (and SOs) not overinterpret or catastrophize what has happened. What really matters is what happens next. Language can make a difference here. Framing resumed use as a "failure," "relapse," "falling off the wagon," and such may add negative emotion but not hope. We are generally inclined to treat it for what it is—behavior and choice—and move on to problem solving.

What's New?

It is also common for resumed use to reflect something new, some kind of change. Were the person's hopes and expectations for abstinence somehow disappointed? Did the person discover that there was something he or she missed about using? Sometimes new feelings or problems emerge with abstinence that had previously been masked by use. Often resumed use occurs when people encounter a new situation for which they were not quite prepared. Here are a few things to consider exploring:

1. What was happening just before the resumed use that might have triggered it? Where was the person, and with whom? What was the person feeling, thinking, and doing? These are not "excuses," but clues to what else may be needed to help the person stay sober.

2. How conscious was the person of making the decision to use? What contributed to that decision? "What were you thinking?" is not for shaming and blaming, but for understanding "apparently irrelevant decisions" and thought processes that increase the risk of recurrence (Cummings et al., 1980).

3. What did the person hope or expect would happen with resumed use? Did it? What if anything did the person enjoy about using (smoking, drinking, etc.)?

4. What, if anything, did the person do at the time to try to avoid using? What else could he or she have done, but didn't?

5. What are the client's other hunches about the resumed use? Is there anything else happening in the person's life that made substance use look more attractive?

6. How did the person react to the initial use? What did he or she think, feel, do after violating the plan?

7. Perhaps most important, what's next? What does the person want, hope for, and choose to do now?

What's Needed?

A period of abstinence can reveal feelings or situations that previously triggered substance use, and for which alcohol/drug use was an attempt to cope. Perhaps substance use was the only tool that the person knew for handling a particular feeling or situation (which is a working definition of psychological dependence). Here again it can be useful to conduct the "new roads" functional analysis of the person's use described in Chapter 7, an exercise that can also be done with groups. The point is to identify different ways for the person to respond to the "trigger" situation, and better ways to get from there to a desired outcome without using substances.

KEY POINTS

📌 Resumed use is common following addiction treatment (as in the care of any chronic condition) and need not be characterized pejoratively as a "relapse."

📌 Even among people who do not maintain perfect abstinence from alcohol, posttreatment drinking is normally reduced by 87% on average.

📌 During maintenance (Phase 4 treatment), people need strategies to retain the good changes they have made, which may be different from what helped them initially.

🖈 Recurrence of substance use and problems is a reason to resume or intensify treatment, not withdraw it.

🖈 Maintain follow-up contact with people who have been under your care and keep the door open for ongoing consultation.

REFLECTION QUESTIONS

🔎 Think about a change you have made and then maintained. What have you done to maintain it?

🔎 How could you arrange to make routine follow-up calls or checkup visits with people who have completed Phase 3 treatment?

🔎 What are your personal reactions when someone you have treated has a recurrence of substance use?

CHAPTER 20

Working with Groups

O ne of the earliest formal treatments for alcohol dependence was group psychotherapy (Voegtlin & Lemere, 1942), which continues to be the most common form of treatment for alcohol and other drug problems in both inpatient and outpatient treatment settings. In Chapter 14 we discussed mutual help groups such as AA. In this chapter we turn to group work led by a designated therapist.

Group therapy is not itself a kind of treatment, but simply a context in which to deliver a particular treatment method with two or more unrelated individuals at the same time. Group therapy can also be done with couples or families (Chapters 11 and 13), but our primary focus in this chapter is on groups of unrelated individuals.

RATIONALE FOR GROUP TREATMENT

One of the factors maintaining the popularity of a group format is the increasing demand for cost-effective treatment delivery. Group therapy allows one or two health care professionals to work with a group of people simultaneously rather than one-to-one. This permits more efficient use of professional time and can also decrease individual cost per session. Another practical advantage is the decreased impact of individual no-shows since the group continues and the professional's time is thus occupied. Given these advantages, if group and individual therapy have comparable outcomes, group delivery would be more cost-effective.

In addition to the economic advantages, group therapy allows clients to learn from each other's experiences. Certain types of treatment, such as social skills training (Chapter 12), may be particularly appropriate to group formats. Furthermore, there are aspects of addiction that may render group therapy advantageous. It is common for people with alcohol/drug problems to feel and to be disconnected from others. As addiction progresses, there is a tendency to detach from important relationships and activities. This detachment was one of the criteria used to make a diagnosis of substance dependence in the DSM (see Chapter 2). In AA, a familiar term is "terminal uniqueness," describing someone's perception of extreme alienation and separateness from peers. If addiction involves isolation from others, it seems intuitive that a group therapeutic approach would offer a foundation for relatedness.

There are potentially powerful curative forces unique to group therapy: the feeling of community, encouragement, hope and optimism, and the sense of commonality and belonging that a group can foster. People who are averse to authority may find it easier to receive information and feedback from peers than from a therapist. One of the underpinnings of 12-step mutual help programs (Chapter 14) is that members benefit from interacting with others who have had similar experiences. The process of cooperating and being useful to others also facilitates the transition from being dependent to being dependable and helping others.

RESEARCH ON THE EFFECTIVENESS OF GROUP THERAPIES

The fact that a treatment approach is practical, economical, and commonly used does not mean that it is effective. Given group therapies' widespread use in addiction treatment, it is surprising that they have been far less studied than individual approaches. This is due in part to some unique methodological challenges in evaluating group treatment. In clinical trials with closed groups, for example, one must recruit enough participants to fill groups before they begin, which can delay the start of treatment and thus endanger retention. If open groups are used, the constantly evolving membership imposes significant challenges in treatment and interpretation (as discussed later in this chapter). Another difficulty is that the interdependence of group members makes data analytic approaches more challenging. For instance, imagine how the presence of one highly disruptive group member might change the dynamics of a whole group, affecting others' participation, retention, and outcomes. Such factors make it difficult to determine whether group therapies are effective and what factors influence outcomes.

Nevertheless, there is a growing body of clinical research to help guide evidence-based practice in group therapy. As with individual treatment methods, it is already apparent that all group therapies are

All group therapies are not equally effective.

not equally effective. Less is known about the impact of particular therapists, but current evidence suggests that as in individual treatment, it matters who provides group treatment.

Evidence on Specific Group Therapies

A wide variety of psychotherapies have been tried in the treatment of addictions, including psychodynamic (Khantzian et al., 1990), confrontational (Yablonsky, 1965), educational/didactic and client-centered (Ends & Page, 1957), gestalt (Browne-Miller, 1993), group process (Yalom & Leszcz, 2005), interpersonal (Weissman, Markowitz, & Klerman, 2000), cognitive (Beck et al., 2001), motivational (Ingersoll, Wagner, & Gharib, 2000; Sobell & Sobell, 2001; Velasquez, Maurer, Crouch, & Diclemente, 2001), and behavioral (Kouimtsidis, Reynolds, Drummond, Davis, & Tarrier, 2007; Monti et al., 2002). There is also wide variability in the evidence base for these various approaches. Some approaches have fairly solid evidence of efficacy. Others have been well supported when delivered as individual therapy, but have not yet been properly evaluated in group format. Still others have little evidence of efficacy in any delivery format (Miller & Wilbourne, 2002; Miller, Wilbourne, et al., 2003).

One long-standing approach is the didactic group, typically using educational lectures and films to convey information about addiction, such as the harmful short-term and long-term effects of substance use. In a large review of 381 clinical trials of alcohol treatment efficacy (Miller, Wilbourne, et al., 2003), such educational approaches were found to be the *least* effective of the 48 treatment methods studied. Of 39 published trials, 34 showed no beneficial effects. Similarly, insight-oriented psychotherapy ranked 46th, and all published studies were negative for both confrontational counseling (ranked 45th) and process group therapy (27th).

Given the broad popularity of educational/didactic groups in particular, it is worth considering why so many studies would find no benefit, or occasionally worse outcomes, with therapies that are intended to provide knowledge, insight, or confrontation. One possibility is that addiction is simply not due to a lack of knowledge, insight, or contact with reality. Another is that any benefit of relatively inert treatment methods may be offset by the effects of exposure to others acting in a similarly unhealthy or destructive manner. Particular concern has been raised about the potentially adverse effects of exposing adolescents to deviant peers in a group format (Dishion, McCord, & Poulin, 1999). While meta-analytic reviews suggest that peer influences outside treatment are much more significant than within-group influences (Weiss et al., 2005), it is still important to understand that negative peer influences are a risk inherent to the group format, particularly if the treatment being offered is relatively weak.

So what does work? The most strongly supported approach for group therapy of addictions focuses on teaching cognitive-behavioral coping skills to prevent a return to substance use and improve drug-free life quality (Carroll & Rounsaville, 2005; Miller, Wilbourne, et al., 2003). Studies of such behavioral skill training report outcomes from group formats to be at least as good as those from individual behavior therapy (e.g., Graham, Annis, Brett, & Venesoen, 1996; Marques & Formigoni, 2001; Miller & Taylor, 1980). Indeed, some studies report better outcomes from group formats when compared to individual behavioral therapy. McKay, for example, found that individuals treated in groups had higher rates of abstinence at 6 months than those treated individually (McKay et al., 1997). Cognitive-behavioral groups seem to reduce the intensity of a return to drinking or drug use and appear to be most effective for those who have more severe substance use, greater levels of negative affect, and greater perceived deficits in coping skills (Carroll, 1996). Given this level of empirical support, we offer some guidance about cognitive-behavioral group therapy later in this chapter.

In between evidence-based cognitive-behavioral groups and the less promising methods described earlier is an intermediate set of group approaches. These are methods that have been reasonably well supported as individual therapies, but less is known about their efficacy in group format. In each case there has been some research on group treatment, but not enough evidence yet to be confident that they work reliably in group contexts. Nevertheless, it is encouraging that they are effective in individual format, and that research more generally suggests similar outcomes from group and individual therapies. These include interpersonal (Weissman et al., 2000), behavioral couples (McCrady & Epstein, 2009a; O'Farrell & Fals-Stewart, 2006), and motivational groups (Ingersoll et al., 2000; Velasquez et al., 2001).

PRACTICAL DECISIONS

Having considered the evidence base for a variety of group approaches, we turn now to a discussion of some decisions that must be made regardless of the group approach used. There are quite a few such decisions to be made with any group, and the choices that you make are important. How many people will be in the group? Can people join along the way? Is it acceptable for people in the same group to be working toward different goals? These are some of the questions we discuss in this section. Some group therapy approaches have specific guidelines for these decisions, while others may be determined by your own agency or personal preference. In any event, it is helpful to think these issues through before you begin a group.

Duration and Frequency of Treatment

Research suggests that most client improvement as a result of group therapy occurs in a relatively brief period, typically around 2–3 months (Garvin, Reid, & Epstein, 1976). There may also be managed care or treatment program guidelines that will determine the length of treatment. In the United States, for example, most outpatient treatment programs provide 8–20 sessions and most inpatient programs are limited to 2–4 weeks. The number of sessions per week is also typically determined by program goals and constraints. It may, for instance, be feasible to have sessions multiple times per week for people in residential or intensive day treatment, whereas a once-per-week format may make more sense for employed people in outpatient treatment. Depending on the content covered in the group, sessions might last between 45 and 120 minutes. A shorter length is typical for cognitive-behavioral groups, while a longer session might be more appropriate for a process group.

Where Groups Are Held

Accessibility is an important element for outpatient groups. A place that is difficult to find and is logistically complicated (e.g., lack of easy parking or public transportation) creates challenges for clients and can decrease their motivation to attend the sessions. Ensuring that the location is safe is another important consideration. What is the neighborhood like? Are group members safe walking to and from the group? A telephone should be available for emergencies.

Group Size

Groups can range from two people to a large audience attending a didactic group. Skills training groups, for example, require a manageable group size so that members can practice the skills they are taught and group members can receive adequate attention and feedback from the facilitator. With the presence of a cofacilitator, the group size can be somewhat larger.

Leaders

A group can be led by one individual, co-led by two facilitators, or led by one primary facilitator with the presence of a secondary facilitator. Two leaders are able to provide different social role models and can share in problem solving during challenging sessions. An added benefit is that coleadership allows for the group to meet even if one leader is unavailable. Additionally, a cofacilitator can provide immediate support if an individual group member is in crisis while the other leader continues the group.

Treatment Goals

Another issue is whether individual treatment goals within the group are homogeneous. Suppose, for example, that clients are at different levels of motivation for change. Should you form groups of people with similar readiness (e.g., contemplation vs. action stage groups) or is it better to have heterogeneity? Those who are at earlier stages of readiness or recovery may benefit from interacting with others who are farther along. Such a mixed membership also removes the need for clients to change groups as they progress. On the other hand, the differing needs and interests of people at varying stages can be frustrating, particularly for clients who are farther along. There are similar issues when deciding whether a group focuses only on one particular problem (such as substance use), or addresses a broader range of life concerns.

Another topic regards the treatment goal of abstinence. Clients vary with regard to what they want to do about their substance use. Some choose total abstinence as their immediate and lifetime goal. Others are initially willing to reduce their use or to choose less risky drugs or routes of administration, but do not embrace lifelong abstinence as their immediate goal. It is also common for clients to have different goals for different drugs; for example, abstinence from heroin, maintenance on methadone, and reduction in alcohol use (Abellanas & McLellan, 1993). Does a therapy group encompass people with such differing goals? Some programs, by virtue of their treatment philosophy or clientele (e.g., probation), accept only total abstinence from alcohol and all illicit drugs as a treatment objective. Other programs seek to serve a broader spectrum of clients and work with harm reduction goals for those who choose not to abstain. In the latter case, you need to decide whether to construct groups that have homogeneous or heterogeneous individual goals. Homogeneous groups may increase focus and diminish discomfort or confusion related to differing goals. Heterogeneous groups allow people to learn from each other and remove the need to change groups if treatment goals change.

Physical Contact

What are the standards about touch within the group? Some people find a hug or a hand on a shoulder to be comforting during a difficult discussion or at the end of the session. Personal histories and cultural backgrounds may also contribute to different interpretations of what touch means. While physical violence is explicitly prohibited, the group should discuss feelings related to physical contact and establish group rules related to appropriate and inappropriate behaviors within the group.

Contact Outside of the Group

Development of intimate relationships between members of ongoing therapy groups is generally discouraged, if not prohibited. In some models of group therapy, any personal contact outside of the group is discouraged. This is another decision for you as a group leader: whether to encourage supportive networks among group members, discourage them, or take a neutral stance. Whatever you decide, of course, group members may still choose to communicate outside the group.

Open versus Closed Groups

With open or revolving group membership, people enter whenever they are ready for the clinical interventions provided in the group. Revolving membership groups are frequently found in short-term residential treatment programs because as people are admitted and discharged, membership of the group changes. In closed-enrollment groups, by contrast, all members are enrolled before the group begins and membership remains constant.

There are pros and cons to both closed and open groups. In open-enrollment groups, members are permitted to initiate treatment at different times. An open-group format removes the need for a waiting list and also decreases problems due to attrition. A practical problem with open groups is that new people may enter at each meeting, so that membership is constantly changing, which can affect group dynamics and trust. If the group has a structured cycle of content, people are also entering that cycle at different points, and it is thus difficult to build on content from one meeting to the next. Closed enrollment minimizes the disruptive effects of changing group membership and capitalizes on group cohesion and also permits a developmental sequence within the group. Attrition is common in addiction treatment, however, so membership in a closed group can wane over time. A closed format also requires new members to wait until a new group is formed. Both of these problems can be alleviated by periodically admitting new members to an otherwise closed group.

Time Limited versus Ongoing

A further decision regards time-limited versus ongoing groups. Time-limited groups meet for a predetermined number of sessions, whereas ongoing groups typically continue within the structure of a treatment program and offer people access for an indefinite period. Time-limited groups are particularly appropriate when there is a certain amount of content to be covered. (Remember, though, that educational/didactic lectures generally have very little impact on outcome.)

Therapist Self-Disclosure

How much should therapists reveal about themselves within group therapy? Individual styles vary, ranging from little or no self-disclosure (as is common within a psychodynamic framework) to a high level of spontaneous participation (as in a humanistic or encounter group). Our rule of thumb is to use a level of personal disclosure that will facilitate the work of the group at that moment in time. Rachman (1990) distinguished between judicious self-disclosures (appropriate level of detail, focus remains on the client) and excessive self-disclosures (those that shift the focus to the therapist). There is also a distinction between revealing things about your own *past history* (such as telling a story from your own life or recovery) and sharing your immediate reactions to clients or observations about group process *in the present moment*. In general, have a clear, conscious, strategic reason for whatever self-disclosure you offer.

Talking Rules

Each group has formal or informal rules about who may talk when. In a didactic group, for example, participants might raise their hand to indicate when they want to ask a question or make a comment. Some groups have a formal turn-taking process, such as going around so that each participant has a chance to talk (or pass). Others use a "talking stick" that is passed from person to person (not necessarily in a fixed order) that designates the holder as the person who has the floor. The most open format allows anyone to talk at any time.

Groups also have formal or informal rules about what members are to say, and how to say it. One such issue is "cross-talk"—whether members may comment on (criticize, agree or disagree, correct, suggest, confront, etc.) what another member has said. Cross-talk is discouraged in most 12-step groups, where members are expected to focus on their own experience. In some types of groups, however, cross-talk can be an important part of therapy. Group members may have suggestions for how a person could make a change, or see a connection between someone's current comment or dilemma and another area in which the person has been successful. A potential downside of cross-talk is the tendency for people to get off the subject or interrupt other group members to insert their own feelings/thoughts about an issue. Group members should be generally encouraged to talk in ways that are not critical, demeaning, or confronting.

In certain types of group therapy, particularly in ongoing or closed groups, members may be taught certain ways of responding to one another. In a person-centered or MI group, for example, the therapist may respond primarily with "OARS" (Chapter 4): Open questions, Affirmations, Reflections, and Summaries. Clients can also learn to respond in these same basic ways to others in the group, and of course these skills can carry over into everyday relationships.

Diversity

Another important decision regards the extent to which a group should be homogeneous or heterogeneous on certain characteristics, such as gender. Women may fare better and be more likely to stay in same-sex groups than in mixed-gender groups, whereas men appear to do equally well in mixed or all-male groups (Stevens, Arbiter, & Glider, 1989). This may be related to additional barriers that women face in engaging and remaining in treatment, including balancing family responsibilities with their own treatment needs, safety issues, and greater stigma. Another possible explanation for why women have better outcomes in same-gender groups is the high co-occurrence of substance use and traumatic events in women (Simpson & Miller, 2002). Often the perpetrators were male partners, family members, or acquaintances. Women are typically more willing to disclose and discuss their victimization (and its relation to their substance use) in same-gender groups. Women may also generally defer and talk less in mixed-gender groups where men dominate the conversation.

Another diversity issue has to do with race, ethnicity, and culture. Some professionals believe that it's better for all members of a group including the therapist(s) to be from the same or similar ethnic-cultural background. Certainly language is important in clear communication, but beyond this there is little evidence that therapists have better outcome with clients of the same cultural background, or that racial-ethnic uniformity improves group outcomes (Salvendy, 1999). People with the same skin tone or socio-economic background are otherwise quite diverse in many ways. For this reason, a client-centered approach (see Chapter 4) is useful, regarding each person as unique and the expert on his or her own life. In determining the outcomes of the group and its members, the overall spirit of the interaction (openness, respect, autonomy) is far more important than a priori matching on client characteristics (Brooks, 1998).

Nevertheless, it is important to be sensitive to people who are different from the majority of the other participants in some way. One example of cultural differences may be the concept of time. In Native American culture, for example, there is a tendency to have a relaxed attitude about time. How will you work with people who are late to groups? How might you find ways to accommodate traditions such as socializing or rituals involving food, music, or prayer? Think and ask about ways in which others' backgrounds or experiences may influence their participation in the group and affect the group dynamic. For example, people approach issues like anger and assertiveness in very different ways depending on their cultural background and individual experiences.

One more issue for group uniformity or diversity is stage of change. Some groups have been designed specifically for clients at an early stage of change (e.g., precontemplation or contemplation). Should stage of change be a factor determining group placement? There are some advantages and disadvantages in trying to structure a group in this way. Having group members who are all at a similar stage of change (e.g., precontemplation or contemplation) allows you to focus on the issues appropriate to that stage (e.g., ambivalence). On the other hand, homogeneity at the precontempla-tion level could encourage group alliances to resist change. It is also important to keep in mind that people may move back and forth among the stages of readiness, even within a single therapy session (Roll-nick, 1998).

> People may move back and forth among the stages of readiness, even within a single therapy session.

Intoxication

Most providers and programs do not permit clients to participate in a group session if they are visibly under the influence of alcohol or another drug. Certainly coming to treatment intoxicated can interfere with the individu-al's and group's ability to benefit. A possible policy here is that the person may not attend group when intoxicated, but can come back or make up the session when sober. If someone comes to the group under the influence of alcohol or drugs, the person should be asked in a nonjudgmental manner to leave and to return for the next session in a condition appropriate for participation.

It is important to have clear standards for how intoxication is deter-mined to avoid arguments about whether or not the person is under the influence. For alcohol, an on-the-spot breath test is feasible, and some instant urine test cups for multiple drug classes are also available. The final criterion, however, is your own judgment as the group leader. You can announce this procedure in advance, with apologies for any "false positive" errors you may make.

It is also important to ensure the individual's safety by helping the group member find a safe way home. Coordinate backup assistance with other providers, a cofacilitator, or support staff in your agency should this occur, to minimize disruption within the group. Having a brief discussion regarding feelings and thoughts this situation triggered for group partici-pants is an appropriate focus for a small portion of the session.

Resistance

Responding effectively to resistance is an important skill in doing group therapy. The material covered in Chapter 16 is all pertinent here, paralleling processes that occur in individual therapy. Because resistance is interpersonal behavior, the opportunities for it to arise are multiplied in group therapy. Remember that resistance occurs in response to communications from you or other group participants. It may appear as anger, interrupting, defensiveness, arguing, ignoring, shutting down, or even leaving the room. Such client behaviors predict poorer treatment outcome, and so it is important to respond effectively without strengthening or further increasing resistance.

A further complication is the possibility of collusion of resistance in a group format. Clients may elicit arguments against change from each other, mutually reinforcing resistance. We have had this experience, for example, in alcohol-focused groups with members of university fraternities, who readily fall into swapping drinking stories and minimizing the risks. The outcomes if this behavior occurs can be worse than no treatment at all, entrenching maladaptive substance use by normalizing it. Group resistance can also appear as a power struggle between the leader and a subset of clients. The easiest way to make this happen is to begin arguing with your clients, reacting defensively, and taking responsibility to argue for the "good" points. The best way to defuse it is to suppress your natural urge to argue back and instead roll with the resistance by practicing reflective listening and acknowledging client autonomy (see Chapters 4 and 16).

It is normal for alliances to develop among clients within groups, and they can be beneficial as mutual support. A group leader does need skill, however, for managing alliances that work against change, as when some group members join in opposition to you. Beyond the methods described in Chapter 16, one group dynamic strategy is to comment in a nonconfrontational way on this alliance, validate the concerns, and shift to a problem-solving focus (e.g., "John commented that this group doesn't seem to be helping him get better and then Sam and Bill said they were feeling the same way. The three of you seem to be feeling pretty stuck, and it seems like we need to find a way to make this work better").

A different problem is presented when group members respond to each other in unhelpful ways and thus elicit defensiveness. It can feel like a tug-of-war if you are using an empathic style that seems to be overshadowed by confrontational comments made by other group participants. Prohibiting cross-talk is one way to prevent this behavior. Another strategy is to teach group members specific ways of communicating with other group members (e.g., listening and "I" messages only).

GETTING THE GROUP STARTED

Once you have thought about these practical details and you have a plan for the size, length, membership, and nature of the group, it remains to

BOX 20.1. Group Structure Checklist

How often will the group meet?

How long will group meetings last?

Will membership be open or closed?

How will clients be screened, admitted, and oriented to the group?

If an open group, how will new members be introduced and integrated?

Will the group be of predetermined length (number of sessions) or ongoing?

Will there be a fixed sequence of topics to be covered?

Will meetings be held in a safe and accessible location?

How large will the group be (number of participants)?

Who will be the group leader(s)?

Will membership be homogeneous or heterogeneous with regard to:

   Gender?

   Stage of readiness?

   Treatment goals?

   Other client characteristics?

What is not allowed (weapons, drugs, violence, etc.) in the group?

What will be the norms and rules with regard to:

   Arriving on time (or late)?

   Privacy and confidentiality?

   Use of cell phones?

   Missed sessions?

   Physical touch?

   Contact outside of group sessions?

   Talking (e.g., raise hand, turn taking, no restrictions)?

   Reasons for termination from the group?

How will you handle:

   Self-disclosure?

   Resistance?

   Cross-talk?

   A member coming to group intoxicated?

What will the leader(s) be required to report (to courts, threats, child abuse, etc.)?

decide how people will be screened, admitted, and oriented to the group. If you work within an agency, there are probably procedures in place for connecting individuals with treatment options, and we offer here some general considerations for integrating clients into a group.

Screening Interview

We recommend that you, as group leader, meet individually at least once with each prospective group member prior to his or her entry to the group. This allows you to introduce yourself, get to know a bit about the person, and provide information about the purpose and rules of the group. A general question to consider together is whether this group is a good fit for this client's needs and goals. The individual pregroup interview is also an opportunity to build motivation to change (Chapter 10). It is useful to ask about any prior experiences with group therapy and the person's hopes and concerns about participation in the group. There are some practical issues to troubleshoot at this point as well. Does the meeting time and place of the group conflict with other responsibilities? Are there transportation problems or other obstacles to participation? You are also evaluating how this person is likely to function in and benefit from a group format in general. Some characteristics of people who may not be a good fit with group therapy include:

- Refusal or lack of interest in the group.
- Strong personal discomfort in groups.
- Severe impulse or anger control problems.
- Unwillingness to respect group rules, including confidentiality.
- Suicidal or in acute crisis.
- Language difficulties that make it hard to follow the conversation.
- Youth who may be adversely influenced by group contact with deviant peers.

If the group format isn't a good fit, what other options are available to the person? If the person is unsure about his or her willingness or desire to be in a group format, ask open questions followed by reflective listening statements (Chapter 4) to understand this person's situation and consider whether this is a good fit for both the individual and the group.

Admission to the Group

If this is a closed group and all participants are starting at the same time, you can introduce and orient everyone in the first meeting. When new members join an ongoing group, consider how they will be introduced to the group. Will you simply introduce them by first name and ask the group to welcome them? Do new participants tell a bit about their story? Do all members of the group introduce themselves to the new person in some way? Perhaps each person would say how long they have been in the group and what they have gained from it thus far. In your individual pregroup screening interview, you can explain these group entry procedures and expectations.

Orientation

Each participant needs to be oriented to the group. When all members are beginning a closed group together, this is done in the first session. With open groups, however, each new member needs an orientation before entry. Typically you won't want to take up much group time to do this for every new member, so most of it is accomplished in the individual pregroup interview.

One element of orientation is to explain the practical aspects of the group, in essence the decisions that you made about the issues discussed in the preceding section of this chapter and listed in Box 20.1 on page 324. It can be wise to prepare a written group agreement that states the group rules and conditions, for each member to sign prior to or at the beginning (essentially an informed consent to treatment). The rules contained in such an agreement should be clearly stated, particularly with regard to specific consequences of violations. The content of this agreement is informed by agency policy, applicable laws, and appropriate legal counsel. Some leaders develop the group agreement through a collaborative approach, allowing group members to contribute to its creation, which may increase adherence as members work toward consensus (Yalom & Leszcz, 2005).

The ethical standards that apply to individual therapy also apply to group therapy (see Chapter 22). While these legal and professional requirements are familiar to you, group members may be unaware of these rules and would benefit from a discussion of what information about them might be shared, under what circumstances, and why. One ethical issue particularly important to the group setting is confidentiality. Members should be admonished not to discuss anything outside of the group that might reveal the identity of other members. Group members will hear private information shared by others, and in order to facilitate an atmosphere of trust, group members need to feel safe enough to disclose their feelings and problems. Other legal requirements that are important to explain include the necessity of reporting instances of child or elder abuse and taking action when people threaten to harm themselves or others. There may also be specific requirements related to reporting missed sessions or premature termination for people who are mandated to treatment.

TERMINATION

There are generally three ways in which clients terminate their participation in group therapy. The first and happiest is successful completion of the group. The second is premature termination, when a client unilaterally decides to drop out of treatment. The third is a decision to terminate for cause, either unilaterally by the therapist or jointly with the client.

Coming to the End of Group Therapy

Termination of individual or group therapy, even when known in advance and expected, can bring up strong feelings for people, and an important part of the closure process in a closed group is to address these issues within therapy as the group's work is coming to an end. Within an open-enrollment group, termination is an ongoing issue as individual members complete the group and leave at different times. Here it may be helpful to have an individual termination session as well as a ritual for the group to say good-bye to completing members.

Premature Termination

As in individual counseling, a member in group therapy may fail to show up without notice. It is important to have clear procedures for responding promptly when this happens, particularly if attendance has been mandated by a court or external agent. In general we recommend taking the initiative after a missed appointment to contact the person as soon as possible by telephone, e-mail, or handwritten letter to ascertain the reason and welcome the person back to the group.

The first month is an especially critical time for retention in addiction treatment (Margolis & Zweben, 1998). Several factors enhance retention and adherence (see Chapter 17). For group therapy, a preparation/role induction session may be particularly important (Zweben et al., 1988) to build readiness and motivation for group work. Another factor that increases retention is the availability of wraparound services such as child care and transportation, barriers that often get in the way of successful treatment engagement. Most of the issues and strategies discussed in Chapter 17 apply in group work as well.

Termination for Cause

Finally, a client may be terminated early from group treatment for specific reasons. Termination may occur by mutual agreement between client and therapist; for example, the client's life circumstances may have changed (obtained or lost a job, moving to another city). A therapist or program may also decide unilaterally to remove a client from a group for a serious violation of the group agreement (e.g., violence during a group session). Such rules apply equally to all group members, and are made clear in advance.

> We do not recommend terminating clients from treatment because of substance use, which is in essence discharging people for the same reason that you admitted them.

As stated earlier, we do not recommend terminating clients from treatment because of substance use, which is in essence discharging people for the same reason that you admitted them. We instead suggest following the example of the 12-step fellowships and welcome people on the basis of their desire for sobriety, not their current pattern of use. If a person comes to group under the influence more than once, consider whether a different form of treatment may be needed.

With any termination, it is also good practice to help people find whatever additional services they need. The completion of a particular treatment is no guarantee that gains will be maintained. Discharge planning considers what continuing support clients may want and need, and includes proactive efforts to link them with services (see Chapters 8 and 19). When clients decide unilaterally to drop out of treatment, you can still communicate an open door policy to welcome them back should they choose or to help them find other services. When it is necessary to remove a person from a group for cause, it is usually possible to continue that person in some other form of treatment. In the situation where a unilateral decision is made to terminate clients from treatment altogether, there is a beneficent responsibility to help them get care elsewhere.

THE GROUP LEADER

What makes an effective group leader? Some of the crucial therapeutic skills are the same ones that characterize a good individual therapist. These common factors, such as empathy, therapeutic alliance, and listening skills, apply in both individual and group formats. An empathic, client-centered communication style is beneficial in group therapy. Conversely, research from the era of encounter groups indicated that having an adversarial, confrontational group leader was associated with higher rates of adverse effects and poor outcomes (Lieberman, Yalom, & Miles, 1973). An empathic style within a group context means being interested in, listening respectfully to, and skillfully reflecting content that is offered by group members. Blaming, criticizing, labeling, and shaming are to be avoided, as one would in individual therapy (Chapter 4).

Group therapy, however, is more complex than individual counseling. In a group setting, the therapeutic alliance involves multiple relationships— member to member, member to group, and member to leader—and the responsibility to maintain rapport within the group is challenging (Burlingame, Fuhriman, & Johnson, 2002). In group therapy, this rapport is often termed "cohesion," describing the benefits of belonging to a healthy environment where the emotional experience is that of acceptance, empathy, support, predictability, and honesty (Moos, Finney, & Maude-Griffin, 1993).

Thus, beyond the skills that you use in individual therapy, group treatment requires some additional know-how. One significant change is that the group environment is more fast-paced than individual therapy, and interactions between group members require increased creativity and spontaneity. The increased number of people also requires more redirection to ensure certain group members do not dominate the interactions or get the group off-track. Self-awareness and monitoring are other important aspects of successful facilitation of group therapy. For example, one common finding is that male group leaders tend to call on male members more than female members. As the leader of the group, be conscious of these tendencies and other thoughts and behaviors that guide your actions.

Yalom (1995) derived a factor analysis of a large number of leader variables for group therapy and categorized them into four basic leadership functions that were related to successful treatment outcome:

1. Acceptance—encouraging members to reflect in safety on their own experience, including maladaptive aspects, and express themselves openly and honestly. (Yalom called this "emotional stimulation," and it obviously overlaps with the clinical skill of accurate empathy.)
2. Caring—warmth, compassion, and genuineness.
3. Meaning attribution—helping clients develop their ability to understand themselves, each other, and people outside the group, as well as what they might do to change things in their lives.
4. Executive function—setting limits, rules, norms, goals, and managing time.

Beyond training in the particular type of psychotherapy (e.g., cognitive-behavioral), Yalom suggested observing experienced group therapists and having intense clinical supervision for the first few groups you conduct.

As group leader, you are also a model for clients in how you respond to others. The first few sessions are a particularly important period in this regard, as you model the behavior that is expected and establish group norms. Depending on the type of group, you may or may not directly teach participants positive skills for responding to each other, but you are always modeling a way of being with others. It is also important to intervene promptly to prevent negative communication patterns from emerging and being normalized in the group.

It is normal human nature to respond to people in different ways and to fluctuate in one's response depending on current mood and recent experience. Within a therapeutic group, however, it is important to respond as consistently and reliably as possible. Respond empathically and respectfully to what clients offer. Avoid favoritism, maintain clear and consistent boundaries, and enforce ground rules for speaking. It can be helpful to record some group sessions and review the recording afterward to listen for consistency in how you respond and for adherence to group rules. This makes it possible to hear things that you may have missed while you were so busy leading the group.

COGNITIVE-BEHAVIORAL SKILLS TRAINING

Beyond these general factors that are relevant to all types of group therapy, we now turn to a more specific consideration of cognitive-behavioral treatment (CBT), the most empirically supported form of group psychotherapy for addictions. CBT groups are intended to develop and strengthen behavioral and cognitive coping skills so that the person is better equipped to have a rewarding life without relying on psychoactive drugs. There is typically emphasis on identifying environmental and intrapersonal risk situations and practicing skills to cope with them successfully (as discussed in Chapters 11–13).

A potential disadvantage of group treatment is that there is less individual attention given to each person, and it can be easy for clients to be passive and tune out. Group treatment is necessarily less individualized, and you may be addressing skills that are already solidly in place for some but not other participants. You can deal with this potential disadvantage by planning activities that engage as many people as possible. Prevent long periods of passivity by having people take turns and work on individual worksheets. Some group approaches have client workbooks (e.g., Daley & Marlatt, 1999; Miller, 2008b; Miller & Mee-Lee, 2010a; Safren, Sprich, Perlman, & Otto, 2005) as well as facilitator guides. Other treatment resources include worksheets and handouts for clients (e.g., Monti et al., 2002; Miller, 2004). A key is to find ways to engage the group in such self-exploration processes rather than simply conducting individual therapy in a group setting. Group CBT can be integrated with motivational approaches (Sobell & Sobell, 2011).

Many CBT groups progress through a cycle of content, covering and practicing a variety of coping skills. This is possible even in open-format groups, where clients enter at different points in the cycle. You can prepare people for this structure in a pregroup individual session, and let them know where in the cycle they are entering. In open groups, people enter anywhere in the cycle and complete the group when it comes back around to the point where they entered.

A typical sequence in introducing a new skill is "tell–show–try." First explain what the skill is and how it works. Next demonstrate it. You go first, and show how the skill looks in practice. It can be fun here to invite participants to do their worst—to give you challenging situations to which you respond with the skill to be learned. It's also OK to struggle a bit here—to make mistakes, stop, and discuss how to do it better. A general social learning principle is that a "coping model" who responds well but imperfectly is generally more effective than a "mastery model" who exudes total competence (Schunk, 1991). Finally, let participants try out the skill. Usually skills are broken down into specific steps that build on each other. When clients are trying out a new skill, don't let other participants be too challenging. It is tempting for clients to pose impossibly difficult scenarios, in part because they are trying to imagine how they themselves might cope. Set it up so that people succeed as they learn a new skill. Take it in small steps, and give lots of positive reinforcement. Comment on what the client did well, perhaps make a small suggestion to try, and then again emphasize positive aspects of what the person did.

KEY POINTS

- On average, outcomes from group or individual counseling are similar.

- Didactic (lecture and film) and confrontational groups appear to have little or no beneficial impact on outcome.

- Many practical issues in group treatment warrant advance consideration and decisions (e.g., size, open vs. closed, duration and frequency, goals, talking rules).

- As in individual treatment, the counseling style of the group leader can have a substantial impact (for better or worse) on client outcomes.

- Cognitive-behavioral skill training is a well-supported form of group treatment.

REFLECTION QUESTIONS

Q How is leading a therapy group different from doing individual counseling?

Q On the list of practical decisions that one must make before beginning a group (Box 20.1), what are your personal preferences? Why?

Q What are the advantages and disadvantages of group versus individual treatment?

CHAPTER 21

Addressing the Spiritual Side

Among special issues that are likely to arise in addiction treatment (assuming you are open to it), spirituality is prominent. There is a widely shared view, especially within the United States, that spirituality is central to understanding and overcoming addiction. Certainly this view lies at the heart of the 12-step program, which is discussed later in this chapter. In a letter to Bill Wilson, cofounder of AA, Carl Jung (1975) quoted the ancient aphorism *spiritus contra spiritum* to mean that there is something mutually exclusive about alcohol (spirits) and healthy spirituality—each tends to drive out the other. Correlational data from a wide variety of studies support this inverse relationship. Religious involvement has been one of the strongest protective factors against the development of alcohol/drug problems, accounting for as much shared variance as family history of addiction (Borders, Curran, Mattox, & Booth, 2010; Gorsuch, 1995; Gorsuch & Butler, 1976; Miller, 1998). People with substance dependence tend to have relatively low levels of current religious and spiritual involvement, compared to the general U.S. population (Hilton, 1991; Larson & Wilson, 1980; Walters, 1957). Indeed, it is characteristic of substance dependence that the drug occupies an increasingly central place in the person's life, gradually displacing any and all prior involvements, relationships, and priorities, including religious ones. Involvement in AA after treatment is modestly but rather consistently associated with sustained abstinence (Emrick et al., 1993; Tonigan et al., 2003).

> Religious involvement has been one of the strongest protective factors against the development of alcohol/drug problems, accounting for as much shared variance as family history of addiction.

Less clear from a scientific perspective is a causal role of spiritual factors in the etiology of and recovery from addiction (Connors, Tonigan, et al., 2001; Miller & Thoresen, 2003; Tonigan, Miller, & Connors, 2001). Spirituality does tend to change and grow over the course of recovery (Brown, 1990; Robinson et al., 2007), as do physical, psychological, and interpersonal health. Whether these spiritual changes are causes, effects, or merely concomitants of abstinence is unclear. Perhaps all of these relationships are true in part.

WHAT IS SPIRITUALITY?

For most of human history, spirituality and religion were equated, a perspective that was evident in William James's (1902) classic volume *The Varieties of Religious Experience*. Within the latter half of the 20th century, however, spirituality came to be differentiated from religion in common usage (Hill et al., 2000). "Spirituality" began to refer to the individual's subjective experience of that which lies beyond the material world, be it of God, a Higher Power, a realm of spirit, meaning in life, or an ultimate reality that transcends human existence. "Religiousness" in turn came to refer to involvement in traditional institutional religion. It thus became meaningful to characterize oneself as "spiritual but not religious," which is also a common description of the 12-step program.

From a scientific perspective, one way to conceptualize spirituality is as a latent construct like personality or health, which has multiple measurable dimensions of belief, behavior, and experience (Miller & Thoresen, 1999, 2003). Within this view, individuals are not characterized as being "spiritual" versus "not spiritual," or as possessing a certain degree of spirituality. Instead, every person is located somewhere along the various dimensions of spirituality. As with health and personality, there is a large scientific literature on reliable measures of spirituality and religiousness (Hill & Hood, 1999; Hill & Pargament, 2003; Hood, Hill, & Spilka, 2009). Involvement in traditional institutional religion is but one aspect of a person's spirituality.

Over 95% of U.S. residents profess belief in a spiritual dimension of reality, be it a supreme God, supernatural beings such as angels, life after death, or ultimate values, and 7 in 10 report membership in a church, synagogue, or mosque (Gallup, 2002; Gallup & Lindsay, 1999). In contrast, the percentage of mental health professionals involved in religion in English-speaking nations tends to be much lower than that of the people they serve (Delaney, Miller, & Bisono, 2007). Through the 20th century, health professions increasingly distanced themselves from their historic roots in religion, and interest in spirituality was very much out of vogue, regarded at times as unprofessional or unscientific. Behavioral health professionals comfortably explored clients' sexuality, finances, family relationships, feelings, and fantasies, but rarely their religion or spirituality (Miller, 1999a). Interestingly, this was less true in addiction treatment, owing in part to the broad influence of the 12-step program, which unapologetically refers to God and emphasizes a spiritual path to recovery (Kurtz, 1991; Miller, 2003).

EXPLORING SPIRITUALITY

Often health professionals have not given much thought to how to ask people about their spiritual/religious side, but it's not difficult. A simple question such as "What role, if any, has religion or spirituality played in your life?" can open up the door to exploring both prior and current religious involvement. The "if any" gives implicit permission for the answer "None." It is also useful to find what exposure a client has had, if any, to AA or another 12-step program because many have at least sampled it. "Have you ever been to an AA meeting?" and if so, "What was that like for you?" (see Chapter 14). Asking, "Do you believe in God?" or "Do you pray?" (90% of Americans say they do; Koenig, Larson, & Weaver, 1998) can give you some indication of the person's potential receptiveness to a 12-step program.

It is also possible to explore spirituality more broadly. In considering what open questions to ask, it can be helpful to have an organizing framework to guide your exploration. One good option proposed by psychologist Paul Pruyser (1976) centers around seven key themes that can be explored in understanding a person's spirituality. Don't misappropriate a diagnostic model here, thinking that you must explore all seven themes or prescribe remedies. Pruyser's themes represent possible content in exploring spirituality, and it is likely that some will be more productive than others. Following are the seven themes, recast somewhat, that highlight core human experiences corresponding to each. It is common for people to use "God language" in talking about these themes, but if religious-sounding language is off-putting for a client, you can ask just as easily about the related core human experiences.

Theme 1: Awareness of the Sacred

Spirituality involves a search for the sacred, the transcendent, and one's relationship to it. What, then, does this person regard with reverence, as sacred or holy? For what does she or he make significant sacrifice, or would be willing to do so? To what, if anything, does this individual acknowledge dependence or ascribe ultimate worth? This can be a significant theme in recovery precisely because dependence on a drug represents progressively giving the drug central and ultimate value in one's life. What will fill the vacuum when substance use is no longer central? A core spiritual experience to explore here is that of awe, reverence, or unspeakable joy. This is a common component of mystical experience and spiritual transformation (Miller & C'de Baca, 2001). When and how has this person felt awe or wonder apart from the use of drugs?

Theme 2: Providence

Whatever the person's conception of the holy, how does he or she understand its disposition or intentions? Is God (or the universe, the world, a higher power) a good and friendly reality, or dark and punishing, or removed and indifferent? What or whom do they trust? What is expected of them, and what is owed to them? In what do they hope? Where (if at all) do they see light and promise? What happens after death? The corresponding core experience here is benevolence. When have they deeply felt benevolent intentions—toward them, or their own toward others? When and whom have they deeply trusted?

Theme 3: Faith

The focus here is not necessarily on "a faith," a particular religion or creed, although certainly this can be important. Rather, what does this person have faith in, believe in? To what is he or she committed? To what extent does the person feel secure and anchored, versus adrift? How inclined is the person to encounter and explore new ideas and perspectives, or does the person seem closed down, with little freedom to move? What is the person's "ultimate concern"? A core human experience here is deep security. This is not to be confused with certainty, the absence of doubt. Rather, in the midst of life's storms, when has the person still felt in some sense safe, grounded? A related experience is the courage of commitment, of devotion to something larger than oneself.

Theme 4: Gratitude

What is the person's experience of feeling blessed (or cursed)? For what is she or he grateful? Is there a sense of sufficiency, of having "enough" (in material goods, recognition, relationships, love) or a tone of deprivation, entitlement, and hunger for more? Has the person "earned" and deserved that which he or she has? There is, of course, the opposite stance of inability to accept grace, of ultimate undeservingness. A core human experience here is unmerited grace. When has the person needed and experienced forgiveness? When has the person extended forgiveness, and why? When has he or she been blessed? Related is the experience of contentment, of *dayenu*—enough—to be satisfied with what one has.

Theme 5: Repentance

To what extent does this person take responsibility for his or her own actions and circumstances? Again there are two extremes. At one extreme, the person experiences excessive remorse and responsibility. At the other, the person perceives little or no responsibility for adversity and assumes a victim role. At issue is conscience, or the self-monitoring and self-dissatisfaction that lead to recognition of a need for change. Related core experiences in this domain include remorse, regret, and contrition—normal human displeasure with self in reaction to actual or perceived guilt or wrongdoing.

Theme 6: Connection

In what ways, if at all, does the person feel connected to fellow human beings, to humanity in general, or to all of creation? At the low end is a "dog-eat-dog" individualism, a sense of being isolated, estranged, disconnected from, or in competition with others. At the higher end is the experience of interconnectedness and interdependence, a sense of community or a mystical experience of oneness with all of humanity or the universe. Core human experiences in this domain include caring for others and being cared for, reverence for life, and union.

Theme 7: Vocation

Finally, what is the person's sense of purpose in life? Is there something that God wants from him or her, or from all human beings? What is it that the person hopes for or is called to do with his or her life? Core experiences in this domain include a calling or a sense of belonging with particular tasks or talents, satisfaction (or dissatisfaction/restlessness) with how one's time is spent, and a sense of meaning and purpose (or lack thereof) in one's life.

Some possible questions for exploring each of these themes are suggested in Box 21.1.

12-STEP SPIRITUALITY

The original 12-step program, Alcoholics Anonymous (AA), grew out of the mutual support of its two cofounders, Bill Wilson and Dr. Bob Smith, and had its origins in a spiritual movement known as the Oxford Group (Kurtz, 1991; Lean, 1985). The structure of 12-step groups is discussed in

BOX 21.1. Some Spiritual Themes, Core Experiences, and Avenues for Exploration

Pruyser's Themes	Core Spiritual Experiences	Possible Open Questions for Exploration
Awareness of the Holy	Awe Reverence Bliss Joy	"What do you regard as sacred or holy?" "What gives you a sense of awe or wonder?" "For what/whom are you willing to make significant sacrifices?" "When in your life have you felt a deep sense of joy?"
Providence	Benevolence Trust Hope	"What do you imagine God is like?" "What image do you have about what happens after death?" "What or whom do you trust?" "What gives you hope?"
Faith	Deep security Safety Courage Commitment	"To what/whom are you most committed in life?" "How safe do you feel in your life?" "What or whom do you believe in, have faith in?" "What things are you anxious about?"
Gratitude	Grace Blessing Forgiveness Contentment	"For what are you most grateful?" "When in your life have you felt truly blessed?" "When has it been hard for you to forgive someone?" "When have you experienced forgiveness from someone?"
Repentance	Remorse Regret Contrition	"In what ways could you be a better person?" "What things in your life have you regretted?" "When have you felt guilty or ashamed?" "When have you seen a need for change in yourself and done it?"
Connection	Belonging Caring Being loved Union	"In what ways do you feel connected to other people?" "Where do you feel most at home, like you belong?" "Whom do you care for?" "Who cares for you?"
Vocation	Meaning Purpose Calling	"How do you understand your purpose in life?" "How do you spend your time? Why?" "What do you want to do with the years of your life?"

Chapter 14; our focus here is on the broad spirituality that serves as their foundation.

AA is unambiguously a spiritual program. It is, in fact, not a treatment but a way of living. Substance use is mentioned only in the first of the 12 steps (see Box 21.2). The rest describe spiritual processes: awareness of and relationship with God, self-examination, confessing shortcomings, openness to being transformed, making amends, prayer and meditation, and conveying the program to others who are still suffering. AA states that abstinence is only a beginning of this lifelong process of spiritual growth

---

BOX 21.2. The 12 Steps of Alcoholics Anonymous

1. We admitted we were powerless over alcohol—that our lives had become unmanageable.
2. Came to believe that a Power greater than ourselves could restore us to sanity.
3. Made a decision to turn our will and our lives over to the care of God *as we understood Him.*
4. Made a searching and fearless moral inventory of ourselves.
5. Admitted to God, to ourselves, and to another human being the exact nature of our wrongs.
6. Were entirely ready to have God remove all these defects of character.
7. Humbly asked Him to remove our shortcomings.
8. Made a list of all persons we had harmed, and became willing to make amends to them all.
9. Made direct amends to such people wherever possible, except when to do so would injure them or others.
10. Continued to take personal inventory and when we were wrong promptly admitted it.
11. Sought through prayer and meditation to improve our conscious contact with God *as we understood Him*, praying only for knowledge of His will for us and the power to carry that out.
12. Having had a spiritual awakening as the result of these steps, we tried to carry this message to others, and to practice these principles in all our affairs.

The 12 steps of AA and a brief excerpt from *Alcoholics Anonymous Comes of Age* (page 341) are reprinted with permission of Alcoholics Anonymous World Services, Inc. ("AAWS"). Permission to reprint these excerpts does not mean that AAWS has reviewed or approved the contents of this publication, or that AAWS necessarily agrees with the views expressed herein. AA is a program of recovery from alcoholism *only*—use of these excerpts in connection with programs and activities which are patterned after AA, but which address other problems, or in any other non-AA context, does not imply otherwise.

toward serenity. There are also 12-step programs that are focused more on illicit drugs (such as Narcotics Anonymous and Cocaine Anonymous).

From a 12-step perspective, the core of addiction lies in *character*. "Selfishness—self-centeredness! That, we think, is the root of our troubles" (Alcoholics Anonymous, 1976, p. 62). Much discussed in 12-step circles are "defects of character" as being at the heart of the pathology of addiction, faults such as obsession with power and control, resentment, dishonesty, defiance, and grandiosity. The long-term remedy, then, is a change of heart, the development of positive virtues such as forgiveness, humility, honesty, patience, responsibility, and wisdom (Peterson & Seligman, 2004; Webb & Trautman, 2010), through ongoing living of the 12-step program.

AA is not affiliated with any religion. The 12-step program, however, has deep roots in Judeo-Christian spirituality and its historic practices of contemplative prayer, confession, and meditative study (Keating, 2009a) to maintain "conscious contact with God" and conformity to God's will. AA is very permissive regarding how the individual understands God or a Higher Power, and the fellowship welcomes atheists and agnostics, who appear to benefit as much as others when they do participate (Tonigan et al., 2002).

Again, AA is not itself a treatment, but rather a spiritual program for living. The program is meant to be internalized and practiced throughout all of one's life (Keating, 2009a). As discussed in Chapters 7 and 14, a manual-guided form of 12-step facilitation (TSF) therapy was developed to encourage clients' entry and engagement in the fellowship of AA (Nowinski & Baker, 1998; Nowinski et al., 1992). TSF was designed to introduce clients to AA, help them work through the first three to five steps of the program, and get established with a sponsor in a home group. Clients assigned at random to TSF on average fared at least as well as those in cognitive-behavioral or motivational-enhancement therapies (Babor & Del Boca, 2003).

Transformational Change

The reference in step 12 to a "spiritual awakening" bespeaks another phenomenon that is observed in recovery, that of sudden transformation. William James (1902) described two kinds of change that occur in human life. The first, more common and familiar, is a step-by-step process of successive approximations that he called the "educational" or "volitional" variety of change. Most people most of the time change in this way: gradually in small steps, like the learning of a new language or skill.

Sudden and seemingly permanent transformations do occur, however. James and his contemporary George Coe documented dozens of these sudden and striking transformations. The occurrence of epiphanies and sudden transformation is familiar in most world religions, and is also found with some frequency in autobiographies (Bidney, 2004; White, 2004). This was certainly the experience of Bill Wilson, who found his own sobriety in this way when from a hospital bed he prayed for help:

> Suddenly the room lit up with a great white light. I was caught up into an ecstasy which there are no words to describe. It seemed to me, in the mind's eye, that I was on a mountain and that a wind not of air but of spirit was blowing. And then it burst upon me that I was a free man. Slowly the ecstasy subsided. I lay on the bed, but now for a time I was in another world, a new world of consciousness. All about me and through me there was a wonderful feeling of Presence, and I thought to myself, "So this is the God of the preachers!" A great peace stole over me and I thought, "No matter how wrong things seem to be, they are all right." (Alcoholics Anonymous World Services, 1957, p. 63; reprinted by permission)

Miller and C'de Baca (2001) interviewed 55 people who had experienced such "quantum change," on average 11 years earlier, with a further 10-year follow-up for a two-decade retrospective (C'de Baca & Wilbourne, 2004), concluding that such transformations appear to be permanent, a kind of one-way door through which people pass. Their experience is quite different from that of the white-knuckle struggle to avoid a return to substance use that is so common in early recovery. Such stories of sudden spiritual transformation are frequently encountered within AA (Forcehimes, 2004), although AA clearly recognizes and honors the gradual "educational" variety of spiritual awakening and recovery as being the more common path.

RECONNECTING WITH RELIGIOUS ROOTS

Recovery from addiction involves reversing the process of isolation through which the person's life became centered on substance use, gradually pushing out other activities, involvements, and relationships. Abstinence creates a vacuum, removing what had been the person's primary use of time, energy, and devotion. It is important therefore for the recovering person to connect or reconnect with other sources of pleasure, meaning, and engagement (see Chapter 11).

It is common for people to have become particularly detached from whatever religious roots they may have had as their substance dependence progressed. Substance use generally competes for the time, talent, energy, and resources that might otherwise be invested in social relationships. Beyond this general trend, people may distance themselves from religion because their substance use and related behavior clash with religious values. Some have experienced outright judgment and rejection from religious quarters, and carry emotional scars. For such people, AA's characterization as being "spiritual but not religious" may make it safer to reexplore spiritual terrain.

For people who have simply drifted away from their religious roots, however, reconnection with their spirituality and a religious community may be a helpful part of recovery. Religious communities and activities typically do not involve drinking or other drug use, and thus they offer an alternative to a prior addictive lifestyle. Like AA, they can also provide a positive social network supportive of sobriety. Also like AA meetings, congregations vary widely in warmth, structure, dogmatism, and acceptance, and it can be useful for a person to sample a number of different ones to find a spiritual home.

Clergy can also be helpful and supportive in the recovery process, particularly those with a loving understanding of addiction. Individual clients may carry heavy baggage from negative religious experiences. In combination with the low self-esteem common in addictions, such experiences may convince a person that he or she is unforgivable, unworthy, unlovable, or is being rejected and punished by God. A loving and knowledgeable pastor, rabbi, imam, or chaplain may be able to help people work through such spiritual obstacles. If the client does not have a home congregation, you could offer referral to clergy you trust. In this regard, it is useful to meet members of the clergy from various religious backgrounds and discuss addiction with them, in order to develop a list of religious professionals to whom you can refer with confidence.

SPIRITUAL DISCIPLINES

In Gallup, New Mexico, there is a unique addiction rehabilitation program, the Na'nizhoozhi Center, Inc. (NCI). It serves primarily Navajo and other Native American people from the surrounding reservations. NCI has integrated evidence-based treatment methods with Native American spirituality (Miller, Meyers, & Hiller-Sturmhofel, 1999). Out in back of the center is a compound with teepees, sweat lodges, and ceremonial dance grounds. For Native people, reconnection with their common spiritual roots can be an important part of recovery.

In most Western treatment settings, however, people come from a wide variety of religious backgrounds. For some, religion is just as central to cultural identify as it is for Native Americans. In Hispanic and African American communities, for example, religion tends to play a major role in cultural life. For such people with religious heritage, what might be the spiritual equivalent of Indian dances, ceremonies, and sweat lodges? It is found, we believe, in the spiritual disciplines of world religions, which have been in practice for centuries if not millennia as paths to spiritual growth. Several of these have a prominent role in 12-step programs: prayer, meditation, surrender, confession, and reconciliation.

One of the most studied spiritual disciplines in the addiction field is mindfulness or transcendental meditation, which has been found to be inversely related to substance use both in the general population and among clients in addiction treatment (Aron & Aron, 1980; Bowen et al., 2006; Marlatt & Marques, 1977; O'Connell & Alexander, 1994). The practice and benefits of meditation can be deepened by, but do not depend on, any particular religious framework, and the basic components for learning it are relatively simple (Benson & Klipper, 1990; Kabat-Zinn, 2006). A sense of relaxation and peacefulness is often experienced quite early in practice, but health benefits tend to occur with sustained practice. Written resources for learning meditation and applying it in addiction recovery are widely available (Bien, 2006; Bien & Bien, 2002; Bowen, Chawla, & Marlatt, 2010; Kabat-Zinn, 2006; Keating, 2009b), as are more general guides for the practice of spiritual disciplines (Foster, 1998; Moore, 1994; Thompson, 2005). Much has also been written by professionals on spirituality (e.g., Guenther, 1992; Merton, 1986; Miller, 1999b; Pargament, Murray-Swank, Magyar, & Ano, 2005; Richards & Bergin, 1997; Thorne, 1998).

Is it effective to promote the practice of spiritual disciplines during the stabilization and rehabilitation phases of addiction treatment? The sizeable correlational literature showing the inverse relationship of addiction and spiritual practice is encouraging in this regard. To find out, we offered individual direction in the use of spiritual disciplines to people during and following residential treatment for substance use disorders. Clients who were interested and willing to participate were randomly assigned to receive or not receive up to 12 sessions of spiritual direction in addition to treatment as usual. In two separate studies, contrary to our expectations, we found absolutely no benefit, whether the additional sessions were offered by professional spiritual directors or by treatment program staff (Miller, Forcehimes, O'Leary, & LaNoue, 2008). Even on spiritual health measures, we saw no change. In retrospect, our expectations were rather naïve. These people had just completed detoxification and had a plethora of pressing life concerns to deal with: finding jobs, a place to live, safety, and child care, in addition to maintaining their newfound sobriety. On Maslow's (1943, 1970) hierarchy of needs, they were down at the bottom of the pyramid addressing basic needs, and we were up at the top talking about spirituality and meaning in life. Furthermore, spiritual development is a lifelong process, and not one to be addressed in a few sessions. Although the whole 12-step program is spiritual, the disciplined practice of prayer and meditation appears later, at step 11. We concluded that a better time to work on spiritual disciplines may be in the maintenance phase, rather than early in stabilization or rehabilitation (see Chapter 7).

EXPLORING VALUES

> Another aspect of the spiritual side of human nature is that which people value, or what is of "ultimate concern" to them.

Another aspect of the spiritual side of human nature is that which people value, or what is of "ultimate concern" to them (Emmons, 2003; Tillich, 1973). What is most important or sacred to this person sitting across from you? What do your clients most want in life for themselves and those they love? What are the values that guide them? In substance dependence, the drug itself gradually becomes the person's ultimate concern, the center of life, displacing all that was dear and sacred before. The process of recovery and a life of sobriety involve discovering or rediscovering the sacred—that which is of ultimate importance.

It can be useful, therefore, to help your clients clarify what matters most to them. Various tools have been developed for this purpose (Rokeach, 1973; Simon, Howe, & Kirschenbaum, 1995). A simple but effective tool is a values card sort, which consists of a set of cards each describing something that may be important to people. Various lists have been developed for different populations, or you can develop your own. The list in Box 21.3 consists of a hundred cards from which to choose. You may wish to use fewer cards and modify the language for the populations you serve. Typically, the client sorts the cards into three to five piles based on their personal importance. If the highest importance pile is large, you can ask the person to choose from it the 5 to 10 values that are most important, most central to his or her identity. These can then be rank-ordered from most important (1) on down. Finally, interview the person about these core values. Some open questions that can be helpful here are:

"Why did you choose this as a central value for you?"
"In what ways is this important to you?"
"How have you shown this core value in your daily life?"
"In what ways could you be even more true to this value?"

Such a conversation about the client's 5 to 10 core values—asking open questions and following with reflective listening (Chapter 4)—can teach you much about the person's hopes, aspirations, and guiding principles for living. It also can strengthen your understanding and working alliance.

Having elicited a client's core values, it is further possible to ask how alcohol/drug use affects the person's living out of each of these core values. Has it helped the person be consistent with this value? Has it hindered living out the value? Or is it irrelevant? You need not draw conclusions for the client; the answer is usually obvious, but asking about substance use in relation to what the person holds dearest can sometimes crystallize motivation for change (Baumeister, 1994).

BOX 21.3. A Values Card Sort

William R. Miller, Janet C'de Baca, Daniel B. Matthews, and Paula L. Wilbourne

These values are usually printed onto individual cards that people can sort into three to five piles such as "Most Important," "Very Important," "Important," "Somewhat Important," and "Not Important." It is wise also to provide a few empty cards so that people can add values of their own. These items are in the public domain and may be copied, adapted, or used without further permission.

1. ACCEPTANCE	to be accepted as I am
2. ACCURACY	to be correct in my opinions and beliefs
3. ACHIEVEMENT	to have important accomplishments
4. ADVENTURE	to have new and exciting experiences
5. ART	to appreciate or express myself in art
6. ATTRACTIVENESS	to be physically attractive
7. AUTHORITY	to be in charge of others
8. AUTONOMY	to be self-determined and independent
9. BEAUTY	to appreciate beauty around me
10. BELONGING	to have a sense of belonging, being part of
11. CARING	to take care of others
12. CHALLENGE	to take on difficult tasks and problems
13. COMFORT	to have a pleasant and comfortable life
14. COMMITMENT	to make enduring, meaningful commitments
15. COMPASSION	to feel and act on concern for others
16. COMPLEXITY	to embrace the intricacies of life
17. COMPROMISE	to be willing to give and take in reaching agreements
18. CONTRIBUTION	to make a lasting contribution in the world
19. COOPERATION	to work collaboratively with others
20. COURAGE	to be brave and strong in the face of adversity
21. COURTESY	to be considerate and polite toward others
22. CREATIVITY	to create new things or ideas
23. CURIOSITY	to seek out, experience, and learn new things
24. DEPENDABILITY	to be reliable and trustworthy
25. DILIGENCE	to be thorough and conscientious in whatever I do
26. DUTY	to carry out my duties and obligations
27. ECOLOGY	to live in harmony with the environment
28. EXCITEMENT	to have a life full of thrills and stimulation

(cont.)

BOX 21.3. *(cont.)*

29. FAITHFULNESS	to be loyal and true in relationships
30. FAME	to be known and recognized
31. FAMILY	to have a happy, loving family
32. FITNESS	to be physically fit and strong
33. FLEXIBILITY	to adjust to new circumstances easily
34. FORGIVENESS	to be forgiving of others
35. FREEDOM	to be free from undue restrictions and limitations
36. FRIENDSHIP	to have close, supportive friends
37. FUN	to play and have fun
38. GENEROSITY	to give what I have to others
39. GENUINENESS	to act in a manner that is true to who I am
40. GOD'S WILL	to seek and obey the will of God
41. GRATITUDE	to be thankful and appreciative
42. GROWTH	to keep changing and growing
43. HEALTH	to be physically well and healthy
44. HONESTY	to be honest and truthful
45. HOPE	to maintain a positive and optimistic outlook
46. HUMILITY	to be modest and unassuming
47. HUMOR	to see the humorous side of myself and the world
48. IMAGINATION	to have dreams and see possibilities
49. INDEPENDENCE	to be free from depending on others
50. INDUSTRY	to work hard and well at my life tasks
51. INNER PEACE	to experience personal peace
52. INTEGRITY	to live my daily life in a way that is consistent with my values
53. INTELLIGENCE	to keep my mind sharp and active
54. INTIMACY	to share my innermost experiences with others
55. JUSTICE	to promote fair and equal treatment for all
56. KNOWLEDGE	to learn and contribute valuable knowledge
57. LEADERSHIP	to inspire and guide others
58. LEISURE	to take time to relax and enjoy
59. LOVED	to be loved by those close to me
60. LOVING	to give love to others
61. MASTERY	to be competent in my everyday activities
62. MINDFULNESS	to live conscious and mindful of the present moment
63. MODERATION	to avoid excesses and find a middle ground
64. MONOGAMY	to have one close, loving relationship

(cont.)

BOX 21.3. *(cont.)*

65.	MUSIC	to enjoy or express myself in music
66.	NONCONFORMITY	to question and challenge authority and norms
67.	NOVELTY	to have a life full of change and variety
68.	NURTURANCE	to encourage and support others
69.	OPENNESS	to be open to new experiences, ideas, and options
70.	ORDER	to have a life that is well ordered and organized
71.	PASSION	to have deep feelings about ideas, activities, or people
72.	PATRIOTISM	to love, serve, and protect my country
73.	PLEASURE	to feel good
74.	POPULARITY	to be well liked by many people
75.	POWER	to have control over others
76.	PRACTICALITY	to focus on what is practical, prudent, and sensible
77.	PROTECT	to protect and keep safe those I love
78.	PROVIDE	to provide for and take care of my family
79.	PURPOSE	to have meaning and direction in my life
80.	RATIONALITY	to be guided by reason, logic, and evidence
81.	REALISM	to see and act realistically and practically
82.	RESPONSIBILITY	to make and carry out responsible decisions
83.	RISK	to take risks and chances
84.	ROMANCE	to have intense, exciting love in my life
85.	SAFETY	to be safe and secure
86.	SELF-ACCEPTANCE	to accept myself as I am
87.	SELF-CONTROL	to be disciplined in my own actions
88.	SELF-ESTEEM	to feel good about myself
89.	SELF-KNOWLEDGE	to have a deep and honest understanding of myself
90.	SERVICE	to be helpful and of service to others
91.	SEXUALITY	to have an active and satisfying sex life
92.	SIMPLICITY	to live life simply, with minimal needs
93.	SOLITUDE	to have time and space where I can be apart from others
94.	SPIRITUALITY	to grow and mature spiritually
95.	STABILITY	to have a life that stays fairly consistent
96.	TOLERANCE	to accept and respect those who differ from me
97.	TRADITION	to follow respected patterns of the past
98.	VIRTUE	to live a morally pure and excellent life
99.	WEALTH	to have plenty of money
100.	WORLD PEACE	to work to promote peace in the world

KEY POINTS

🔖 Spiritual/religious involvement is a consistent predictor of lower risk for substance use disorders.

🔖 People who develop substance dependence are often disconnected or even alienated from their spiritual/religious traditions and community (if they had one).

🔖 The program of AA and other 12-step groups is strongly spiritual but not affiliated with any religion and welcomes all who desire sobriety regardless of belief.

🔖 Sudden transformational changes that release people from addictions are well documented, though most people change in a more gradual manner.

🔖 Exploring a person's core values can clarify what are often regarded as spiritual or meaning-in-life motivations for change.

REFLECTION QUESTIONS

💬 How would you describe your own spirituality?

💬 What role (if any) do you think spirituality has in recovery from addiction?

💬 How do you understand the widely reported phenomenon of sudden transformational changes (like that of Bill W.) that release people from addiction?

CHAPTER 22

Professional Ethics

In Greek mythology, the Sphinx guarded the entrance to the city of Thebes and asked a riddle of those who wished to enter, devouring travelers who failed to answer correctly (Hamilton, 1999). One reported version of the riddle is: "What creature goes on four feet in the morning, on two at noonday, and on three in the evening?" The right answer was "man," who early in life crawls on all fours, then learns to walk upright on two feet, and in later years walks with a stick. Francis Bacon (1992) regarded this myth as an allegory for the scientist's search for truth.

In treating addictions, we are confronted daily with puzzling riddles, fitting together the pieces of a puzzle to find what seems to be the best answer for the people we serve. One of our goals in this book is to provide the knowledge to solve some of these puzzles, but a different kind of riddle in clinical practice comes in the form of ethical questions to which there may not be black-and-white answers, yet which may need to be decided quickly. Getting one of these riddles wrong can indeed devour you in lawsuits, loss of license, or even criminal charges.

Sometimes an applicable law does mandate a clear answer. An example is found in laws that require professionals to break client confidentiality in order to protect people from clear and imminent danger, or to report child or elder abuse (Kalichman, 1999; Welfel, Danzinger, & Santoro, 2000). In many cases, however, the ethical dilemma falls within a legally permissive gray area where more than one answer could be argued to be the right one. Additional guidance may be provided by the code of ethics for your profession, although general ethical codes may not factor in the unique and specific circumstances that can muddle professional decision making (Pope & Vasquez, 2007). How then does one decide what is the right thing to do?

Ethics is the branch of philosophy that is about values for defining what is right and wrong in human actions and decisions. It is not an area in which answers come from the memorization of facts. Ethics is a different sort of beast, a different kind of riddle. It is more about judgment and critical thinking than retrieval of information. The kind of riddle posed by the Sphinx was not one for which the answer could be retrieved from memory. It required thoughtful reflection to arrive at the right answer.

Ethical decision making is also not an appropriate arena for trial and error. It is not like scientific hypothesis testing. There isn't much room for "Whoops! I guess that was the wrong decision. Oh well. I'll now know what to do differently in the future." The ethical Sphinx gives us one chance to get it right, to make the best decision with the information that we have available at this particular moment, in a specific set of circumstances that we may never encounter again. Once this kind of decision has been made, we cannot take it back. Once done, a breach of confidentiality, misrepresentation, or a sexual boundary violation cannot be undone.

WHAT IT MEANS TO BE A PROFESSIONAL

Why do we have to answer the Sphinx's questions at all? It is in part because we have unique access to the road on which they arise, and so we must decide how to respond when they do. Unlike a job, in which one may travel alone and operate independently, the nature of a profession is to have privileged work that interfaces with and impacts the lives of others. Ethical decision making is part of our duty as clinical professionals.

Different standards exist for professions such as law, medicine, counseling, and clergy because particular values are attached to these professions, but there is also commonality. Professionals have unique specialized knowledge that gives them significant influence over the lives of others. With this role and knowledge come respect, trust, and credibility to the public. Degrees and licenses are symbols that people can trust us even though they don't know us personally. Clients come to us in vulnerability, and expect competent professional treatment. They place in our hands their trust, sensitive private information, and significant influence. A professional relationship is inherently one of uneven power.

> A professional relationship is inherently one of uneven power.

A BRIEF HISTORY OF ETHICS

Ethics have been debated for thousands of years. The professional oath for physicians that is attributed to Hippocrates dates from the fourth century

B.C.E. and contains a variety of ethical principles including "first of all, to do no harm." Formal ethical standards of professional conduct, however, are surprisingly recent in origin. It was the Nazi medical experiments during World War II that prompted the development of formal safeguards to protect human participants in research. Principles of voluntary participation with informed consent arose from the Nuremberg trials in a 1948 code that required a balancing of the potential benefits of research against its risks. It took even longer to implement ethical principles systematically in clinical care.

A 1979 document known as the Belmont Report (*www.hhs.gov/ohrp/ policy/belmont.htm*) set forth three basic consensus principles as a moral basis for responsible conduct in research. The first of these is *autonomy/ respect for persons*, meaning that individuals should be treated as self-determining agents and that people with diminished autonomy are entitled to additional protections. The second principle is *beneficence*, which means that participants should not be harmed and research should maximize possible benefits and minimize possible risks. The third principle is *justice*, meaning that the benefits and risks of research should be distributed fairly. These principles provided a way of thinking about professional ethical responsibilities in terms of obligations and duties. A fourth principle of nonmaleficence (do no harm) has subsequently been differentiated from beneficence, leading to a practical four-principle approach for ethical decision making known as *principlism* (Beauchamp & Childress, 2001). These four basic principles represent a minimum consensus of what should guide providers' ethical decision making.

Nonmaleficence

The principle of nonmaleficence is that clinical providers should not cause harm. The Hippocratic Oath places this even before doing good. Unpleasant though it is to contemplate, what we do in our work with clients is not inert and so has the potential to harm people. Delivering an ineffective treatment may leave clients feeling hopeless, as though nothing will help them. A confrontational counseling style is particularly liable to do harm, especially with more vulnerable clients (Annis & Chan, 1983; Lieberman et al., 1973; MacDonough, 1976; White & Miller, 2007). Protecting confidentiality is an important part of preventing harm from disclosure of information.

It is also possible to do harm by inaction. Is it ethical, for example, to allow an intoxicated client to drive away? A colleague who is a trauma surgeon asked herself whether it was ethical for her to treat only the physical injuries resulting from alcohol-related crashes and indiscretions, but do nothing to encourage a change in drinking. People who come into an emergency room or a trauma center with alcohol-related injuries are at substantially increased risk for future morbidity and mortality because of their drinking. Is it ethical, then, to do nothing to try to change the behavior that caused the injury?

Beneficence

In addition to preventing harm, providers should actively promote clients' welfare. The treatment services that we provide should be those most likely to benefit and least likely to harm clients. This is a clear argument for offering the best evidence-based treatment methods at our disposal. It is what we expect of our own health care providers.

Autonomy

As much as possible, people should have choices, freedom, and adequate understanding when making decisions about treatment. The principle of autonomy is a reminder of our clients' inherent worth as human beings and the need to respect their own values and goals. Whatever clinicians may do, it is ultimately the client who decides whether, when, and how to change. In that sense, telling clients that they "can't" or "must" is not actually accurate. Honoring autonomy certainly involves telling people the truth about their options, and having an open discussion about choices. These are fundamental to informed consent. It is also truth telling to acknowledge that only the client can decide whether or not to make changes.

> Telling clients that they "can't" or "must" is not actually accurate.

Justice

The principle of justice primarily has to do with an equal distribution of benefits and burdens. One important issue here is *access* to treatment. Ideally, effective treatment should be available on demand to anyone who wants and needs it, without regard to their personal characteristics or ability to pay. The perspective of "There but for fortune" is helpful here—that we don't deserve whatever advantages we happen to have, and by the luck of the draw could be sitting in the client's chair instead (Rawls, 1999).

Promoting justice of course includes ensuring that our services are fairly available and provided without discrimination. A sliding scale that adjusts fees to clients' ability to pay is one common approach in a fee-for-service context, as is providing some pro bono work for those who can't afford treatment. Another example is taking appropriate caution when using assessment and treatment procedures with populations other than those with whom they have been developed and tested.

Ethical Balance

There are times when these four principles conflict with each other, and ethical navigation involves finding the right balance of considerations (Beauchamp & Childress, 2001). An ethical situation (see Box 22.1) may require giving greater weight to one of the principles while balancing with the others as much as possible given the particular dilemma under consideration.

For example, two principles that often clash with each other are beneficience and nonmaleficence. In the process of trying to do good, there is a risk that some harm may be done. For example, the efficacy of some medications is directly related to the presence of risk and unpleasant side effects. To use a behavioral example, treating PTSD with exposure therapy necessarily causes the person to experience short-term distress.

Taleff (2009) recommended these steps as a process for evaluating ethical dilemmas:

BOX 22.1. An Ethical Puzzle

Consider what you might do in the following situation: You are treating a 30-year-old woman named Vanessa, who is on probation for a drug-related offense. She reenrolled in community college, maintained a B+ average in her first semester courses, earned a scholarship, and found a steady job working as a waitress. Vanessa knows that her probation officer, who referred her to treatment, requires regular updates from you regarding her progress, and specifically asked to be informed of any drug use. For the past 6 months she has been coming regularly for counseling, and all urine screens have been drug-free. Now with only a few weeks left in her second semester back in college, she is going into her finals with an A average. Vanessa arrives for this week's session on time and tearfully informs you that she made a terrible mistake and used cocaine once after receiving tragic news that her mother was diagnosed with pancreatic cancer and has only a few weeks to live. This is the first time Vanessa has used drugs since she was put on probation, and her urine drug screen was again clear. She is ashamed and tells you that she just wanted to be open and honest with you and work on the skills needed to maintain her sobriety and find alternative ways to cope with stress. She pleads with you to not tell her probation officer, knowing that she will not be able to complete the semester, will lose her job and scholarship, and could not spend the last few weeks with her mother if her probation is revoked and she is sent back to jail.

What do you do? How would you balance the four principles of nonmaleficence, benevolence, autonomy, and justice? What would affect your decision?

1. Collect yourself and settle down. Take some deep breaths and get some emotional distance.
2. Clearly identify the ethical dilemma. Is there something wrong? An injustice done? A right violated? Someone harmed?
3. Start gathering your facts and evidence. What do you already know? What do you need to know, but don't? Who exactly is involved? How reliable are your facts?
4. Consult with relevant guidelines, codes, or authorities. What do national and regional ethical guiding principles/codes have to say about the situation? With whom might you consult as reliable colleagues with good ethical judgment?
5. Look at the identified problem through various ethical perspectives. What are the issues from the perspective of nonmaleficence? Beneficence? Autonomy? Justice?
6. Look at the problem through critical thinking principles. If you could form an argument regarding this situation, what would be your premises and conclusions?
7. Weigh the arguments and evidence and make a first probable course of judgment and action. How would the judgment direct a course of action?
8. Rest and reflect. Focus on other things for a while (unless a decision needs to be made immediately).
9. Revisit your first judgment and first course of action by going through steps 1–7 again, and refine as necessary.
10. If your assessment reveals that your first judgment/decision seems to be the best thing to do, then it's time for action. Make a decision and act on it.

PRACTICAL GUIDELINES

With this background, we turn now to some specific practical issues, beginning with two common ones—informed consent and confidentiality—that illustrate how such issues may be complicated when treating addictions.

Informed Consent

Informed consent is a formal procedure that is required before people participate in research, and similar (though sometimes less formal) procedures are used in treatment. In primary care, this is often a generic consent to receive treatment, without specifying what treatment procedures will be used. More specific informed consent may be required with particular specialist procedures, such as surgery, and with experimental treatments.

Often consent is thought of as a one-time event occurring before treatment, but the consenting process can also be ongoing and revisited from time to time as needs, goals, and plans change. It may be necessary to obtain consent in formal written format, or in other circumstances it may be verbal and documented in case notes. In addiction treatment, the consent process can be compromised by short-term (intoxication or withdrawal) or long-term neurobiological changes related to drug use. This is another reason to revisit consent after Phase 2 stabilization.

There are three primary elements of informed consent, the first of which is *competence*. The consenting person must have the ability to make a decision that is in his or her own best interest (Van Staden & Krüger, 2003). In court, this is a legal determination made by specified criteria. In practice, it is a judgment call whether the person is able to understand the situation and make an informed choice. When a person is legally incapable of giving informed consent, then permission is typically obtained from a legally authorized person except when immediate emergency care is required. As much as possible with clients who cannot themselves give consent (e.g., minors), still inform them of what is happening, consider their preferences and best interests, and seek their assent to treatment.

Comprehension, a second requirement for informed consent, implies the capacity to understand the information presented. The information should be presented in language that the client can understand. Because of the possible acute and long-term effects of substance use, educational level is not itself a sufficient indicator of comprehension. It is wise therefore to check for comprehension of key points. With written consents, we have asked clients to read a key paragraph of the consent form in order to ensure reading ability. The person is always offered time to ask questions, and it is also reasonable to ask clients to tell you what they understood about key points, to make sure they comprehend. Some of the information commonly included in a consent process includes:

- A clear description of the treatment to be provided.
- A fair and balanced disclosure of what is known about the efficacy of the treatment, and of known risks and side effects.
- The expected duration of treatment and conditions for termination.
- The alternatives that are available besides the proposed treatment, whether or not you yourself can provide them.
- The qualifications of treatment staff to provide the treatment.
- The protections and limits of confidentiality.
- Financial aspects of treatment, such as fees and policies regarding missed or cancelled appointments.

Given all of this, a written and signed consent form offers some advantages. The original can be retained in the client's file, and the client can also be given a copy.

In addition to competence and comprehension, a third essential element for informed consent is *freedom of choice*. The person should freely choose to participate in the research or treatment without any coercion or undue influence (such as excessive incentives). The consent must be clearly expressed, documented, and witnessed, and maintained in the person's records.

Confidentiality and Its Limitations

Confidentiality implies an explicit contract or promise not to reveal anything about your client except under certain circumstances agreed to by both parties. Even the fact that a person is being treated is itself confidential information. This is both a standard component of professional ethics (not to discuss or disclose to anyone a client's private information without permission) and a stipulation of applicable laws. U.S. federal regulations require an even higher than normal level of confidentiality protection for client records of treatment for substance use disorders.

Privilege is a legal term describing certain specific types of relationships that enjoy protection from legal proceedings. In many jurisdictions, people don't have privilege unless they specifically ask for it in an explicit way. Therefore, it is wise in your consent form or elsewhere in client records to document that the person expected and requested confidentiality.

We advise our trainees to observe paranoid standards in protecting client confidentiality. Imagine that there are people actively trying to find out private information about your client. There are some commonsense practical things to do. Close the door whenever you are discussing private information with or about a client. Keep client records in locked cabinets in a locked room with restricted access. *Never* discuss clients in a hallway or public place, even without using names or identifying information. If someone calls for information about a client, do not even acknowledge whether or not the person is in treatment without a written release of information. If you have such a release, ensure that you are talking to the appropriate person before disclosing any information. Technological innovations have challenged traditional confidentiality protections, so be particularly aware of how the use of cell phones, answering systems, fax machines, e-mail, and the Internet may impact client confidentiality.

People with substance use disorders are particularly stigmatized, so there are extra safeguards in place when working with this population. Inadvertent disclosure of treatment information could cause someone to lose a job, insurance, a security clearance, or a relationship, and to experience discrimination by other health care professionals. A U.S. federal rule (42 CFR, part 2) provides special protection for the confidentiality of patients suffering from or seeking evaluation for substance-related problems. This rule applies to any treatment program receiving direct or indirect federal funding or a tax-exempt status and requires substance-related problems to be kept separate from other health information and protected from subpoena or warrant if the records are requested.

Group therapy (Chapter 20) presents some ethical complexities with regard to confidentiality because information is shared within the group. The standard way to address this issue is to establish the ethical ground rule that anything shared in the group remains within the group, and neither the group's membership nor its content are to be discussed with others. Each participant in the group should explicitly agree to this. A tradition in some 12-step groups is to recite this reminder at the end of each meeting: "Who you see here, what you hear here, stays here!" Clients, of course, are not bound by the same ethical and legal requirements that guide your professional practice, so you cannot guarantee the same level of anonymity and confidentiality as would apply in individual treatment.

What happens to confidentiality if your client is deceased? You might be asked, for example, for information that is relevant in settling a disputed estate or that would be helpful to an insurance company in determining whether the client's death was a suicide. However, a client's death does not negate confidentiality, nor can next of kin authorize release of information. You are not obliged to release information without a court ordering you to do so. Even in this case, federal law (described above) may protect your records from subpoena.

Duty to Protect

There are important exceptions to confidentiality. Some issues are required by law to be disclosed. Know your regional laws and contact your licensing or certification board for direction if you are unsure of requirements about breaking confidentiality. As we discussed earlier, any threats that are imminent, foreseeable, and dangerous (usually understood as suicide, homicide, or grave bodily harm to others) are reportable. For example, a client planning on running up his credit card bills and then declaring bankruptcy is not "dangerous" in this sense.

Professionals also have a duty to warn an intended victim or the police when a client divulges intent to kill (see Box 22.2). Even in this case, you can still protect the client's confidentiality by not revealing the fact that the person is being treated for a substance use disorder or other unnecessary private information (Gendel, 2004).

Child or elder abuse is another exception to confidentiality regulations. Regional laws typically require the reporting of disclosed abuse for the protection of the client's victim. State laws also mandate the reporting of certain infectious diseases, such as STDs and TB, to public health authorities. Again, disclose only the information that is necessary to protect the welfare of your client or others. In the case of health care providers,

---

BOX 22.2. The *Tarasoff* Case

Prosenjit Poddar came to the University of California Berkeley from India as a graduate student. There he met Tatiana Tarasoff. The two students had differing views of the relationship. Tarasoff felt that it was casual and she continued to date other men, while Poddar felt a serious monogamous relationship existed. Poddar was angered by her lack of commitment and began to stalk her. Poddar began to experience a severe mental crisis and eventually sought psychological help and told his psychologist of his intent to kill Tarasoff. The psychologist requested that the campus police detain Poddar and suggested that he be committed as a dangerous person. Rather than follow this suggestion, however, the campus police detained Poddar only briefly. A few months later, Poddar stopped treatment with the psychologist he had been seeing. Neither Tarasoff nor her parents had received any warning of the threat. Several months later, Poddar went through with the plan he had told his psychologist about and stabbed Tarasoff to death.

The question in the *Tarasoff* case was whether the psychologist had the responsibility to directly warn the intended victim. The original 1974 decision mandated warning the threatened individual, but a 1976 rehearing of the case by the California Supreme Court called for a "duty to protect" the intended victim. Therefore, this duty can be interpreted in several ways, including notifying police, warning the intended victim, and/or taking other reasonable steps to protect the threatened individual.

---

it can be important to inform them of the patient's substance use disorder diagnosis and prognosis. Health care providers may need this information to determine appropriate treatment and to avoid drug interactions. People with high tolerance for alcohol or other sedatives, for example, may require higher doses of anesthesia. Medical emergencies are another exception to confidentiality. For example, if a patient presents to the hospital with chest pain but without a history of heart problems, knowledge that the patient is a stimulant user would be important information for the medical team to have.

Identifying a pregnant woman as a substance user does not generally imply an obligation to report to child protection or law enforcement agencies, though state laws may differ in this regard. There is, of course, good reason to work with pregnant women to abstain from alcohol, tobacco, and other psychoactive drugs, and the motivational approach described in Chapter 10 is a good option. Pregnant women have a right to confidential or anonymous HIV counseling and testing, and also a right to refuse it. Also, as long as the woman has custody of her infant, her consent is required for the infant to be tested.

Addiction treatment confidentiality is also tricky because illicit drug use is illegal. It is vital to be clear, with clients and with anyone to whom you report information, what you will and will not disclose. Clients who are mandated to treatment usually come with conditions for reporting. In most cases, disclosure is limited to reporting on treatment attendance and progress in treatment, which allows you to establish trust with your client while still giving the courts the information they need.

Confidentiality When Working with Minors

When working with children or adolescents, confidentiality means something different because parents do have rights with regard to some information. Children younger than a certain age (e.g., 14) cannot themselves agree to treatment without parental consent. Know your regional laws regarding the age at which the child's own assent or consent is required. Under most conditions, you have an option to deny parents access to treatment records if you believe that harm may come from it. It is wise, of course, to explain these conditions to both children and parents in advance before you begin treatment.

More generally, it is important to explain to the client and the family in their first session the standards of confidentiality. For example, make sure to inform adolescents that if they place themselves at risk of physical harm either deliberately or accidentally, you will have to let their parents know. It's helpful to give scenarios, but don't agree to tight limits such as "I will only tell if you are using these IV drugs" or "I will only tell if you are drinking and driving." If a need to inform parents arises, it is usually better to have the child inform the parent him- or herself (with you ensuring that it does happen) or for you to tell the parent with the child present.

Boundary Issues

A professional relationship includes maintaining clear boundaries. "Boundary crossings" are more minor, but nevertheless important, infringements of professional courtesy (see Box 22.3). Some examples of inappropriate boundary crossings include arriving late for sessions, starting sessions late or ending them too early, having social contact with clients outside the session, or giving too much special attention to one of your clients. "Boundary violations," as compared to boundary crossings, are major transgressions that exploit or harm the client. Examples include a dual relationship, such as any sexual contact with a client, or engaging in any business dealings with clients. Other boundary violations include giving or receiving significant gifts, or inappropriately violating confidentiality.

BOX 22.3. Personal Reflection: An Ethical Choice

I had to look through my files to recover his research ID number, but I remembered him well, though I hadn't seen him for 3 months. Jack (whose name and identifying details have been changed to preserve anonymity) had been the second volunteer from AA to participate in a qualitative study on transformational change (Forcehimes, 2004).

The first question we had asked everyone who participated in the study was, "Tell me about your experience; how it was before, during, and after." There was an even divide between those who would delve right into the story with a succinct description and others who would go into copious detail. Jack was of the latter type; his story took 3 hours the first day and 90 minutes the second.

Jack had a troubled background, including sexual and physical abuse, exposure to gang violence, heavy drug and alcohol use, and financial struggles. He was a frequent drunk driver, but had never been arrested. His transforming experience was a dream, which to him was more real than any dream he had ever experienced. In his mind's eye, he saw himself driving on the freeway after a long night of drinking. His car hit the guard rail, then spun and collided head-on with another car. He got out of his car, uninjured, to examine the damages. In the other car, he saw the bloody wreckage of a family of four. The mother in the passenger seat was the only one breathing. Two small children had been thrown from the car, their small bodies distorted on the pavement, surrounded by pools of blood. The father had not been wearing his seatbelt and his head had gone through the windshield. He watched in horror as the dazed mother got out of the car to examine the remains of her family. His dream flashed forward and he saw himself in court, tortured by the agony of watching the mother sobbing. Then he saw himself in prison, unable to handle the misery he had inflicted on this family, hanging himself in his cell. Just as he was losing consciousness in his dream, he awoke in a cold sweat and vowed to never drink again. Ten years later he continued to keep that promise to himself.

Three months after I met with Jack, I was in an AA club recruiting volunteers for another study. In the meeting room, tables were arranged in a square formation and Jack was directly across from where I was sitting. In the tradition of AA, members each spoke for a few minutes about issues related to recovery as well as particular difficulties they were experiencing. When it was Jack's turn, his eyes filled with tears and he began explaining his present hardship. He expressed how alone he felt in the world and said that he felt like life wasn't worth living anymore.

After the meeting, I decided to forgo my recruiting efforts and instead talk with Jack. I told him that I was worried about him and that I thought it would be a good idea for him to talk to someone about his problems. I listened to the difficulties he was experiencing, and although he did not seem to be imminently suicidal, I gave him some local crisis numbers. As I turned to walk away, he said, "Hey, can you be my therapist?"

Ethical decision making is not always guided by absolute rules, and there are not always clear-cut answers. I began to think of the pros and cons: I knew about his history, he needed someone to talk with, and he obviously felt comfortable

(cont.)

BOX 22.3. *(cont.)*

talking to me. Also, he was feeling particularly rejected and my declining might feel like yet another abandonment, and I wanted to help him. On the other hand, I was just beginning the qualitative analyses of stories from our study, and the additional experience of being his therapist would clearly alter my interpretation of his story. There was also just something that felt not quite right about having these two different relationships with him: researcher and therapist. I've learned to pay attention to those "not quite right" feelings, even and especially when they conflict with something I want.

As Jack detailed what he was struggling with, I told him that I would rather refer him to someone who had more experience in treating his particular issues, and that I would help him find the right therapist. He did begin therapy, and a few months later he called to say that he was doing much better.

—A. A. F.

Technology

With the growth of technology in the workplace come both opportunities and dangers. If you use electronic means to communicate with clients, it is essential to ensure security at both sending and receiving points. If a consent form or other private information is to be e-mailed or faxed, who has access to the receiving machine? Electronic billing and other communication involves significant risk of inadvertent disclosure of sensitive information to unintended recipients. Electronic storage of client information in your office requires robust protection against hackers. If you record sessions for later review or supervision purposes (which we encourage for continued feedback and professional development), written consent is advisable, and there should be a clear stated agreement about when and how such recordings will be destroyed.

Will you communicate with clients by e-mail? Some providers will accept information from clients by e-mail, but do not send out messages to clients in this way in order to avoid unintended disclosure. It is wise to have clear policies and procedures for when e-mail is appropriate, who can read the e-mails, and who may respond to them. You should also inform your clients about what information and types of discussions are appropriate for e-mail and those that are not (e.g., emergencies), how long a response might take, and not including identifying information. If this is used often in your practice, this should be in your informed consent. It should also explain some of the risks of using this form of communication. For example, what if you receive your e-mail messages on your cell phone in addition to your firewalled computer? What if you happened to leave your phone at a restaurant?

Self-Disclosure

How much personal information should you disclose to your client? When is it appropriate to disclose? Some professionals struggle with wanting to disclose when the client's situation resonates with them personally. An important consideration here is *why* you would disclose. The normal rules of social reciprocity (you tell me something, and I tell you something) do not apply in professional relationships. You are not expected to divulge personal information about yourself. If you choose to do so, be conscious of your intention. Here are some possibilities:

• To build relationship. Perceived similarity is one source of alliance in relationship. In social conversation, it is common to look for points of common experience and discuss them. Such "chat" is generally off-topic in professional service contexts, but some professionals do choose modest self-disclosure in hopes of building rapport.

• Solidarity in recovery. If you are yourself in recovery from a substance use disorder, there is a decision to make as to whether and when to disclose this. As mentioned earlier, personal recovery status is unrelated to a counselor's effectiveness in treating substance use disorders. Some clients do feel more understood if they know that their counselor is also in recovery. These clients will tend to ask. If you are in recovery and have not told your client, there is a risk of being inadvertently "outed" elsewhere, for example, at a mutual help meeting.

• Answering client questions. Another reason to disclose is in answer to a client's question. "Are you in recovery?" "Did you ever use drugs?" Again, the decision is yours, and you are not required to answer. With binary questions like this, one possibility is to say, "I'm willing to tell you, but first I'd like to understand what it will mean to you if the answer is 'Yes,' and what it will mean if the answer is 'No.'" Discussing this first can address concerns or traps that underlie the question.

• Desire to be forthcoming. In client-centered counseling, for example, such "congruence" is regarded as a necessary therapeutic condition. Congruence, however, typically has to do with one's immediate reaction to a client within the session, and not the recounting of past personal history.

A caution to keep in mind with any self-disclosure is to avoid *identification* with clients. A professional helping relationship is not a mutual help group. It is between unique individuals. Identification can impede your ability to see clients as separate individuals and to help them without becoming over-invested in their choices. Identification is an appropriate issue to discuss in supervision.

Limits of Professional Expertise

Another standard aspect of professionalism is to practice within but not beyond your areas of expertise. A desire to be helpful and to have answers can lead to giving inadequate advice on issues outside your expertise (e.g., medical issues, legal issues, co-occurring disorders, case management problems). In other words, practicing outside one's expertise violates the precept to first do no harm. It is common for clients to not understand the differences in training and expertise among various kinds of health professionals.

There are certainly times when the needs for professional expertise intersect. Clients in addiction treatment often bring significant medical and mental health issues as well. A client might be taking a medication like buprenorphine for opioid addiction in addition to counseling. Side effects or feeling like the dose is inadequate may come up in counseling. In this case it is important to have a team approach to treatment where possible, or at least to have in place a professional release to exchange information so that you can communicate and discuss such concerns with professional colleagues.

The lines between addiction and other behavioral health problems also can be blurred. For example, a woman in treatment for drug dependence may bring up feelings related to a history of child abuse and evidence symptoms of PTSD. Should you explore this? It depends on your professional training not just in addiction, but in the treatment of PTSD. Just talking about abuse and PTSD is not very helpful, and runs the risk of reviving traumatic experiences without benefit. Professional practice remains within the bounds of one's expertise.

Professional Honesty

A related issue in most professional codes of ethics is truth telling and the avoidance of misleading statements. What if a client asks you about your "success rate" in treating a particular disorder? In one study, investigators called addiction treatment centers asking this question, and the lowest estimate given was 80% (Miller & Hester, 1986). On further inquiry, none had any data to substantiate their estimate. Representation of one's professional expertise, both verbally and in print and electronic media, should be substantiated by an accurate description of training and experience. Avoid misleading or unsubstantiated statements, even and especially with the desire to impress and comfort clients.

Record Keeping

Client records are legal documents. Even when there are extra legal protections for addiction treatment records, you should not put anything in a client chart that you would not want to defend in court or to clients themselves. A good guideline is to keep client records factual based on what you have observed. Rather than writing "The client used cocaine this week" (which you did not directly observe), it is better to write, "The client reported using cocaine this week." Discreet, objective documentation is particularly important in charting addiction treatment. Avoid judgmental comments or interpretations and embellishment that go beyond the facts.

Some clinicians keep a "shadow chart," a separate set of notes on treatment, apart from the client's official medical record. These might be less formal notes on your thoughts and concerns, things you think of during a session or between sessions to raise on next meeting. Understand, however, that such records are equally subject to subpoena as the official treatment records.

Harm Reduction

To what extent should professionals try to protect clients from the adverse consequences of their own drug use? This is an ethical issue on which there has been much debate. Surely the prevention of harm is a common goal among treatment professionals; disagreements arise over specific methods for doing so (Miller, 2008a).

Less controversial is screening for harm that has already occurred or is occurring. It is sensible to evaluate for common substance-related problems including infections (e.g., hepatitis, HIV, TB, STDs), domestic violence, child abuse/neglect, and suicide risk, and to provide appropriate treatment. What have been more controversial are proactive public health interventions to reduce harm from *future* substance use. One classic example is exchanging used needles for sterile ones to prevent the spread of blood-borne infections among intravenous drug users. Another is vaccinating intravenous drug users against hepatitis (Clark, 2005–2007). Proponents of such measures regard them to be pragmatic and humanitarian efforts to reduce harm to users and to society. Opponents view them as condoning and facilitating continued drug use. Harm reduction is discussed further in Chapter 23 on prevention.

OTHER PROFESSIONAL PRACTICE ISSUES

Supervision

Some addiction treatment personnel are required by law or program policy to work under the supervision of a more highly trained licensed professional who reviews and approves their treatment plans and records. In this case, clients need to be informed about the supervisory arrangement and about who will have access to their case information. Other professionals are licensed for independent practice without ongoing supervision.

In either case, there is great value in regular consultation with colleagues regarding clinical practice. These supervision or peer-consultation meetings can be thought of as a learning community and should not be focused primarily on administrative minutia but on the art and science of clinical care. They offer an important opportunity for continued professional learning, reflection, and practice improvement. Reviewing recorded sessions (with clients' knowledge and permission, of course) together can be particularly valuable. Beyond case presentations and discussion, such regular meetings can also include a "journal club" discussing a clinically relevant article in a scientific or professional journal.

It is particularly important and useful to discuss ethical quandaries with a supervisor or peers. Good ethical decision making involves deliberation, and not just fact retrieval. The sharing of this deliberation affords learning for all, and makes for better decision making.

Special Populations

The term "special populations" originally referred to anyone other than white males, and more generally evokes the challenges of counseling people with a cultural background that is different from one's own. One key justice issue here is equal access to treatment services (Miller, Villanueva, Tonigan, & Cuzmar, 2007). Discrimination in service delivery can occur simply by the way in which services are structured and provided. For example, offering treatment only during weekday work hours makes it more difficult for lower income working people to attend. Fees, child care, and location affect accessibility. Women who seek treatment for addiction tend to have fewer financial resources than men, are more likely to need child care, and tend to be more stigmatized (Lisansky, 1999). There are also comfort issues. Does the treatment setting feel safe? Do clients see other people like themselves on the staff, in pictures on the walls, or among the other clients?

Another issue is how best to proceed when working with clients from a different ethnic or cultural background than your own. A key here is good listening, regarding clients as the experts on themselves. Rather than assuming that you understand, let your clients educate you regarding their own beliefs about addiction and its causes and their hunches about what will work best for them. Assuming that you know how to work with someone *because* of their racial–ethnic background is risky in itself, because there is substantial variability within as well as across cultures.

> Let your clients educate you regarding their hunches about what will work best for them.

It is not assured that treatment methods that work with one population will be effective with others. Nevertheless, evidence-based treatments from another population are a good place to start when considering options, and are arguably preferable to treatment methods with no scientific basis at all. It would, in fact, pose an ethical justice problem to deny delivery of an evidence-based treatment because a client came from a population different from the one in which the research had been done (Miller et al., 2007). Adaptations may be needed to make evidence-based treatments accessible across cultures (Venner, Feldstein, & Tafoya, 2006).

Professional Development and Continuing Education

Staying current with the development of new and effective treatments is an ethical responsibility for addiction professionals, just as one expects this of one's own health care providers (Miller, Zweben, et al., 2005). In North America and the United Kingdom, there is an increasing trend toward reimbursing only for treatments that have been scientifically validated.

This requires effort to keep up with emerging research. In a span of 5 years, literally hundreds of new studies are published that are relevant to practice in treating addictions. Few providers have the time and expertise to read this volume of scientific research critically. The usual way to keep up is through continuing professional education, a certain amount of which is normally required for all licensed health professionals. However, there is rarely any requirement that the content of such materials or workshops reflect current scientific evidence. One can often fulfill the continuing education requirements of licensure without learning anything about evidence-based treatment or new research.

Various informational resources are available for keeping up with new developments. A remarkable source is the public domain Treatment Improvement Protocol (TIP) series, with more than 50 volumes available online from the Center for Substance Abuse Treatment (*www.ncbi.nlm.nih. gov/bookshelf/br.fcgi?book=hssamhsatip*). Another large and free resource is the Clinical Trials Network dissemination library (*ctndisseminationlibrary.org*). For keeping up to date on emerging addiction research that is relevant in health care, the online bimonthly newsletter *Alcohol, Other Drugs, and Health: Current Evidence* is an excellent and free resource (*www.bu.edu/aodhealth*). There are practitioner-friendly journals presenting new research on addiction treatment, including the *Journal of Substance Abuse Treatment*, and the *Brown University Digest of Addiction Theory and Application*. Other journals publish reviews that summarize a body of research for clinicians: examples are *Drug and Alcohol Review* and *Clinical Psychology Review*. Such resources are available by subscription or may be accessible through a local university library.

Simply reading about or even attending a workshop on an evidence-based treatment, however, is unlikely to be enough to change practice behavior significantly, although it may convince participants that they now understand and can use the new method (Miller et al., 2004, 2006). In this way, attending a workshop might even inoculate one against further learning because of the illusion that one has already mastered it (Miller & Mount, 2001). Learning any new complex skill typically takes practice over time with feedback and coaching. This is another way in which a learning community of peers can be helpful, working together to strengthen new skills and improve practice. Again we encourage listening to actual recordings (with client permission) of client sessions. This departs from a long tradition of closeted addiction treatment that occurs in secret behind closed doors, a tradition that deprives clinicians of feedback and opportunities to learn. Even listening to your own sessions can be instructive.

Counselor Impairment

Finally, as clinicians we have an ethical obligation to be sufficiently sound mentally and emotionally to be able to give clients our full and undistorted attention. The acute and cumulative effects of alcohol or other drugs represent only one potential source of professional impairment. Major life changes such as the loss of a loved one, a serious medical condition, or acute family distress can also distract, impairing clinical judgment and ability to provide quality services for those who rely on us for help. It is important to recognize one's own limits and accept the need of a healing break from professional work. This requires a backup plan to ensure the care of clients currently in your care until you are able to resume work with them.

KEY POINTS

🖈 Beyond the usual professional standards, addiction treatment requires additional ethical protections, particularly with regard to record keeping.

🖈 Competence, comprehension, and freedom of choice are three key requirements for informed consent.

🖈 Important ethical responsibilities include confidentiality, professional boundaries and honesty, duty to protect, and practicing within one's expertise.

🖈 While supervision is a legal requirement for some providers, all professionals can benefit from ongoing consultation with knowledgeable colleagues.

🖈 Professionals are responsible to be informed about emerging new knowledge and adjust treatment practices accordingly to provide effective care to clients.

REFLECTION QUESTIONS

Q Of the four ethical principles described (nonmaleficence, beneficence, autonomy, and justice), which one do you ponder most often in treating clients?

Q When you face a difficult ethical issue, what steps do you follow in deciding what to do?

Q What ethics issues regarding addiction treatment most concern you?

CHAPTER 23

Promoting Prevention

W hy should treatment professionals be interested in prevention? For one thing, because no societal epidemic has ever been overcome by treatment alone. Although pulling people out of the river just before or after they go over the waterfall is worthy work, it also makes sense to go upstream and find out why they are falling in. Historically, addiction treatment programs have focused on people at the severe end of substance dependence, who represent a rather small fraction of all those with alcohol and other drug problems. For example, contrary to public stereotype, only a minority of drunk drivers who cause crashes, injuries, and deaths are alcohol-dependent people. Heavy drinkers with no or low dependence are far more numerous than those with alcohol dependence, and although per capita their risk of causing a fatal crash while intoxicated is lower, their sheer number means that they account for a majority of drunk driving incidents and deaths (Institute of Medicine, 1990). This "prevention paradox" means that if we are devoting our efforts primarily to individuals at the severe end of the spectrum, we are missing most of the problem (Babor, 2010).

> If we are devoting our efforts primarily to individuals at the severe end of the spectrum, we are missing most of the problem.

In a way, the difference between prevention and treatment is just a matter of when you intervene. A classic continuum in public health differentiates three levels of preventive intervention: primary (universal), secondary (selective), and tertiary (indicated). Tertiary or indicated prevention is what is often thought of as treatment: intervening with people who are *already* infected or affected by a condition, ideally at an early stage. These are folks who are already caught up in the rapids. Certainly prevention is part of treatment: to prevent recurrence, future suffering, and disability. Secondary or selective prevention moves upstream a bit to work with people who are particularly at risk of developing problems. These might be likened to people swimming upstream in mild current, or balancing on a narrow bridge over the river. The goal here is to intervene with a targeted subpopulation who are more likely, by virtue of risk factors, to fall victim to an illness or condition. Finally, primary or universal prevention intervenes with an entire population—perhaps a whole city or a school district. People are not selected for intervention because of particular risk factors. Rather the goal is to reach *everyone* in the population to reduce the prevalence of a problem.

Consider the example of diabetes. Tertiary (indicated) prevention works with people who are already diagnosed with diabetes, in order to help them manage their glucose levels, prevent long-term adverse consequences and premature mortality, and promote quality of life. Secondary (selective) prevention identifies and intervenes with people particularly at risk for developing diabetes, perhaps by virtue of family history or body mass index. The identification of "prediabetes" metabolic syndrome is an example of finding people who are likely to develop diabetes within a few years to help them make life changes early before the disease emerges fully or results in organ damage. Primary (universal) prevention might involve educating all middle or high school students about the effectiveness of a healthy diet and exercise to reduce risk of diabetes and its consequences. Universal prevention can also be implemented at a point of developmental transition in which risk for substance use disorders is elevated (e.g., transition from high school to postsecondary education; National Institute on Drug Abuse, 2003).

Different intervention strategies are likely to be optimal at different levels of prevention. Educational strategies that are effective in universal prevention of tobacco and alcohol use (e.g., Botvin, Griffin, Paul, & Macaulay, 2003) may be ineffective once nicotine or alcohol dependence is established (Miller & Wilbourne, 2002). Helping heavy drinkers to moderate their alcohol use has become recommended practice (selective prevention) in health care (National Institute on Alcohol Abuse and Alcoholism, 2005). However, once drinkers have passed a certain level of alcohol dependence, it is very difficult at best for them to maintain problem-free moderation (Miller, Leckman, et al., 1992; Miller & Muñoz, 2005), much as a return to moderate smoking is unlikely once nicotine dependence has been established (Cohen et al., 1989).

As is the case with addiction treatment (Institute of Medicine, 1998), there is a wide gap between science-based approaches known to be effective and those actually delivered in universal and selective community programs for the prevention of alcohol/drug use and problems. The fact that something is *called* "prevention" does not mean that it actually decreases risk. Neither

is the fact that a program seems logical, popular, theoretically sound, or commonsense any
guarantee that it has beneficial effects. There
are ample examples in outcome research of
prevention programs that students and teach-

> The fact that something is *called* "prevention" does not mean that it actually decreases risk.

ers liked and rated as effective, the actual result of which was *increased* alcohol or drug use (e.g., Foxcroft, Lister-Sharp, & Lowe, 1997; Gorman, 2003; Hallfors et al., 2006; Institute of Medicine, 1998). Popular universal programs that have been shown to be ineffective, such as the 17-week Drug Abuse Resistance Education (DARE) course for schoolchildren, may nevertheless continue in widespread use (Ennett, Tobler, Ringwalt, & Flewelling, 1994; Rogers, 2002; Rosenbaum & Hanson, 1998).

Another reason for treatment professionals to get involved in prevention efforts is that you already have much more knowledge about substance use disorders than do most people in the general population, in school systems, or in government. There has been an unfortunate disconnect between treatment and prevention professionals, who typically attend different courses and conferences and often work in settings isolated from each other. A public health approach focuses on the entire spectrum of severity (see Box 23.1), with efforts to prevent people from moving to a

---

BOX 23.1. Continuum of Alcohol Use and Problems in the General Population

Prevention efforts are intended to keep people from moving down the funnel.

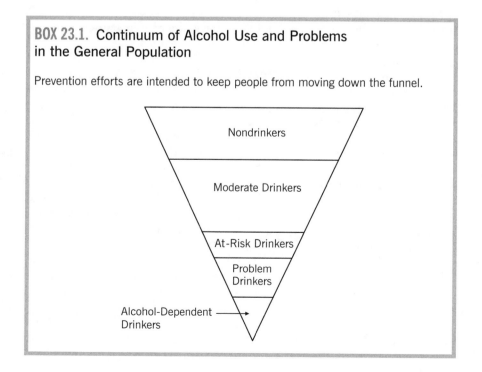

higher level of risk. Prevention efforts may focus on controlling affordability (e.g., through taxation and pricing), availability (e.g., via distribution and marketing), and harmful consequences of substance use in the population (Babor, 2010), issues that can seem remote from the day-to-day world of addiction treatment. All three levels of prevention (including treatment) are needed to address a problem of this scope and seriousness.

UNIVERSAL PREVENTION

A wide variety of population-level primary prevention strategies have been tried and tested. One general strategy has been developmental: to delay the onset of alcohol, tobacco, and other drug use. People who do not begin drinking, smoking, or using illicit drugs before the age of 18 are quite unlikely to develop disorders related to these drugs, although of course there are exceptions. Conversely, producers and distributors who can engage youth in using their products before adulthood may recruit customers for life.

A common distinction in prevention efforts is between *supply-side* and *demand-side* interventions. Supply-side interventions are those designed to reduce or control the availability of a particular drug, such as alcohol or tobacco. Demand-side efforts, in contrast, seek to reduce consumer desire for and use of the drug. It is possible to have effective or ineffective interventions on both sides of this balance.

A clear general finding in universal prevention research is that policies that moderately reduce the affordability and availability of a drug do significantly decrease population use and related problems (Babor, 2010). The word "moderately" is important here, for it is equally clear that large and abrupt interruption of availability tends not only to be unpopular, but also to create problems of its own, as occurred during the American experience with Prohibition. The period of Prohibition following the 1919 ratification of the 18th Amendment to the U.S. Constitution was highly successful in the sense of dramatically reducing the production and consumption of alcohol beverages and their health consequences. The drastic change was so unpopular, however, and generated such widespread disregard, illicit production, sales, and organized crime that it was repealed by yet another amendment (21st) to the Constitution in 1933.

More effective are gradual changes that reduce availability. Both alcohol and tobacco, for example, are relatively *price elastic*, meaning that use and sales decrease as price increases. For this reason, modest tax increases do tend to reduce smoking and drinking, particularly among the young with less discretionary income. Conversely, reduction in price of commodities like alcohol and tobacco can substantially increase use, particularly among the young. Overall reductions in use at a population level are reflected in parallel reductions in social and health problems related to the drug (Babor, 2010).

Other supply-side policies affect outlets through which a drug can be obtained. In general, the more outlets that are available for purchasing a drug, the higher its use and related consequences. This applies even at a local level: the higher the density of alcohol sales outlets, for example, the greater the adverse consequences in the immediate neighborhood. Again, drastic reductions in availability can have unintended consequences. A 1985 Russian policy change dramatically curtailed outlets for vodka sales, with apparently large reductions in alcohol consumption and related morbidity and mortality. However, a drastic drop in government revenues from alcohol taxes prompted revocation of the restrictions 3 years later (McKee, 1999). Some nations have experimented with prescribing and providing heroin to registered users through controlled public clinics, thus undercutting the demand for illicit sales and the need for users to recruit other users in order to finance their own addiction.

Complementary to controls on availability (supply side) are efforts to reduce a population's desire for and consumption of a drug. Both approaches are needed. Education is the most commonly used tool to target population demand. Commercial advertising is, of course, a form of public education intended to increase demand, and therefore controls on advertising (e.g., for alcohol and tobacco) are one form of universal demand-side prevention. Various educational approaches have been tried, particularly with schoolchildren, with the intention of preventing alcohol/drug use and problems, and the results have been highly variable (Foxcroft et al., 1997). This is of concern, in that an entire school district of children may be exposed to a program that has unknown or even harmful results. The educational approach that has shown most promise is one that does not focus primarily on substance use, but rather teaches social skills for coping with life's challenges (Botvin & Griffin, 2004; Botvin et al., 2003). This is an example of a more general strategy, which is to target known risk and protective factors (Hawkins, Catalano, & Miller, 1992).

SELECTIVE PREVENTION

Selective or secondary prevention focuses on those who are at particular risk of developing a disorder, rather than targeting an entire population (universal prevention) or waiting for problems to emerge before intervening (indicated prevention). A prime question, then, is how to identify people who do not yet have but are at higher risk of developing substance use disorders.

Who Is at Risk?

Substance use disorders are widespread, but they are not randomly distributed. Some people are clearly at higher risk than others. Knowing about significant risk and protective factors opens up the possibility of implementing prevention efforts selectively with those who are at greater risk. There are hundreds of studies examining longitudinal risk factors for the development of substance use disorders, many of which focus on predictors of alcohol problems, but there is also a rapidly growing literature on risk factors for nicotine and other drug use disorders. Here are some brief highlights of a complicated field of research.

A good example of a population in urgent need of preventive attention is offenders with a history of substance use disorders, just before and after release from prison. Release is a key transition point, where suddenly restored freedom invites a return to substance use and increased risk of drug-related death (Merrall et al., 2010), in part due to reduced tolerance and inadvertent overdose.

Family History

It is now abundantly clear that the biological relatives of people with substance use disorders are at higher risk themselves. This is true even when children are adopted at birth and did not know their biological parents. In both men and women, shared risk is higher in monozygotic (identical) than in dizygotic twins (Heath et al., 1997). No one or two genes explain hereditary transmission; instead a range of genes contributes to risk and protective factors (Dick & Foroud, 2003).

Religiousness

Another strong predictor of substance use and problems is religiousness, or an active involvement in organized religion. Religious attendance is itself a consistent predictor of low risk for substance use disorders at present or in the future, with an effect size similar to that for family history (see Chapter 21).

Demographics

Worldwide, men are more likely than women to use most psychoactive drugs and to develop related problems and dependence. An exception to this is the misuse of certain prescription medications (Simoni-Wastila, 2004). Age of peak risk for substance use disorders is in the 20s or 30s, although of course onset also can happen before or after this. As mentioned earlier, adolescents who reach the age of 18 without using alcohol or drugs are quite unlikely ever to develop a substance use disorder (Grant & Dawson, 1997; Robins & Przybeck, 1985).

Alcohol Sensitivity

A well-established risk factor is relative insensitivity to alcohol: the ability to "hold your liquor" without feeling or appearing to be as affected as others are (Schuckit & Smith, 2010). This is a heritable trait on which individuals vary influenced by multiple genes (e.g., Joslyn, Ravindranathan, Busch, Schuckit, & White, 2010), a trait that can also be expressed through selective breeding of certain laboratory animals. Human responsiveness to alcohol can be measured at a very fine level. Imagine this: You are given a dose of alcohol and are then asked to stand upright and still inside a metal frame. Spring-loaded cords are pulled from each of four corner posts and attached to your clothing with alligator clips. You are told, "Close your eyes now and stand as still as you can." The tension-loaded cords sensitively measure the amount of sway in your body as you try to stay steady. This is a sensitive measure of tolerance used by Marc Schuckit and his colleagues at the University of California, San Diego (e.g., Eng, Schuckit, & Smith, 2005). Normally alcohol, even in relatively small doses, increases people's body sway when the eyes are closed, which is one component of field sobriety tests for driving under the influence. Some people, however, sway very little. Their bodies are relatively insensitive to alcohol. These low-response people have substantially *greater* risk of developing alcohol dependence. In other words, being able to hold your liquor is not a good thing, not a protection. Rather, it is like lacking a smoke alarm.

Drug Expectancies

People also differ in what they *expect* to happen when they use a drug even before they have had any direct experience with it. As one might anticipate, those who expect more positive and fewer negative effects of drug use are more likely to begin using at an earlier age, to use more heavily, to develop problems and dependence, and to return to using after treatment (Goldman et al., 1999; Jones & McMahon, 1994; Leventhal & Schmitz, 2006). However, it is unclear whether and how preventive interventions may change these expectancies, and if so whether this impacts substance use (Jones et al., 2001).

Comorbidity

Finally, people with certain psychiatric disorders have a significantly higher prevalence of substance use disorders relative to the general population (see Chapter 18). Children with a history of antisocial behavior or conduct disorder are at elevated risk of alcohol/drug use during adolescence and of developing a substance use disorder. ADHD, depression, schizophrenia, PTSD, and other anxiety disorders, and certain personality disorders (e.g., antisocial, borderline) all have high comorbidity with substance use disorders.

Selective Intervention

Although selective (rather than universal) prevention seems a sensible idea, with promise for being more cost-efficient than targeting an entire population, intervening with high-risk individuals and groups is not without its problems and controversies. Here are a few examples.

Stigma

Suppose that a school system were to identify students who are at particularly high risk for later development of alcohol/drug problems, based on a set of predictive factors. They selectively pull these students out of class for an evidence-based preventive intervention. It would be virtually impossible to keep secret the purpose of the program. What do you think the unintended effects might be on the students themselves? On teachers' and administrators' perceptions? On peer perceptions and relationships?

Similarly, there are legitimate reservations about bringing an alcohol/drug prevention intervention to particular high-risk subpopulations. What could be some unintended adverse consequences of singling out for selective prevention, based on known elevated statistical risk for alcohol/drug problems, a particular school? A Native American tribe? Schoolchildren with poorer academic performance? A military base? Smokers within a large company?

Selective Association

There can also be unintended consequences of bringing together a group of high-risk individuals (see Chapter 20). They may encourage or normalize the problem behavior, or teach each other new bad habits. Consider the impact of being arrested for the first time for driving while intoxicated: handcuffed, fingerprinted, jail time, fines, picture in the newspaper. It's humiliating, and does tend to discourage further offenses. But now consider the potential impact of putting that same individual in a classroom full of 150 people who have all done the same thing. Most of them seem pretty normal and friendly, and they get to laughing and joking together, grumbling about the lectures and films, swapping arrest stories, maybe even going out for a drink together afterward.

There are, of course, environments where demographically high-risk people are brought together naturally under conditions that favor problematic use: college, the armed forces, fraternities and sororities, spring break, Octoberfest. Being thrown together with peer models who are using drugs, smoking, or drinking heavily tends to normalize and increase one's own substance use (Schwab, Gmel, Annaheim, Mueller, & Schwappach, 2010), particularly when combined with environmental conditions that favor it (e.g., easy access, stress, expectations, drinking contests).

Self-Fulfilling Prophecy

Both stigma and selective association can contribute to expectancies. Tell people that they have a high probability of a particular behavior problem, and it can become a self-fulfilling prophecy. This is another potential risk of identifying and intervening with people who are at elevated risk for a behavioral disorder.

INDICATED PREVENTION

Finally, tertiary or indicated prevention intervenes with those who are already showing signs and symptoms of a disorder, preferably at an early stage of development. Because substance use disorders occur all along a continuum of severity, it would be ideal to find and intervene with people who are toward the lower end of the severity spectrum.

The vast majority of people who use alcohol are occasional, light, or moderate drinkers who never meet diagnostic criteria for an alcohol use disorder (AUD). However, about 7% of the U.S. population at any given time *do* meet diagnostic criteria for an AUD, most of whom are not alcohol-dependent. These nondependent or low-dependence AUDs are sometimes referred to as "problem drinkers" (Alcoholics Anonymous, 1976), although both "problem drinking" (Cahalan, 1970) and "alcoholism" (Jellinek, 1960) have also been used to describe the full spectrum of AUDs, contributing to the confusion. About 20% of men and 10% of women in the United States drink more than the NIAAA-recommended limits (see Box 23.2), placing them at risk for adverse health or other consequences.

Because treatment was historically conceptualized in the United States as applicable to the disease of alcoholism, the more severe end of the continuum of alcohol dependence, the much larger group of problem drinkers was often thought of as not needing any intervention, an opinion that they generally shared. Indeed, if problem drinkers did decide to seek help, few if any services were available that were designed for and appropriate for them at this lower level of severity (Institute of Medicine, 1990), and they were likely to be labeled "alcoholic" and told they must abstain for life (Hanson & Emrick, 1983). This state of affairs tends to discourage people from seeking help until their drinking and problems become severe.

BOX 23.2. What Is "Heavy" or "At-Risk" Drinking?

The U.S. National Institute on Alcohol Abuse and Alcoholism (NIAAA) recommends upper limits for alcohol consumption. These are:

> No more than four drinks on any day or 14 drinks per week for men.
>
> No more than three drinks on any day or seven drinks per week for women.

Why the lower limit for women? Because women tend to have smaller body size than men, and also metabolize alcohol more slowly than men do. For these reasons, if a man and a woman drink the same amount of alcohol, the woman will have a higher blood alcohol concentration. This is true even if they have the same body weight, because of the difference in alcohol metabolism.

So what counts as a "drink"? NIAAA lists these as having roughly the same amount of alcohol:

12	ounces of	beer	(5% alcohol)
8–9	ounces of	malt liquor	(7% alcohol)
5	ounces of	table wine	(12% alcohol)
3–4	ounces of	fortified wine	(17% alcohol)
2–3	ounces of	liqueur, aperitif, or cordial	(24% alcohol)
1.5	ounces of	distilled spirits, liquor	(40% alcohol)

All of these contain about the same amount of ethyl alcohol: one "standard drink."

From *Rethinking Drinking: Alcohol and Your Health.* Bethesda, MD: National Institutes of Health. Available at *www.rethinkingdrinking.niaaa.nih.gov.*

Again an analogy to diabetes is helpful. The diagnosis of diabetes was once largely restricted to more severe disorders of glucose metabolism, such as would require insulin dependence. Type 1 and Type 2 diabetes were not differentiated until the 1950s. Over the years, however, the threshold for diagnosing diabetes has been decreasing, and a gray area of "prediabetes" insulin resistance is now widely recognized. The trend has been toward earlier recognition of the metabolic syndrome that underlies Type 2 diabetes, which can often be successfully managed or even reversed by health behavior changes (diet, exercise) and/or oral medication without insulin. No one would now insist that only Type 1 diabetes should be treated.

Similarly, it has become widely accepted that health care practitioners should screen for heavy drinking as well as smoking, and offer at least brief intervention to patients at risk (National Institute on Alcohol Abuse and Alcoholism, 2005). Diagnostic criteria now recognize a continuum of substance use disorders, rather than conceptualizing "abuse" and "dependence" as two separate conditions. Research has, however, pointed to two subtypes of AUDs that are interestingly parallel to diabetes: Type I occurring in both men and women, with later onset, more gradual progression, with mild and severe forms, influenced by environmental factors; and Type II with early onset, rapid progression, moderate severity, influenced primarily by genetics, found predominantly in males and often linked to criminality (Cloninger, Sigvardsson, & Bohman, 1996). As with diabetes, different treatment goals and methods are likely to be effective for people at different points along the continuum (e.g., Kiefer, Jimenez-Arriero, Klein, Diehl, & Rubio, 2007).

Why intervene early? A large majority of people in the general population who have diagnosable AUDs will resolve them without formal treatment (Dawson et al., 2005). College students, who are typically in the peak risk years of development, have a high prevalence of AUDs, many of which resolve once they graduate and take on the responsibilities of adult life. Why not simply wait for nature to take its course?

There are at least two broad and persuasive reasons. First, although heavy/problem drinking does often abate over time, a worrisome proportion does not (Vaillant, 1996). Heavy drinking is a gateway, if it continues, to alcohol problems and dependence that can have devastating, even deadly, consequences for drinkers and their loves ones. In a longitudinal study, people who had been binge drinkers during college were six times more likely to be diagnosed with alcohol dependence 10 years later (Jennison, 2004). As with most chronic diseases, AUDs are usually easier to turn around at earlier stages of development, and early treatment is at least as successful as at later stages of development. Recognizing and addressing AUDs early thus can prevent the *later* development of a host of health, social, occupational, financial, and family problems.

A second important reason for intervening early is to prevent tragic early consequences of heavy drinking or other drug use—those that can occur well before dependence sets in (Hingson, Heeren, Winter, & Wechsler, 2005). Alcohol is involved in at least a substantial proportion if not a majority of deaths from drowning, falls, fire, hypothermia, firearms, cancer, stroke, traumatic injury, suicide, vehicular crashes, pedestrian fatalities, and of course overdose (Laslett, Dietze, Matthews, & Clemens, 2004; Stinson & DeBakey, 1992). Taken together, alcohol-related incidents constitute the leading cause of death before the age of 35. Beyond mortality, intoxication also contributes to countless consequences of poor judgment that can have lifelong consequences, including injury-related disability, sexually transmitted infections such as HIV, illicit drug use, marital infidelity, child abuse, sexual assault and other violence, felonies, and fetal alcohol effects. Most of these require only one intoxicated indiscretion. Earlier intervention can thus shorten the window of vulnerability to such tragedies.

The commonly recommended goal for brief intervention with heavy drinkers is to reduce consumption to a moderate low-risk level (see Box 23.2). Of course, abstinence is also a possible choice at any point along the line. People who quit drinking are unlikely to have new problems related to their own alcohol use (although as with ex-smokers, consequences can still crop up later). Abstinence is an available option for drinkers to consider, joining the substantial proportion of the general population who are nondrinkers—about 30% of men and 40% of women in the United States (Falk, Yi, & Hiller-Sturmhöfel, 2006).

An important strategy for indicated prevention, reaching people as early as possible in the course of problem development, is to extend the reach of services (Velicer, Prochaska, & Redding, 2006). This means providing consultation well beyond the traditional bounds of office-based face-to-face counseling. Tobacco quitlines, for example, provide free smoking cessation counseling by telephone throughout the United States (1-800-QUIT-NOW). Such telephone consultation has been found to be as effective as face-to-face services, with considerably easier access (Lichtenstein, Zhu, & Tedeschi, 2010). Online consultation in real time is also feasible, and software programs have been developed to deliver substance use intervention at the user's convenience (e.g., Hester et al., 2005, 2009).

The Drinker's Checkup

The idea of a checkup for drinkers was introduced as a way to encourage people to take a look at their own alcohol use and its consequences (Miller et al., 1988). The availability of a "free checkup for people who wonder whether their drinking may be harming them in any way" was announced in a newspaper article. The checkup offered personal health feedback and was not connected with any treatment program. What participants did with the information was up to them.

| By the time you wonder whether you're drinking too much, you probably are. |

The program attracted a sizeable response (Miller et al., 1993; Miller & Sovereign, 1989). Most people who came had never been treated for an AUD, talked to any professional about it, or been to a mutual help meeting. Most would not go near an addiction treatment program, and yet every one of them had significant alcohol problems. In other words, by the time you wonder whether you're drinking too much, you probably are.

Why had they not gone for treatment? Rarely was it a problem of not knowing where to go, having no access, or believing treatment to be ineffective. Rather they simply believed that their problems weren't really all that serious, that they didn't *need* treatment, and that they could handle it on their own. As it turned out, they were right! So why then had they come for a checkup? The most commonly stated reasons were concern for health (75%), belief that it would help them (48%), concern about problems caused by their drinking (43%), and concern that they might be "alcoholic" (43%; Miller et al., 1988). In other words, they were ambivalent about their drinking.

The checkup consisted of measures sensitive to the earlier (as well as later) adverse psychological, social, physical, and neurocognitive consequences of overdrinking. It was not intended to give a yes/no answer or a diagnosis. Instead, after careful assessment, participants were given individual quantitative feedback about their level of drinking, liver function, alcohol-related problems, dependence symptoms, and cognitive functioning relative to population norms. The counselor responded in the empathic, evocative style of MI (Chapter 10) rather than telling participants what they should do.

Although the initial prediction was that people would be more likely to seek alcohol treatment following the checkup (cf. Chafetz et al., 1962), almost no one did. Instead most people cut back their alcohol use substantially, reducing by more than half on average (Miller et al., 1993), a medically meaningful reduction. The drinker's checkup was subsequently formalized as motivational enhancement therapy (MET; Miller, Zweben, et al., 1992), which has been well supported as an evidence-based intervention (Lundahl & Burke, 2009). The checkup format has subsequently been adapted for marijuana users (Martin, Copeland, & Swift, 2005; Stephens, Roffman, & Curtin, 2000) and families (Cordova et al., 2005; Slavert et al., 2005). A computer-assisted version has been developed and evaluated (Hester, Squires, & Delaney, 2005) and is available to use free of charge at *www.moderation.org/software/drinkerscheckup.shtml.* An online "checkup to go" (CHUG; *www.echeckuptogo.com/usa*) for college students has also been evaluated (Walters, Miller, & Chiauzzi, 2005; Walters, Vader, & Harris, 2007).

Behavioral Self-Control Training

Another type of intervention for less severe AUDs is behavioral self-control training (BSCT), teaching behavioral self-management methods for moderation or abstinence (Sanchez-Craig, 1980; Sanchez-Craig et al., 1996). BSCT has been evaluated in dozens of trials in individual face-to-face counseling, group format, self-help bibliotherapy, and computer-administered versions (e.g., Hester, 2003; Miller, Gribskov, & Mortell, 1981; Miller, Leckman, et al., 1992; Miller et al., 1980). Reductions in drinking have been surprisingly similar, on average, across counselor-delivered and self-administered formats. Common components of BSCT include:

ISSUES IN ADDICTION TREATMENT

- Setting specific individualized goals as upper limits for drinking.
- Self-monitoring alcohol use.
- Implementing specific strategies for slowing down and limiting consumption.
- Self-reinforcing progressive attainment of goals.
- Identifying high-risk situations for overdrinking.
- Developing specific coping strategies for high-risk situations.
- Learning alternative coping skills to replace drinking.

Both client (Levy, 2007; Miller & Muñoz, 2005) and therapist guidelines are available (Hester, 2003; Sanchez-Craig, 1996). The usual course of outpatient counselor-facilitated BSCT is 6 to 10 sessions.

Moderation for Whom?

Perhaps the most decisive factor in treatment goal selection is the client's own choice. We don't get to set other people's goals for them. Said another way, it's not a change goal until it's the client's goal. Clients feel equally free to disregard a treatment goal that someone else has set for them, be it abstinence or moderation (Graber & Miller, 1988).

There is, however, quite a sizeable research literature to draw on in helping clients make informed choices. Naturalistic longitudinal studies (e.g., Dawson et al., 2005) as well as evaluations of abstinence-oriented (e.g., Armor, Polich, & Stambul, 1978) and moderation-oriented treatment (Miller, Leckman, et al., 1992) have reached similar conclusions about who does and does not maintain stable problem-free moderation. The more severe the alcohol problems and dependence, the less likely it is that moderation will last, and abstinence is the better choice. Conversely, at the lower end of the continuum of AUDs, moderation is more likely than abstention to be the stable outcome. There are exceptions at both ends (Dawson et al., 2005), but that's the general trend (see Box 23.3).

Any health care system intending to serve the full spectrum of AUDs should include moderation-oriented options for people who are drinking too much. There is no scientific evidence that the availability of or publicity about moderation programs endangers the sobriety of abstinent people, although this is a common worry among professionals. Counselors are also sometimes concerned that they might be liable if a client with whom they were working toward a moderation goal were to overdrink with tragic or fatal consequences. We know of no such legal case, and it would be equally plausible to hold a therapist accountable in such circumstances for insisting on abstinence with a client for whom moderation was a more feasible goal. In either case, the client would have violated the goal of treatment.

BOX 23.3. Is Moderation a Reasonable Goal?

The U.S. NIAAA published the following specific guidelines for considering a treatment goal of moderate drinking (Miller et al., 1992), based on 3- to 8-year outcomes in four studies of moderation-oriented treatment (Miller, Leckman, et al., 1992). Two pretreatment measures of problem severity were used as predictors: the Michigan Alcoholism Screening Test (MAST; Selzer, 1971) and the Alcohol Dependence Scale (ADS; Skinner & Horn, 1984). The charts below show the relative probabilities, within four different severity score ranges, that clients at follow-up would be totally abstaining versus drinking moderately without problems. In all cases, the probability of moderation is shown relative to that for abstinence (set at 1.0).

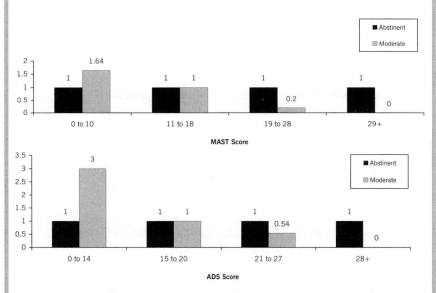

The pattern is the same on both measures. At low severity, clients were more likely to become moderate nonproblem drinkers than to abstain totally. At the highest level of severity, no one in these studies managed to maintain moderate problem-free drinking.

PREVENTING HARM

This opens up the larger controversial issue of harm reduction, which in some quarters has fueled a furor similar to that inspired by "controlled drinking" in the 1980s. It is self-evident that those of us who work in addiction treatment hope that our lives and efforts will diminish the harm and suffering so frequently caused by substance use disorders. That much is uncontroversial (see Chapter 22).

The pragmatic question is this: If clients do not accept our own aspiration for their total abstention from all drugs of abuse, is it ethical to do (or to not do?) whatever we can to at least prevent harm to themselves or others from their drug use? What are some of the possible reasons why a professional might reject such attempts to prevent harm? Here are some arguments that have been expressed:

- Such harm reduction efforts only prolong the client's addiction by removing its natural negative consequences.
- It enables and implicitly condones illegal behavior.
- Anything but total abstinence from all drugs of abuse will ultimately lead to relapse, deterioration, and death.
- Drug abuse is self-inflicted, and people deserve whatever they get if they don't stop it.
- Harm reduction is just a foot in the door for the legalization of drugs.

Absolute opinions for or against harm reduction in general tend to be polemical, and in a way it comes down to what a provider, program, or system decides to do (or not do) in day-to-day practice with actual clients. For many clinicians, some measures to reduce risk of potential harm and suffering are reasonable (even if not comfortable), whereas others are unacceptable. The term "harm reduction" can cover a wide array of possible professional practices. Box 23.4 offers some examples that have been implemented in various locations. How acceptable to you is each of the described services?

A broader challenge in indicated prevention is finding and reaching those in need, most of whom do not readily seek treatment. This requires thinking beyond the confines of "treatment" in order to reach people where they are. Internet-based interventions represent a promising avenue for such outreach (Hester et al., 2005, 2009; T. G. Miller & Sønderlund, 2010). An ideal combination is to offer screening and services in places where people with alcohol/drug problems already are, making these resources as accessible and barrier-free as possible (Institute of Medicine, 1990; National Institute on Drug Abuse, 2010).

> Offer screening and services in places where people with alcohol/drug problems already are.

BOX 23.4. Would You?

How acceptable to you would each of the following services be?

This is unacceptable or unethical to me.				It's OK with me if I don't have to do it myself.				I would be willing to do this myself.		
0	1	2	3	4	5	6	7	8	9	10

_____ Operate a free needle exchange program to provide clean syringes to injection drug users and safely dispose of their used needles.

_____ Provide heroin users with naloxone rescue kits, similar to those used in emergency rooms, to inject if witnessing a heroin overdose. (Many heroin overdose deaths happen in the presence of at least one other drug user, who is often reluctant to call for help.)

_____ Offer free testing of drugs with unknown content, to identify for users or parents what's in them.

_____ Provide a substitution drug like buprenorphine if the person is willing to taper off toward abstinence.

_____ Provide a safer maintenance drug like buprenorphine or methadone for longer-term use instead of heroin.

_____ Help a client gradually taper down his or her use of a drug toward an ultimate goal of abstinence. (Does it make a difference to you if the drug is nicotine, alcohol, marijuana, or cocaine?)

_____ Provide free condoms for people in addiction treatment. (Does it make a difference to you if the client is an adult or an adolescent?)

_____ Encourage heroin-dependent adults to register with a medical service that dispenses heroin to be injected on-site, if you know that doing so would reduce (1) overdose deaths, (2) property crime, (3) the need to recruit other users in order to support one's own habit, (4) medical consequences of using drugs of unknown strength and purity, (5) violence associated with buying from drug dealers, and (6) the market for illegal sale of heroin.

_____ Work with a marijuana user who is currently unwilling to quit, to try cutting down and see how it goes.

If an injection polydrug user is willing to come to treatment sessions but is not willing to accept a goal of total abstinence, would you be willing to work with this person to:

_____ Get HIV testing?

_____ Use only clean needles from a needle exchange and never share needles?

_____ Switch to a less risky route of administration (e.g., from injection to snorting)?

_____ Quit using some drugs (e.g., methamphetamine, heroin) but not others (e.g., alcohol, marijuana, tobacco)?

_____ Focus on quitting one drug at a time (e.g., methamphetamine, alcohol, nicotine)?

KEY POINTS

📌 Three levels of preventive intervention are primary (universal), secondary (selective), and tertiary (indicated). Indicated prevention encompasses most addiction treatment efforts.

📌 Universal prevention targets an entire community or population and is often differentiated into supply-side and demand-side interventions.

📌 Selective prevention targets a group with higher risk of developing, but who do not yet have, substance use disorders.

📌 Indicated prevention targets individuals who already have a substance use disorder, ideally at an early stage, to arrest or reverse its development.

📌 Harm reduction is a form of tertiary prevention, intended to reduce substance-related harm to the user or others.

REFLECTION QUESTIONS

💬 What is your own inclination with regard to harm reduction efforts? Of the interventions listed in Box 23.4, which are you willing to consider?

💬 In what service systems within your community are people with alcohol and other drug problems likely to turn up? Where might it make sense to implement screening?

💬 What in your mind are the pros and cons of helping heavy drinkers moderate their alcohol use? Is this a service that you are willing to provide?

Looking Forward

A. Thomas McLellan

I t is the authors' stated hope that *Treating Addiction: A Guide for Professionals* will lead to greater understanding and willingness to treat substance use disorders on the part of clinicians in many related fields of health care and social services. I am sure the book will; it is an excellent source of practical knowledge and expert clinical practice in the field of substance use disorders.

Because of the stature of the authors and the extraordinary range of clinical, research, and teaching experience, I was prepared for a book that would extend and advance the knowledge and understanding of even the most seasoned professionals. To be sure, this is the case, but two special features of this book are likely to extend its impact in important ways.

The first of these features is its presentation. The book has an especially clear and welcoming writing style, which makes it understandable to a wide range of readers, from introductory students through experienced professionals. Even complicated theoretical distinctions, mechanisms of action for medications and other interventions, and sophisticated experimental evidence are described very clearly. This is an important feature because the authors had to synthesize and clarify a very broad range of scientific advances in treating and managing the addiction-related behaviors that are so troubling to affected individuals, their families, and society as a whole.

A. Thomas McLellan, PhD, is Professor, Department of Psychiatry, University of Pennsylvania School of Medicine and Director, The Penn Center for Substance Abuse Solutions, Philadelphia, Pennsylvania.

But it is the second feature of this book—its public health orientation—that is likely to change thinking and action in the substance abuse field.

The use of a public health approach to substance use problems is most significant. This approach extracts the issue from the moral, military, and justice domains where it has been catalogued for so long and brings it into the public health arena. That is a very good start. The authors describe the roles of agent, host, and environment in explaining how substance use problems develop in an individual and spread through a community. They provide a clear strategy for individuals, families, and communities to share responsibility and informed effort to control substance use problems through prevention, early intervention, treatment, and recovery support.

A public health understanding of substance abuse has been a long time coming. This country has tried to scare, scold, stigmatize, interdict, punish, and incarcerate our way out of alcohol, tobacco, and other substance use problems. Only in the past decade has public recognition of the costs and consequences of simplistic, punitive policies been combined with research advances to create a willingness to try something new. As Winston Churchill famously said, "You can always count on the Americans to do the right thing . . . after they have tried everything else!"

Part of the appeal of these earlier strategies was that each attributed substance use problems to just one or two causal agents, thereby absolving most of society from responsibility or action. Usually the solutions were the responsibility of someone wearing a uniform—a soldier who eradicated crops and interdicted smuggled drugs, a policeman who arrested sellers and users, and/or a judge who sentenced and incarcerated those convicted. The public health approach is fundamentally different in that it requires much broader involvement, understanding, and particularly responsibility on the part of individuals, families, and agencies within our communities. For this reason, and despite the importance of treatment methods, the many advances in medications and behavioral interventions treatment are not likely by themselves to control society's alcohol and drug problems. Controlling substance use problems will likely require shared responsibility and coordinated, informed actions on the part of virtually all members of society.

As suggested in the book, a public health approach offers a way of treating substance abuse that is fundamentally different from the traditional "rehab program" approach that has remained virtually unchanged since the 1960s. This approach changes the very concept of treatment from a time-limited, single treatment episode provided within a clinical setting, to a continuum of interventions, medications, therapies, social services, and community supports delivered to individuals and families by health care, faith, and social service agencies. The need for a broader continuum of clinical services and better access to early care for substance use problems has been recognized in the recent historic health care reform legislation.

This law expands and integrates treatments for substance use disorders into mainstream health care as part of an overall effort to improve general health care quality, efficiency, and effectiveness. Specialty care providers will of course continue to be necessary—likely more than ever—for severe and complicated forms of addiction. But the law creates a national requirement for clinicians to learn and practice screening and brief interventions with emerging cases of harmful or hazardous substance use, and also to become proficient with office-based monitoring and managing and medicating mild to moderate cases of substance abuse and dependence.

Sharing responsibility and working together may be among the most unnatural of human acts, so the public health approach is by no means an easy or quick fix. But if a new, collaborative, and informed public health approach is initiated, there is reason for real optimism. So I believe that *Treating Addiction: A Guide for Professionals* will achieve the authors' laudable goals of fostering greater understanding and willingness of clinicians from many areas of health care and social services to treat substance use disorders. If clinicians learned how and when to implement the many clearly and rationally described evidence-based clinical practices in this book, we would have come a long way toward achieving the kind of effective treatment system we all envisage and need.

References

Abbott, P. J., Moore, B., & Delaney, H. (2003). Community reinforcement approach and relapse prevention: 12 and 18-month follow-up. *Journal of Maintenance in the Addictions, 2*(3), 35–50.

Abbott, P. J., Quinn, D., & Knox, L. (1995). Ambulatory medical detoxification for alcohol. *American Journal of Drug and Alcohol Abuse, 21*(4), 549–563.

Abbott, P. J., Waller, S. B., Delaney, H. D., & Moore, B. A. (1998). Community reinforcement approach in the treatment of opiate addicts. *American Journal of Drug and Alcohol Abuse, 24*, 17–30.

Abellanas, L., & McLellan, A. T. (1993). "Stages of change" by drug problem in concurrent opioid, cocaine and cigarette users. *Journal of Psychoactive Drugs, 25*, 307–313.

Abraham, A. (2010). *Implementation of alcohol pharmacotherapies in specialty AUD treatment settings: How are programs using medication in routine treatment practice?* Paper presented at the symposium *Adopting Alcoholism Pharmacotherapy in Clinical Practice: Barriers and Facilitators*, 33rd Annual Scientific Meeting of the Research Society on Alcoholism, San Antonio, TX.

Agostinelli, G., Brown, J. M., & Miller, W. R. (1995). Effects of normative feedback on consumption among heavy drinking college students. *Journal of Drug Education, 25*, 31–40.

Ait-Daoud, N., & Johnson, B. A. (2003). Medications for the treatment of alcoholism. In B. A. Johnson, P. Ruiz, & M. Galanter (Eds.), *Handbook of clinical alcoholism treatment* (pp. 119–130). Philadelphia: Lippincott, Williams, & Wilkins.

Aktan, G. B., Calkins, R. F., Ribisl, K. M., Kroliczak, A., & Kasim, R. M. (1997). Test–retest reliability of psychoactive substance abuse and dependence diagnoses in telephone interviews using a modified Diagnostic Interview Schedule substance abuse module. *American Journal of Drug and Alcohol Abuse, 23*, 229–248.

Al-Anon Family Group Headquarters. (1976). *Living with an alcoholic with the help of Al-Anon.* New York: Author.

Albanese, A. P., Gevirtz, C., Oppenheim, B., Field, J. M., Abels, I., & Eustace, J. C. (2000). Outcome and six month follow up of patients after ultra rapid opiate detoxification (URODsm). *Journal of Addictive Diseases, 19*(2), 11–28.

Alcoholics Anonymous. (1976). *Alcoholics Anonymous: The story of how many thousands of men and women have recovered from alcoholism* (3rd ed.). New York: Alcoholics Anonymous World Services.

Alcoholics Anonymous General Service Office. (2002). *Memo on participation of A.A. members in research and other non-A.A. surveys.* New York: Alcoholics Anonymous World Services.

Alcoholics Anonymous World Services. (1957). *Alcoholics Anonymous.* New York: Author.

Alcoholics Anonymous World Services. (2001). *Alcoholics Anonymous: The story of how many thousands of men and women have recovered from alcoholism* (4th ed.). New York: Author.

Alcoholics Anonymous World Services. (2008). *Alcoholics Anonymous 2007 membership survey.* New York: Author.

Alexander, J. A., Pollack, H., Nahra, T., Wells, R., & Lemak, C. H. (2007). Case management and client access to health and social services in outpatient substance abuse treatment. *Journal of Behavioral Health Services Research, 34,* 221–236.

Alterman, A., O'Brien, C. P., McLellan, A. T., August, D. A., Snider, E., Drobra, M., et al. (1994). Effectiveness and costs of inpatient versus day hospital cocaine rehabilitation. *Journal of Nervous and Mental Disease, 182*(3), 157–163.

Alterman, A., Snider, E., Caccioia, J., May, D., Parikh, G., Maany, I., et al. (1996). A quasi-experimental comparison of the effectiveness of 6- versus 12-hour per week outpatient treatments for cocaine dependence. *Journal of Nervous and Mental Disease, 184,* 54–56.

American Psychiatric Association. (1952). *Diagnostic and statistical manual of mental disorders.* Washington, DC: Author.

American Psychiatric Association. (1968). *Diagnostic and statistical manual of mental disorders* (2nd ed.). Washington, DC: Author.

American Psychiatric Association. (1980). *Diagnostic and statistical manual of mental disorders* (3rd ed.). Washington, DC: Author.

American Psychiatric Association. (1987). *Diagnostic and statistical manual of mental disorders* (3rd ed., rev). Washington, DC: Author.

American Psychiatric Association. (1994). *Diagnostic and statistical manual of mental disorders* (4th ed.). Washington, DC: American Psychiatric Association.

American Psychiatric Association. (2000). *Diagnostic and statistical manual of mental disorders* (4th ed., text rev.). Washington, DC: Author.

American Society of Addiction Medicine. (1996). *Patient placement criteria for the treatment of substance-related disorders* (2nd ed.). Chevy Chase, MD: Author.

American Society of Addiction Medicine. (2001). *Patient placement criteria for the treatment of substance-related disorders (PPC-2R)*. Chevy Chase, MD: Author.

Amrhein, P. C. (1992). The comprehension of quasi-performance verbs in verbal commitments: New evidence for componential theories of lexical meaning. *Journal of Memory and Language, 31*, 756–784.

Amrhein, P. C., Miller, W. R., Yahne, C. E., Palmer, M., & Fulcher, L. (2003). Client commitment language during motivational interviewing predicts drug use outcomes. *Journal of Consulting and Clinical Psychology, 71*, 862–878.

Angarita, G. A., Reif, S., Pirard, S., Lee, S., Sharon, E., & Gastfriend, D. (2007). No-show for treatment in substance abuse patients with comorbid symptomatology: Validity results from a controlled trial of the ASAM patient placement criteria. *Journal of Addiction Medicine, 1*, 79–87.

Annis, H. M., & Chan, D. (1983). The differential treatment model: Empirical evidence from a personality typology of adult offenders. *Criminal Justice and Behavior, 10*, 159–173.

Annis, H. M., & Graham, J. M. (1988). *Situational Confidence Questionnaire (SCQ-39) user's guide*. Toronto, ON: Addiction Research Foundation.

Annis, H. M., & Graham, J. M. (1991). *Inventory of Drug-Taking Situations (IDTA) user's guide*. Toronto, ON: Addiction Research Foundation.

Annis, H. M., Graham, J. M., & Davis, C. D. (1987). *Inventory of Drinking Situations: User's guide*. Toronto, ON: Addiction Research Foundation.

Anton, R. F., Lieber, C., Tabakoff, C., & CDTect Study Group. (2002). Carbohydrate deficient transferrin (CDT) and gamma glutamyltransferase for the detection and monitoring of alcoholics. *Alcoholism: Clinical and Experimental Research, 26*(8), 1215–1222.

Anton, R. F., Litten, R. A., & Allen, J. P. (1995). Biological assessment of alcohol consumption. In J. P. Allen & M. Columbus (Eds.), *Assessing alcohol problems: A guide for clinicians and researchers* (pp. 31–39). Rockville, MD: National Institute on Alcohol Abuse and Alcoholism.

Anton, R. F., O'Malley, S. S., Ciraulo, D. A., Couper, D., Donovan, D. M., Gastfriend, D. R., et al. (2006). Combined pharmacotherapies and behavioral interventions for alcohol dependence. The COMBINE study: A randomized controlled trial. *Journal of the American Medical Association, 295*, 2003–2017.

Apodaca, T. R., & Longabaugh, R. (2009). Mechanisms of change in motivational interviewing: A review and preliminary evaluation of the evidence. *Addiction, 104*, 705–715.

Apodaca, T. R., & Miller, W. R. (2003). A meta-analysis of the effectiveness of bibliotherapy for alcohol problems. *Journal of Clinical Psychology, 59*, 289–304.

Armor, D. J., Polich, J. M., & Stambul, H. B. (1978). *Alcoholism and treatment*. New York: Wiley.

Aron, A., & Aron, E. N. (1980). The transcendental meditation program's effect on addictive behavior. *Addictive Behaviors, 5*, 3–12.

Azrin, N. H. (1976). Improvements in the community-reinforcement approach to alcoholism. *Behaviour Research and Therapy, 14*, 339–348.

Azrin, N. H., & Besalel, V. A. (1982). *Finding a job*. Berkeley, CA: Ten Speed Press.

Azrin, N. H., Sisson, R. W., Meyers, R. J., & Godley, M. (1982). Alcoholism treatment by disulfiram and community reinforcement therapy. *Journal of Behavior Therapy and Experimental Psychiatry, 13,* 105–112.

Babor, T. F. (2010). *Alcohol: No ordinary commodity: Research and public policy* (2nd ed.). Oxford, UK: Oxford University Press.

Babor, T. F., & Del Boca, F. K. (Eds.). (2003). *Treatment matching in alcoholism.* Cambridge, UK: Cambridge University Press.

Babor, T. F., & Grant, M. (1989). From clinical research to secondary prevention: International collaboration in the development of the Alcohol Use Disorders Identification Test (AUDIT). *Alcohol Health and Research World, 13,* 371–374.

Babor, T. F., & Higgins-Biddle, J. C. (2000). Alcohol screening and brief intervention: Dissemination strategies for medical practice and public health. *Addiction, 95*(5), 677–686.

Babor, T. F., Higgins-Biddle, J. C., Saunders, J. B., & Monteiro, M. G. (2001). *The Alcohol Use Disorders Identification Test: Guidelines for use in primary care* (2nd ed.). Geneva: World Health Organization.

Bacon, F. (1992). *The wisdom of the ancients.* London: Kessinger. (Original work published 1619)

Baer, J. S., Kivlahan, D. R., Blume, A. W., McKnight, P., & Marlatt, G. A. (2001). Brief intervention for heavy-drinking college students: 4-year follow-up and natural history. *American Journal of Public Health, 91,* 1310–1316.

Baker, A., Heather, N., Wodak, A., Dixon, J., & Holt, P. (1993). Evaluation of a cognitive behavioral intervention for HIV prevention among injecting drug users. *AIDS, 7,* 247–256.

Baker, A., Kochan, N., Dixon, J., Heather, N., & Wodak, A. (1994). Controlled evaluation of a brief intervention for HIV prevention among injecting drug-users not in treatment. *AIDS Care, 6*(5), 559–570.

Baker, A., Turner, A., Kay-Lambkin, F. J., & Lewin, T. J. (2009). The long and the short of treatments for alcohol or cannabis misuse among people with severe mental disorders. *Addictive Behaviors, 34,* 852–858.

Ball, S. A., Martino, S., Nich, C., Frankforter, T. L., van Horn, D., Crits-Christoph, P., et al. (2007). Site matters: Multisite randomized trial of motivational enhancement therapy in community drug abuse clinics. *Journal of Consulting and Clinical Psychology, 75,* 556–567.

Bamatter, W., Carroll, K. M., Añez, L. M., Paris, M. Jr., Ball, S. A., Nich, C., et al. (2010). Informal discussions in substance abuse treatment sessions with Spanish-speaking clients. *Journal of Substance Abuse Treatment, 39,* 353–363.

Bandura, A. (1997). *Self-efficacy: The exercise of control.* New York: Freeman.

Barber, J. G., & Crisp, B. R. (1995). Social support and prevention of relapse following treatment for alcohol abuse. *Research on Social Work Practice, 5*(3), 283–296.

Barber, J. G., & Gilbertson, R. (1997). Unilateral interventions for women living with heavy drinkers. *Social Work, 42,* 69–78.

Barber, W. S., & O'Brien, C. P. (1999). Pharmacotherapies. In B. S. McCrady & E. E. Epstein (Eds.), *Addictions: A comprehensive guidebook* (pp. 347–369). New York: Oxford University Press.

Barnett, P. G., Trafton, J. A., & Humphreys, K. (2010). The cost of concordance with opiate substitution treatment guidelines. *Journal of Substance Abuse Treatment, 39*(2), 141–149.

Batki, S. L., Kauffman, J. F., Marion, I., Parrino, M. W., & Woody, G. E. (2005). *Medication-assisted treatment for opioid addiction in opioid treatment programs* (Vol. 43, Treatment Improvement Protocol [TIP] series). Rockville, MD: Center for Substance Abuse Treatment.

Baumeister, R. F. (1994). The crystallization of discontent in the process of major life change. In T. F. Heatherton & J. L. Weinberger (Eds.), *Can personality change?* (pp. 281–297). Washington, DC: American Psychological Association.

Baumeister, R. F., Heatherton, T. F., & Tice, D. M. (1994). *Losing control: How and why people fail at self-regulation.* New York: Academic Press.

Beauchamp, T. L., & Childress, J. F. (2001). *Principles of biomedical ethics* (5th ed.). New York: Oxford University Press.

Beck, A. T., Wright, F. D., Newman, C. F., & Liese, B. S. (2001). *Cognitive therapy of substance abuse.* New York: Guilford Press.

Becker, H. C. (1998). Kindling in alcohol withdrawal. *Alcohol Health and Research World, 22*, 25–33.

Becker, H. C., & Hale, R. L. (1993). Repeated episodes of ethanol withdrawal potentiate the severity of subsequent withdrawal seizures: An animal model of alcohol withdrawal "kindling." *Alcoholism: Clinical and Experimental Research, 17*, 94–98.

Beckman, L. J. (1993). Alcoholics Anonymous and gender issues. In B. S. McCrady & W. R. Miller (Eds.), *Research on Alcoholics Anonymous: Opportunities and alternatives* (pp. 319–348). New Brunswick, NJ: Rutgers Center of Alcohol Studies.

Beckman, L. J., & Amarno, H. (1986). Personal and social difficulties faced by women and men entering alcoholism treatment. *Journal of Studies on Alcohol, 47*, 135–145.

Benshoff, J. J., & Janikowski, T. P. (2000). *The rehabilitation model of substance abuse counseling.* Belmont, Canada: Wadsworth.

Benson, H., & Klipper, M. Z. (1990). *The relaxation response.* New York: Avon.

Berglund, M., Thelander, S., Salaspuro, M., Franck, J., Andreasson, S., & Ojehagen, A. (2003). Treatment of alcohol abuse: An evidence-based review. *Alcoholism: Clinical and Experimental Research, 27*, 1645–1656.

Berman, A. H., Bergman, H., Palmstierna, T., & Schlyter, F. (2005). Evaluation of the Drug Use Disorders Identification Test (DUDIT) in criminal justice and detoxification settings and in a Swedish population sample. *European Addiction Research, 11*(1), 22–31.

Bernstein, E., Bernstein, J., Feldman, J., Fernandez, W., Hagan, M., Mitchell, P., et al. (2007). An evidence-based alcohol screening, brief intervention and referral to treatment (SBIRT) curriculum for emergency department (ED) providers improves skills and utilization. *Substance Abuse, 28*(4), 79–92.

Bernstein, E., Bernstein, J., & Levenson, S. (1997). Project ASSERT: An ED-based intervention to increase access to primary care, preventive services and the substance abuse treatment system. *Annals of Emergency Medicine, 30*, 181–189.

Bernstein, E., Edwards, E., Dorfman, D., Heeren, T., Bliss, C., & Bernstein, J. (2009). Screening and brief intervention to reduce marijuana use among youth and young adults in a pediatric emergency department. *Academic Emergency Medicine, 16*(11), 1174–1185.

Bernstein, J., Bernstein, E., Tassiopoulos, K., Heeren, T., Levenson, S., & Hingson, R. (2005). Brief motivational intervention at a clinic visit reduces cocaine and heroin use. *Drug and Alcohol Dependence, 77,* 49–59.

Beutler, L. E., Harwood, T. M., Michelson, A., Song, X., & Holman, J. (2011). Resistance/reactance level. *Journal of Clinical Psychology: In Session, 67*(2), 133–142.

Beutler, L. E., Machado, P. P. P., & Neufeldt, S. A. (1994). Therapist variables. In A. E. Bergin & S. L. Garfield (Eds.), *Handbook of psychotherapy and behavior change* (4th ed., pp. 229–269). New York: Wiley.

Bickel, W. K., Amass, L., Higgins, S. T., Badger, G. J., & Esch, R. A. (1997). Effects of adding behavioral treatment to opioid detoxification with buprenorphine. *Journal of Consulting and Clinical Psychology, 65,* 803–810.

Bickel, W. K., Christensen, D. R., & Marsch, L. A. (2011). A review of computer-based interventions used in the assessment, treatment, and research of drug addiction. *Substance Use and Misuse, 46*(1), 4–9.

Bidney, M. (2004). Epiphany in autobiography: The quantum changes of Dostoevsky and Tolstoy. *Journal of Clinical Psychology, 60,* 471–480.

Bien, T. (2006). *Mindful therapy: A guide for therapists and helping professionals.* Somerville, MA: Wisdom.

Bien, T., & Bien, B. (2002). *Mindful recovery: A spiritual path to healing from addiction.* New York: Wiley.

Bien, T. H., & Bien, B. (2003). *Finding the center within: The healing way of mindfulness meditation.* Hoboken, NJ: Wiley.

Bien, T. H., Miller, W. R., & Boroughs, J. M. (1993). Motivational interviewing with alcohol outpatients. *Behavioural and Cognitive Psychotherapy, 21,* 347–356.

Bien, T. H., Miller, W. R., & Tonigan, J. S. (1993). Brief interventions for alcohol problems: A review. *Addiction, 88,* 315–336.

Bischof, G., Grothues, J. M., Reinhardt, S., Meyer, C., John, U., & Rumpf, H.-J. (2008). Evaluation of a telephone-based stepped care intervention for alcohol-related disorders: A randomized controlled trial. *Drug and Alcohol Dependence, 93*(3), 244–251.

Blount, A. (1998). Introduction to integrated primary care. In A. Blount (Ed.), *Integrated primary care: The future of medical and mental health collaboration* (pp. 1–43). New York: Norton.

Bobo, J. K., McIlvain, H. E., Lando, H. A., Walker, D., & Leed-Kelly, A. (1998). Effect of smoking cessation counseling on recovery from alcoholism: Findings from a randomized community intervention trial. *Addiction, 93,* 877–887.

Bohart, A. C., & Greenberg, L. S. (Eds.). (1997). *Empathy reconsidered: New directions in psychotherapy.* Washington, DC: American Psychological Association.

Bohart, A. C., & Tallman, K. (1999). *How clients make therapy work: The process of active self-healing.* Washington, DC: American Psychological Association.

Borders, T. F., Curran, G. M., Mattox, R., & Booth, B. M. (2010). Religiousness among at-risk drinkers: Is it prospectively associated with the development or maintenance of an alcohol-use disorder? *Journal of Studies on Alcohol and Drugs, 71,* 136–142.

Botvin, G. J., & Griffin, K. W. (2004). Life skills training: Empirical findings and future directions. *Journal of Primary Prevention, 25,* 211–232.

Botvin, G. J., Griffin, K. W., Paul, E., & Macaulay, A. P. (2003). Preventing tobacco and alcohol use among elementary students through life skills training. *Journal of Child and Adolescent Substance Abuse, 12,* 1–17.

Bowen, M. (1991). Alcoholism as viewed through family systems theory and family psychotherapy. *Family Dynamics of Addiction Quarterly, 1*(1), 94–102.

Bowen, S., Witkiewitz, K., Dilworth, T. M., Chawla, N., Simpson, T. L., Ostafin, B. D., et al. (2006). Mindfulness meditation and substance use in an incarcerated population. *Psychology of Addictive Behaviors, 20,* 343–347.

Bowen, S., Chawla, N., & Marlatt, G. A. (2010). *Mindfulness-based relapse prevention for addictive behaviors.* New York: Guilford Press.

Bowman, K. M., & Jellinek, E. M. (1941). Alcohol addiction and its treatment. *Quarterly Journal of Studies on Alcohol, 2,* 98–176.

Brady, J. V., & Lucas, S. E. (1984). *Testing drugs for physical dependence potential and abuse liability.* Washington, DC: U.S. Government Printing Office.

Brandsma, J. M., Maultsby, M., & Welsh, R. J. (1980). *The outpatient treatment of alcoholism: A review and comparative study.* Baltimore: University Park Press.

Brehm, S. S., & Brehm, J. W. (1981). *Psychological reactance: A theory of freedom and control.* New York: Academic Press.

Brewer, C. (1992). Controlled trials of Antabuse in alcoholism: The importance of supervision and adequate dosage. *Acta Psychiatrica Scandinavica, 86*(Suppl. 369), 51–58.

Bringhurst, D. L., Watson, C. W., Miller, S. D., & Duncan, B. L. (2006). The reliability and validity of the Outcome Rating Scale: A replication study of a brief clinical measure. *Journal of Brief Therapy, 5*(1), 23–30.

Brooks, A. C., Ryder, D., Carise, D., & Kirby, K. C. (2010). Feasibility and effectiveness of computer-based therapy in community treatment. *Journal of Substance Abuse Treatment, 39,* 227–235.

Brooks, G. R. (1998). Group therapy for traditional men. In W. S. Pollack & R. F. Levant (Eds.), *New psychotherapy for men* (pp. 83–96). Hoboken, NJ: Wiley.

Brown, H. P. Jr. (1990). Values and recovery from alcoholism through Alcoholics Anonymous. *Counseling and Values, 35,* 63–68.

Brown, J. M. (1998). Self-regulation and the addictive behaviors. In W. R. Miller & N. Heather (Eds.), *Treating addictive behaviors* (2nd ed., pp. 61–74). New York: Plenum Press.

Brown, J. M., & Miller, W. R. (1993). Impact of motivational interviewing on participation and outcome in residential alcoholism treatment. *Psychology of Addictive Behaviors, 7,* 211–218.

Brown, R. L., & Rounds, L. A. (1995). Conjoint screening questionnaires for alcohol and drug abuse. *Wisconsin Medical Journal, 94,* 135–140.

Brown, S. A., Christiansen, B. A., & Goldman, M. S. (1987). The Alcohol Expectancy Questionnaire: An instrument for the assessment of adolescent and adult alcohol expectancies. *Journal of Studies on Alcohol, 85,* 483–491.

Brown, S. A., Goldman, M. S., Inn, A., & Anderson, L. R. (1980). Expectations of reinforcement from alcohol: Their domain and relation to drinking problems. *Journal of Consulting and Clinical Psychology, 48,* 419–426.

Browne-Miller, A. (1993). *Gestalting addiction: The addiction-focused group therapy of Dr. Richard Louis Miller.* New York: Ablex.

Buckland, P. R. (2008). Will we ever find the genes for addiction? *Addiction, 103*(11), 1768–1776.

Budney, A. J., Higgins, S. T., Radonovich, K. J., & Novy, P. L. (2000). Adding voucher-based incentives to coping skills and motivational enhancement improves outcomes during treatment for marijuana dependence. *Journal of Consulting and Clinical Psychology, 68,* 1051–1061.

Burke, B. L., Arkowitz, H., & Dunn, C. (2002). The efficacy of motivational interviewing and its adaptations: What we know so far. In W. R. Miller & S. Rollnick, *Motivational interviewing: Preparing people for change* (2nd ed., pp. 217–250). New York: Guilford Press.

Burke, B. L., Arkowitz, H., & Menchola, M. (2003). The efficacy of motivational interviewing: A meta-analysis of controlled clinical trials. *Journal of Consulting and Clinical Psychology, 71,* 843–861.

Burke, B. L., Dunn, C. W., Atkins, D. C., & Phelps, J. S. (2004). The emerging evidence base for motivational interviewing: A meta-analytic and qualitative inquiry. *Journal of Cognitive Psychotherapy: An International Quarterly, 18*(4), 309–322.

Burke, B. L., Vassilev, G., Kantchelov, A., & Zweben, A. (2002). Motivational interviewing with couples. In W. R. Miller & S. Rollnick, *Motivational interviewing: Preparing people for change* (2nd ed., pp. 217–250). New York: Guilford Press.

Burlingame, G. M., Fuhriman, A., & Johnson, J. E. (2002). Cohesion in group psychotherapy. In J. C. Norcross (Ed.), *Psychotherapy relationships that work: Therapist contributions and responsiveness to patients* (pp. 71–87). New York: Oxford University Press.

Burnett, G. B., & Reading, H. W. (1970). The pharmacology of disulfiram in the treatment of alcoholism. *British Journal of Addiction, 65,* 281–288.

Burns, L., & Teesson, M. (2002). Alcohol use disorders comorbid with anxiety, depression and drug use disorders: Findings from the Australian National Survey of Mental Health and Well Being. *Drug and Alcohol Dependence, 68*(3), 299–307.

Butler, S. F., Budman, S. H., Goldman, R. J., Newman, F. L., Beckley, K. E., Trottier, D., et al. (2001). Initial validation of a computer-administered Addiction Severity Index: The ASI-MV. *Psychology of Addictive Behaviors, 15,* 4–12.

C'de Baca, J., Miller, W. R., & Lapham, S. C. (2001). A multiple risk factor approach to predicting DWI recidivism. *Journal of Substance Abuse Treatment, 21,* 207–215.

C'de Baca, J., & Wilbourne, P. (2004). Quantum change: Ten years later. *Journal of Clinical Psychology, 60,* 531–541.

Cahalan, D. (1970). *Problem drinkers.* San Francisco: Jossey-Bass.

Calsyn, D. A., Hatch-Maillette, M., Tross, S., Doyle, S. R., Crits-Christoph, P., Song, Y. S., et al. (2009). Motivational and skills training HIV/sexually transmitted infection sexual risk reduction groups for men. *Journal of Substance Abuse Treatment, 37*(2), 138–150.

Campbell, T. C., Hoffman, N. G., Madson, M. B., & Melchert, T. P. (2003). Performance of a brief assessment tool. *Addictive Disorders and Their Treatment, 2*, 13–17.

Cantor-Graae, E., Nordström, L. G., & McNeil, T. F. (2001). Substance abuse in schizophrenia: A review of the literature and a study of correlates in Sweden. *Schizophrenia Research, 48*(1), 69–82.

Carbonari, J. P., & DiClemente, C. C. (2000). Using transtheoretical model profiles to differentiate levels of alcohol abstinence success. *Journal of Consulting and Clinical Psychology, 68*(5), 810–817.

Cardenas, H. L., & Ross, D. H. (1976). Calcium depletion of synaptosomes after morphine treatment. *British Journal of Pharmacology, 57*(4), 521–526.

Carey, K. B., & Carey, M. P. (1990). Enhancing the treatment attendance of mentally ill chemical abusers. *Journal of Behavior Therapy and Experimental Psychiatry, 21*(3), 205–209.

Carr, L. A. (1993). The pharmacology of mood-altering drugs of abuse. *Primary Care, 20*(1), 19–31.

Carr, S. (2011). *Scripting addiction: The politics of therapeutic talk and American sobriety.* Princeton, NJ: Princeton University Press.

Carroll, K. M. (1996). Relapse prevention as a psychosocial treatment: A review of controlled clinical trials. *Experimental and Clinical Psychopharmacology, 4*, 46–54.

Carroll, K. M. (1997a). *Improving compliance with alcoholism treatment (Project MATCH Monograph Series Vol. 6).* Rockville, MD: National Institute on Alcohol Abuse and Alcoholism.

Carroll, K. M. (1997b). Integrating psychotherapy and pharmacotherapy to improve drug abuse outcomes. *Addictive Behaviors, 22*, 233–245.

Carroll, K. M. (1999). Behavioral and cognitive behavioral treatments. In B. S. McCrady & E. E. Epstein (Eds.), *Addictions: A comprehensive guidebook.* (pp. 250–267). New York: Oxford University Press.

Carroll, K. M., Ball, S. A., Nich, C., Martino, S., Frankforter, T. L., Farentinos, C., et al. (2006). Motivational interviewing to improve treatment engagement and outcome in individuals seeking treatment for substance abuse: A multisite effectiveness study. *Drug and Alcohol Dependence, 81*, 301–312.

Carroll, K. M., Fenton, L. R., Ball, S. A., Nich, C., Frankforter, T. L., Shi, J., et al. (2004). Efficacy of disulfiram and cognitive behavior therapy in cocaine-dependent outpatients: A randomized placebo-controlled trial. *Archives of General Psychiatry, 61*, 264–272.

Carroll, K. M., Nich, C., Ball, S. A., McCance, E., & Rounsaville, B. (1998). Treatment of cocaine and alcohol dependence with psychotherapy and disulfiram. *Addiction, 93*, 713–728.

Carroll, K. M., & Rounsaville, B. J. (2005). Behavioral therapies: The glass would be half full if only we had a glass. In W. R. Miller & K. M. Carroll (Eds.), *Rethinking substance abuse: What the science shows, and what we should do about it* (pp. 223–239). New York: Guilford Press.

Carroll, K. M., Ziedonis, D., O'Malley, S., McCance-Katz, E., Gordon, L., & Rounsaville, B. (1993). Pharmacologic interventions for alcohol- and cocaine-abusing individuals: A pilot study of disulfiram vs. naltrexone. *American Journal of Addictions, 2,* 77–79.

Carruth, B. E., & Mendenhall, W. E. (1989). *Co-dependency: Issues in treatment and recovery.* New York: Hayworth Press.

Casteneda, C. (1985). *The teachings of Don Juan: A Yaqui way of knowledge.* New York: Washington Square Press.

Cermak, T. L. (1991). Co-addiction as a disease. *Psychiatric Annals, 21*(5), 266–272.

Chafetz, M. E. (1961). A procedure for establishing therapeutic contact with the alcoholic. *Quarterly Journal of Studies on Alcohol, 22,* 325–328.

Chafetz, M. E., Blane, H. T., Abram, H. S., Golner, J. H., Hastie, E. L., & Meyers, W. (1962). Establishing treatment relations with alcoholics. *Journal of Nervous and Mental Disease, 134,* 395–409.

Chamberlain, P., Patterson, G., Reid, J., Kavanagh, K., & Forgatch, M. S. (1984). Observation of client resistance. *Behavior Therapy, 15,* 144–155.

Chapman, P. L. H., & Huygens, I. (1988). An evaluation of three treatment programmes for alcoholism: An experimental study with 6- and 18-month follow-ups. *British Journal of Addiction, 83,* 67–81.

Cherpitel, C. J. (1995). Analysis of cut points for screening instruments for alcohol problems in the emergency room. *Journal of Studies on Alcohol and Drugs, 56,* 695–700.

Cherpitel, C. J. (2006). Screening for alcohol problems in the U.S. general population: Comparison of the CAGE, RAPS4, and RAPS4–QF by gender, ethnicity, and service utilization. *Alcoholism: Clinical and Experimental Research, 26,* 1686–1691.

Chi, F. W., Kaskutas, L. A., Sterling, S., Campbell, C. I., & Weisner, C. (2009). Twelve-step affiliation and 3-year substance use outcomes among adolescents: Social support and religious service attendance as potential mediators. *Addiction, 104*(6), 927–939.

Chick, J., Anton, R., Checinski, K., Croop, R., Drummond, D. C., Farmer, R., et al. (2000). A multicentre, randomized, double-blind, placebo-controlled trial of naltrexone in the treatment of alcohol dependence or abuse. *Alcohol and Alcoholism, 35,* 587–593.

Chick, J., Howlett, H., Morgan, M. Y., Ritson, B., & Investigators, t. U. (2000). United Kingdom multicentre acamprosate study (UKMAS): A 6-month prospective study of acamprosate versus placebo in preventing relapse after withdrawal from alcohol. *Alcohol and Alcoholism, 35,* 176–187.

Chick, J., Ritson, B., Connaughton, J., Stewart, A., & Chick, J. (1995). Advice versus extended treatment for alcoholism: A controlled study. *British Journal of Addiction, 83*(2), 159–170.

Christo, G., & Franey, C. (1995). Drug users' spiritual beliefs, locus of control and the disease concept in relation to Narcotics Anonymous attendance and six-month outcomes. *Drug and Alcohol Dependence, 38,* 51–56.

Clark, D. B., Gordon, A. J., Ettaro, L. R., Owens, J. M., & Moss, H. B. (2010). Screening and brief intervention for underage drinkers. *Mayo Clinic Proceedings, 85,* 380–391.

Clark, H. W. (2005–2007). Center for Substance Abuse Treatment (CSAT), Substance Abuse and Mental Health Services Administration (SAMHSA): News from the Director, CSAT. *Journal of Maintenance in the Addictions, 3*(2–4), 13–16.

Cloninger, C. R., Sigvardsson, S., & Bohman, M. (1996). Type I and Type II alcoholism: An update. *Alcohol Health and Research World, 20,* 18–23.

Cohen, S., Lichtenstein, E., Prochaska, J. O., Rossi, J. S., Gritz, E. R., Carr, C. R., et al. (1989). Debunking myths about self-quitting: Evidence from 10 prospective studies of persons who attempt to quit smoking by themselves. *American Psychologist, 44,* 1355–1365.

Colby, S. M., Monti, P. M., Barnett, N. P., Rohsenow, D. J., Weissman, K., Spirito, A., et al. (1998). Brief motivational interviewing in a hospital setting for adolescent smoking: A preliminary study. *Journal of Consulting and Clinical Psychology, 66,* 574–578.

COMBINE Study Research Group. (2003). Testing combined pharmacotherapies and behavioral interventions in alcohol dependence: Rationale and methods. *Alcoholism: Clinical and Experimental Research, 27,* 1107–1122.

Compton, W. M., Thomas, Y. F., Stinson, F. S., & Grant, B. F. (2007). Prevalence, correlates, disability, and comorbidity of DSM-IV drug abuse and dependence in the United States: Results from the National Epidemiologic Survey on alcohol and related conditions. *Archives of General Psychiatry, 64,* 566–576.

Connors, G. J., & Dermen, K. H. (1996). Characteristics of participants in Secular Organizations for Sobriety (SOS). *American Journal of Drug and Alcohol Abuse, 22,* 281–295.

Connors, G. J., Donovan, D. M., & DiClemente, C. C. (2001). *Substance abuse treatment and the stages of change: Selecting and planning interventions.* New York: Guilford Press.

Connors, G. J., & Maisto, S. A. (1988). Alcohol expectancy construct: Overview and clinical applications. *Cognitive Therapy and Research, 12,* 487–504.

Connors, G. J., Tonigan, J. S., & Miller, W. R. (2001). Religiosity and responsiveness to alcoholism treatments. In R. Longabaugh & P. W. Wirtz (Eds.), *Project MATCH hypotheses: Results and causal chain analyses* (Vol. 8, pp. 166–175). Bethesda, MD: National Institute on Alcohol Abuse and Alcoholism.

Connors, G. J., Walitzer, K. S., & Dermen, K. H. (2002). Preparing clients for alcoholism treatment: Effects on treatment participation and outcomes. *Journal of Consulting and Clinical Psychology, 70,* 1161–1169.

Conrad, K. J., Hultman, C. I., Pope, A. R., Lyons, J. S., Baxter, W. C., Daghestani, A., et al. (1998). Case managed residential care for homeless addicted veterans: Results of true experiment. *Medical Care, 36*(1), 40–53.

Cooney, N. L., Zweben, A., & Fleming, M. F. (1995). Screening for alcohol problems and at-risk drinking in health care settings. In R. K. Hester & W. R. Miller (Eds.), *Handbook of alcoholism treatment approaches: Effective alternatives* (2nd ed., pp. 45–60). New York: Allyn & Bacon.

Copeland, J. (1997). A qualitative study of barriers to formal treatment among women who self-managed change in addictive behaviours. *Journal of Substance Abuse Treatment, 14,* 183–190.

Corcoran, J. (2004). *Building strengths and skills: A collaborative approach to working with clients.* New York: Oxford University Press.

Cordova, J. V., Scott, R. L., Dorian, M., Mirgain, S., Yeager, D., & Groot, A. (2005). The marriage checkup: An indicated preventive intervention for treatment-avoidant couples at risk for marital deterioration. *Behavior Therapy, 36*, 301–309.

Cox, G. B., Walker, D., Freng, S. A., Short, B. A., Meijer, L., & Gilchrist, L. (1998). Outcome of a controlled trial of the effectiveness of intensive case management for chronic public inebriates. *Journal of Studies on Alcohol, 59*, 523–532.

Cucchia, A. T., Monnat, M., Spagnoli, J., Ferrero, F., & Bertschy, G. (1998). Ultra-rapid opiate detoxification using deep sedation with oral midazolam: Short and long-term results. *Drug and Alcohol Dependence, 52*(3), 243–250.

Cummings, C. C., Gordon, J. R., & Marlatt, G. A. (1980). Relapse: Prevention and prediction. In W. R. Miller (Ed.), *The addictive behaviors: Treatment of alcoholism, drug abuses, smoking and obesity* (pp. 291–321). New York: Pergamon Press.

Daeppen, J. B., Bertholet, N., & Gaume, J. (2010). What process research tells us about brief intervention efficacy. *Drug and Alcohol Review, 29*, 612–616.

Daley, D. C., & Marlatt, G. A. (1999). *Managing your drug or alcohol problem: Client workbook*. New York: Academic Press.

Dallery, J., & Raiff, B. R. (2011). Contingency management in the 21st century: Technological innovations to promote smoking cessation. *Substance Use & Misuse, 46*(1), 10–22.

Dattilio, F. M. (2009). *Cognitive-behavioral therapy with couples and families: A comprehensive guide for clinicians*. New York: Guilford Press.

Dawson, D. A., Grant, B. F., Stinson, F. S., & Chou, P. S. (2006). Estimating the effect of help-seeking on achieving recovery from alcohol dependence. *Addiction, 101*, 824–834.

Dawson, D. A., Grant, B. F., Stinson, F. S., Chou, P. S., Huang, B., & Ruan, W. J. (2005). Recovery from DSM-IV alcohol dependence: United States 2001–2002. *Addiction, 100*, 281–292.

Day, E., & Strang, J. (2011). Outpatient versus inpatient opioid detoxification: A randomized controlled trial. *Journal of Substance Abuse Treatment, 41*(1), 56–66.

Deci, E. L., & Ryan, R. M. (1985). *Intrinsic motivation and self-determination in human behavior*. New York: Plenum Press.

Deci, E. L., & Ryan, R. M. (2008). Facilitating optimal motivation and psychological well-being across life's domains. *Canadian Psychology, 49*, 14–23.

Delaney, H. D., Miller, W. R., & Bisono, A. M. (2007). Religiosity and spirituality among psychologists: A survey of clinician members of the American Psychological Association. *Professional Psychology: Research and Practice, 38*, 538–546.

Dench, S., & Bennett, G. (2000). The impact of brief motivational intervention at the start of an outpatient day programme for alcohol dependence. *Behavioural and Cognitive Psychotherapy, 28*, 121–130.

DeShazer, S., Dolan, Y., Korman, H., Trepper, T., McCollum, E., & Berg, I. K. (2007). *More than miracles: The state of the art of solution-focused brief therapy*. Binghamton, NY: Haworth Press.

DeWeert-Van Oene, G. H., Schippers, G. M., De Jong, C. A., & Schrijvers, G. J.

(2001). Retention in substance dependence treatment: The relevance of in-treatment factors. *Journal of Substance Abuse Treatment, 20,* 253–261.

Diaz, R. M., & Fruhauf, A. G. (1991). The origins and development of self-regulation: A developmental model on the risk for addictive behaviours. In N. Heather, W. R. Miller, & J. Greeley (Eds.), *Self-control and the addictive behaviours* (pp. 83–106). Sydney: Maxwell Macmillan Publishing Australia.

Dick, D. M., & Foroud, T. (2003). Candidate genes for alcohol dependence: A review of genetic evidence from human studies. *Alcoholism: Clinical and Experimental Research, 27,* 868–879.

DiClemente, C. C., Carbonari, J. P., Montgomery, R. P. G., & Hughes, S. O. (1994). The Alcohol Abstinence Self-Efficacy Scale. *Journal of Studies on Alcohol, 55,* 141–148.

DiClemente, C. C., Doyle, S. R., & Donovan, D. (2009). Predicting treatment seekers' readiness to change their drinking behavior in the COMBINE study. *Alcoholism: Clinical and Experimental Research, 33*(5), 879–892.

DiClemente, C. C., & Hughes, J. R. (1990). Stages of change profiles in outpatient alcoholism treatment. *Journal of Substance Abuse, 2,* 217–235.

DiClemente, C. C., & Velasquez, M. W. (2002). Motivational interviewing and the stages of change. In W. R. Miller & S. Rollnick, *Motivational interviewing: Preparing people for change* (2nd ed., pp. 217–250). New York: Guilford Press.

Dillard, J. P., & Shen, L. (2005). On the nature of reactance and its role in persuasive health communication. *Communication Monographs, 72*(2), 144–168.

Dishion, T. J., McCord, J., & Poulin, F. O. (1999). When interventions harm: Peer groups and problem behavior. *American Psychologist, 54*(9), 755–764.

Ditman, K. S., Crawford, G. G., Forgy, E. W., Moskowitz, H., & MacAndrew, C. (1967). A controlled experiment on the use of court probation for drunk arrests. *American Journal of Psychiatry, 124,* 160–163.

Dodge, K., Krantz, B., & Kenny, P. J. (2010). How can we begin to measure recovery? *Substance Abuse Treatment, Prevention & Policy, 5*(31).

Donohue, B., Azrin, N., Allen, D. N., Romero, V., Hill, H. H., Tracy, K., et al. (2009). Family behavior therapy for substance abuse and other associated problems: A review of its intervention components and applicability. *Behavior Modification, 33*(5), 495–519.

Donovan, D. M. (1995). Assessments to aid in the treatment planning process. In J. P. Allen & M. Columbus (Eds.), *Assessing alcohol problems: A guide for clinicians and researchers* (pp. 75–122). Rockville, MD: National Institute on Alcohol Abuse and Alcoholism.

Donovan, D. M. (1999). Assessment strategies and measures in addictive behaviors. In B. S. McCrady & E. E. Epstein (Eds.), *Addictions: A comprehensive guidebook* (pp. 187–215). New York: Oxford University Press.

Donovan, D. M., Hague, W. H., & O'Leary, M. R. (1975). Perceptual differentiation and defense mechanisms in alcoholics. *Journal of Clinical Psychology, 31,* 356–359.

Donovan, D. M., & Rosengren, D. B. (1999). Motivation for behavior change and treatment among substance abusers. In J. A. Tucker, D. M. Donovan, & G. A. Marlatt (Eds.), *Changing addictive behavior: Bridging clinical and public health strategies* (pp. 127–159). New York: Guilford Press.

Donovan, D. M., Rosengren, D. B., Downey, L., Cox, G. B., & Sloan, K. L. (2001). Attrition prevention with individuals awaiting publicly funded drug treatment. *Addiction, 96*, 1149–1160.

Doyle, S. R., Donovan, D. M., & Simpson, T. L. (in press). Validation of a nine-dimensional measure of drinking motives for use in clinical applications: The Desired Effects of Drinking Scale. *Addictive Behaviors.*

Drake, R. E., Mueser, K. T., Brunette, M. F., & McHugo, G. J. (2004). A review of treatments for people with severe mental illnesses and co-occurring substance use disorders. *Psychiatric Rehabilitation Journal, 27*(4), 360–374.

Dunn, C., Deroo, L., & Rivara, F. P. (2001). The use of brief interventions adapted from motivational interviewing across behavioral domains: A systematic review. *Addiction, 96*, 1725–1742.

Dunn, C. W., & Ries, R. (1997). Linking substance abuse services with general medical care: Integrated, brief interventions with hospitalized patients. *American Journal of Drug and Alcohol Abuse, 23*, 1–13.

Durbeej, N., Berman, A. H., Gumpert, C. H., Palmstierna, T., Kristiansson, M., & Alm, C. (2010). Validation of the Alcohol Use Disorders Identification Test and the Drug Use Disorders Identification Test in a Swedish sample of suspected offenders with signs of mental health problems: Results from the Mental Disorder, Substance Abuse and Crime study. *Journal of Substance Abuse Treatment, 39*, 364–377.

Dutcher, L. W., Anderson, R., Moore, M., Luna-Anderson, C., Meyers, R. J., Delaney, H. D., et al. (2009). Community reinforcement and family therapy (CRAFT): An effectiveness study. *Journal of Behavior Analysis in Health, Sports, Fitness and Medicine, 2*(1), 80–90.

Edwards, G. (1986). The alcohol dependence syndrome: A concept as stimulus to enquiry. *British Journal of Addiction, 81*, 171–183.

Edwards, G., & Gross, M. M. (1976). Alcohol dependence: Provisional description of a clinical syndrome. *British Medical Journal, 1*, 1058–1061.

Edwards, G., Orford, J., Egert, S., Guthrie, S., Hawker, A., Hensman, C., et al. (1977). Alcoholism: A controlled trial of "treatment" and "advice." *Journal of Studies on Alcohol, 38*, 1004–1031.

Edwards, P., Harvey, C., & Whitehead, P. C. (1973). Wives of alcoholics: A critical review and analysis. *Quarterly Journal of Studies on Alcohol, 34*(1, Pt. A), 112–132.

Ellis, A., & Velten, E. (1992). *Rational steps to quitting alcohol: When AA doesn't work for you.* New York: Barricade Books.

Emmons, R. A. (2003). *The psychology of ultimate concerns: Motivation and spirituality in personality.* New York: Guilford Press.

Emrick, C. D., Tonigan, J. S., Montgomery, H., & Little, L. (1993). Alcoholics Anonymous: What is currently known? In B. S. McCrady & W. R. Miller (Eds.), *Research on Alcoholics Anonymous: Opportunities and alternatives* (pp. 41–76). New Brunswick, NJ: Rutgers Center of Alcohol Studies.

Ends, E. J., & Page, C. W. (1957). A study of three types of group psychotherapy with hospitalized inebriates. *Quarterly Journal of Studies on Alcohol, 18*, 263–277.

Eng, M. Y., Schuckit, M. A., & Smith, T. L. (2005). The level of response to alcohol in daughters of alcoholics and controls. *Drug and Alcohol Dependence, 79*, 83–93.

Ennett, S. T., Tobler, N. S., Ringwalt, C. L., & Flewelling, R. L. (1994). How effective is drug abuse resistance education?: A meta-analysis of Project DARE outcome evaluations. *American Journal of Public Health, 84*, 1394–1401.

Ernst, D., MIller, W. R., & Rollnick, S. (2007, October–December). Treating substance abuse in primary care: A demonstration project. *International Journal of Integrated Care*, (7).

Ewing, J. A. (1984). Detecting alcoholism: The CAGE questionnaire. *Journal of the American Medical Association, 252*, 1905–1907.

Falk, D. E., Yi, H., & Hiller-Sturmhöfel, S. (2006). An epidemiologic analysis of co-occurring alcohol and tobacco use disorders: Findings from the National Epidemiologic Survey on alcohol and related conditions. *Alcohol Health and Research World, 29*, 162–171.

Fals-Stewart, W., & Kennedy, C. (2005). Addressing intimate partner violence in substance-abuse treatment. *Journal of Substance Abuse Treatment, 29*(1), 5–17.

Fals-Stewart, W., & Lam, W. K. K. (2008). Brief behavioral couples therapy for drug abuse: A randomized clinical trial examining clinical efficacy and cost-effectiveness. *Families, Systems, and Health, 26*(4), 377–392.

Fals-Stewart, W., & O'Farrell, T. J. (2003). Behavioral family counseling and naltrexone for male opioid-dependent patients. *Journal of Consulting and Clinical Psychology, 71*(3), 432–442.

Fals-Stewart, W., O'Farrell, T. J., & Birchler, G. R. (1997). Behavioral couples therapy for male substance-abusing patients: A cost outcomes analysis. *Journal of Consulting and Clinical Psychology, 65*(5), 789–802.

Faris, A. S., Cavell, T. A., Fishburne, J. W., & Britton, P. C. (2009). Examining motivational interviewing from a client agency perspective. *Journal of Clinical Psychology, 65*, 955–970.

Feighner, J. P., Robins, E., Guze, S. B., Woodruff, R. A., Winokur, G., & Munoz, R. (1972). Diagnostic criteria for use in psychiatric research. *Archives of General Psychiatry, 26*, 57–63.

Feldstein, S. W., & Miller, W. R. (2007). Does subtle screening for substance abuse work?: A review of the Substance Abuse Subtle Screening Inventory (SASSI). *Addiction, 102*, 41–50.

Feldstein Ewing, S. W., Filbey, F. M., Sabbineni, A., & Hutchinson, K. E. (2011). How psychological alcohol interventions work: A preliminary look at what fMRI can tell us. *Alcoholism: Clinical & Experimental Research, 35*(4), 643–651.

Fingarette, H. (1988). *Heavy drinking: The myth of alcoholism as a disease.* Berkeley and Los Angeles: University of California Press.

Finkelstein, N. B., & Mora, J. (2009). *Addressing the specific needs of women* (Vol. 51, Treatment Improvement Protocol Series). Rockville, MD: Center for Substance Abuse Treatment.

Fiorentine, R., Nakashima, J., & Anglin, M. D. (1999). Client engagement in drug treatment. *Journal of Substance Abuse Treatment, 17*(3), 199–206.

First, M. B., Spitzer, R. L., Gibbon, M., & Williams, J. B. W. (1997). *User guide for the Structured Clinical Interview for DSM-IV axis I disorders: Clinician version.* Washington, DC: American Psychiatric Press.

Fleming, M. (2002). Identification and treatment of alcohol use disorders in older adults. In A. M. Gurnack, R. Atkinson, & N. J. Osgood (Eds.), *Treating alcohol and drug abuse in the elderly* (pp. 85–108). New York: Springer.

Fleming, M. F., Lund, M. R., Wilton, G., Landry, M., & Scheets, D. (2008). The Healthy Moms Study: The efficacy of brief alcohol intervention in postpartum women. *Alcoholism: Clinical and Experimental Research, 32*(9), 1600–1606.

Fleming, M. F., & Manwell, L. B. (1999). Brief intervention in primary care settings: A primary treatment method for at-risk, problem, and dependent drinkers. *Alcohol Research and Health, 23*(2), 128–137.

Forcehimes, A. A. (2004). De profundis: Spiritual transformations in Alcoholics Anonymous. *Journal of Clinical Psychology, 60*(5), 503–517.

Forcehimes, A. A., Tonigan, J. S., Miller, W. R., Kenna, G. A., & Baer, J. S. (2007). Psychometrics of the Drinker Inventory of Consequences (DrInC). *Addictive Behaviors, 32*, 1699–1704.

Fortney, J., Booth, B., Zhang, M., Humphrey, J., & Wiseman, E. (1998). Controlling for selection bias in the evaluation of Alcoholics Anonymous as aftercare treatment. *Journal of Studies on Alcohol, 59*, 690–697.

Foster, R. J. (1998). *Celebration of discipline: The path to spiritual growth.* San Francisco: Harper.

Foxcroft, D. R., Lister-Sharp, D., & Lowe, G. (1997). Alcohol misuse prevention for young people: A systematic review reveals methodological concerns and lack of reliable evidence of effectiveness. *Addiction, 92*, 531–537.

Frankl, V. E. (1969). *The will to meaning.* New York: World.

Frisman, L. K., Mueser, K. T., Covell, N. H., Lin, H.-J., Crocker, A., Drake, R. E., et al. (2009). Use of integrated dual disorder treatment via assertive community treatment versus clinical case management for persons with co-occurring disorders and antisocial personality disorder. *Journal of Nervous and Mental Disease, 197*(11), 822–828.

Fromme, K., Stroot, E. A., & Kaplan, D. (1993). Comprehensive effects of alcohol: Development and psychometric assessment of a new expectancy questionnaire. *Psychological Assessment, 51*, 19–26.

Fuller, R. K., & Gordis, E. (2004). Does disulfiram have a role in alcoholism treatment today? *Addiction, 99*, 21–24.

Futterman, S. (1953). Personality trends in wives of alcoholics. *Journal of Psychiatric Social Work, 23*, 37–41.

Galanter, M., Egelko, S., & Edwards, H. (1993). Rational Recovery: Alternative to AA for addiction? *American Journal of Drug and Alcohol Abuse, 19*, 499–510.

Gallup, G. H. Jr. (2002). *The Gallup Poll: Public opinion 2001.* Wilmington, DE: Scholarly Resources.

Gallup, G. H. Jr., & Lindsay, D. M. (1999). *Surverying the religous landscape.* Harrisburg, PA: Morehouse.

Garbutt, J. C. (2009). The state of pharmacotherapy for the treatment of alcohol dependence. *Journal of Substance Abuse Treatment, 36*(1), S15–S23.

Garbutt, J. C., Kranzler, H. R., O'Malley, S. S., Gastfriend, D. R., Pettinati, H.

M., Silverman, B. L., et al. (2005). Efficacy and tolerability of long-acting injectable naltrexone for alcohol dependence. *Journal of the American Medical Association, 293*, 1617–1625.

Garbutt, J. C., West, S. L., Carey, T. S., Lohr, K. N., & Crews, F. T. (1999). Pharmacological treatment of alcohol dependence. *Journal of the American Medical Association, 281*, 1318–1325.

Garcia-Rodriguez, O., Secades-Villa, R., Higgins, S. T., Fernandez-Hermida, J. R., Carballo, J. L., Errasti Perez, J. M., et al. (2009). Effects of voucher-based intervention on abstinence and retention in an outpatient treatment for cocaine addiction: A randomized controlled trial. *Experimental and Clinical Psychopharmacology, 17*(3), 131–138.

Garner, B. R. (2009). Research on the diffusion of evidence-based treatments within substance abuse treatment: A systematic review. *Journal of Substance Abuse Treatment, 36*(4), 376–399.

Garvin, C. D., Reid, W., & Epstein, L. (1976). A task-centered approach. In R. W. Roberts & H. Northen (Eds.), *Theories of social work with groups* (pp. 238–267). New York: Columbia University Press.

Gastfriend, D. (2003). *Addiction treatment matching: Research foundations of the American Society of Addiction Medicine (ASAM) criteria.* Binghamton, NY: Haworth Medical Press.

Gaume, J., Bertholet, N., Faouzi, M., Gmel, G., & Daeppen, J. B. (2010). Counselor motivational interviewing skills and young adult change talk articulation during brief motivational interventions. *Journal of Substance Abuse Treatment, 39*, 272–281.

Gendel, M. H. (2004). Forensic and medical legal issues in addiction psychiatry. *Psychiatric Clinics of North America, 27*, 611–626.

George, W. H., Frone, M. R., Cooper, M. L., Russell, M., Skinner, J. B., & Windle, M. (1995). A revised Alcohol Expectancy Questionnaire: Factor structure confirmation, and invariance in a general population sample. *Journal of Studies on Alcohol, 56*, 177–185.

Glaser, F. B. (1993). Matchless?: Alcoholics Anonymous and the matching hypothesis. In B. S. McCrady & W. R. Miller (Eds.), *Research on Alcoholics Anonymous: Opportunities and alternatives* (pp. 379–395). New Brunswick, NJ: Rutgers Center of Alcohol Studies.

Glasgow, R. E., Whitlock, E. E., Eakin, E. G., & Lichtenstein, E. (2000). A brief smoking cessation intervention for women in low-income planned parenthood clinics. *American Journal of Public Health, 90*, 786–789.

Glynn, L. H., & Moyers, T. B. (2010). Chasing change talk: The clinician's role in evoking client language about change. *Journal of Substance Abuse Treatment, 39*, 65–70.

Godley, S. H., Smith, J. E., Meyers, R. J., & Godley, M. D. (2009). Adolescent Community Reinforcement Approach (A-CRA). In D. W. Springer & A. Rubin (Eds.), *Substance abuse treatment for youth and adults: Clinician's guide to evidence-based practice* (pp. 109–201). Hoboken, NJ: Wiley.

Goldberg, L. R. (1970). Man versus model of man: A rationale plus evidence for a method of improving clinical inferences. *Psychological Bulletin, 73*, 422–432.

Goldman, M. S., Del Boca, F. K., & Darkes, J. (1999). Alcohol expectancy theory:

The application of cognitive neuroscience. In H. T. Blane & K. E. Leonard (Eds.), *Psychological theories of drinking and alcoholism* (2nd ed., pp. 203–246). New York: Guilford Press.

Gollwitzer, P. M. (1999). Implementation intentions: Simple effects of simple plans. *American Psychologist, 54*, 493–503.

Gollwitzer, P. M., & Schaal, B. (1998). Metacognition in action: The importance of implementation intentions. *Personality and Social Psychology Review, 2*, 124–136.

Gordon, T. (1970). *Parent effectiveness training.* New York: Wyden.

Gordon, T., & Edwards, W. S. (1997). *Making the patient your partner: Communication skills for doctors and other caregivers.* New York: Auburn House Paperback.

Gorman, D. M. (2003). Alcohol and drug abuse: The best of practices, the worst of practices: The making of science-based primary prevention programs. *Psychiatric Services, 54*, 1087–1089.

Gorsuch, R. L. (1995). Religious aspects of substance abuse and recovery. *Journal of Social Issues, 51*, 65–83.

Gorsuch, R. L., & Butler, M. C. (1976). Iniial drug abuse: A review of predisposing social psychological factors. *Psychological Bulletin, 83*, 120–137.

Gossop, M., Stewart, D., & Marsden, J. (2007). Attendance at Narcotics Anonymous and Alcoholics Anonymous meetings, frequency of attendance and substance use outcomes after residential treatment for drug dependence: A 5-year follow-up study. *Addiction, 103*, 119–125.

Gottheil, E., Sterling, R. C., & Weinstein, S. P. (1997a). Outreach engagement efforts: Are they worth the effort? *American Journal of Drug and Alcohol Abuse, 23*(1), 61–66.

Gottheil, E., Sterling, R. C., & Weinstein, S. P. (1997b). Pretreatment dropouts: Characteristics and outcomes. *Journal of Addictive Diseases, 16*(2), 1–14.

Gottman, J. M. (1994). *Why marriages succeed or fail.* New York: Simon & Schuster.

Gottman, J. M., Gottman, J. S., & Declaire, J. (2007). *Ten lessons to transform your marriage: America's love lab experts share their strategies for strengthening your relationship.* New York: Three Rivers Press.

Gottman, J. M., & Silver, N. (2000). *The seven principles for making marriage work: A practical guide from the country's foremost relationship expert.* New York: Three Rivers Press.

Graber, R. A., & Miller, W. R. (1988). Abstinence or controlled drinking goals for problem drinkers: A randomized clinical trial. *Psychology of Addictive Behaviors, 2*, 20–33.

Graham, K., Annis, H. M., Brett, P. J., & Venesoen, P. (1996). A controlled field trial of group versus individual cognitive-behavioural training for relapse prevention. *Addiction, 91*(8), 1127–1140.

Grant, B. F., & Dawson, D. A. (1997). Age at onset of alcohol use and its association with DSM-IV alcohol abuse and dependence: Results from the National Longitudinal Alcohol Epidemiologic Survey. *Journal of Substance Abuse, 9*, 103–110.

Grant, B. F., Dawson, D. A., Stinson, F. S., Chou, P. S., Kay, W., & Pickering, R. (2003). The Alcohol Use Disorder and Associated Disabilities Interview

Schedule-IV (AUDADIS-IV): Reliability of alcohol consumption, tobacco use, family history of depression and psychiatric diagnostic modules in a general population sample. *Drug and Alcohol Dependence, 71*, 7–16.

Grant, B. F., Dawson, D. A., Stinson, F. S., Chou, S. P., Dufour, M. C., & Pickering, R. P. (2004). The 12-month prevalence and trends in DSM-IV alcohol abuse and dependence: United States, 1991–1992 and 2001–2002. *Drug and Alcohol Dependence, 74*(3), 223–234.

Grant, B. F., Hasin, D. S., Stinson, F. S., Dawson, D. A., Chou, S. P., Ruan, W. J., et al. (2005). Co-occurrence of 12-month mood and anxiety disorders and personality disorders in the US: Results from the National Epidemiologic Survey on Alcohol and Related Conditions. *Journal of Psychiatric Research, 39*(1), 1–9.

Greenberger, R. S. (1983). Sobering methods: Firms are confronting alcoholic executives with threat of firing, *The Wall Street Journal*, pp. 1, 26.

Greenfield, S. F., Brooks, A. J., Gordon, S. M., Green, C. A., Kropp, F., McHugh, R. K., et al. (2007). Substance abuse treatment entry, retention, and outcome in women: A review of the literature. *Drug and Alcohol Dependence, 86*(1), 1–21.

Griffiths, R. R., Richards, W. A., Johnson, M. W., McCann, U. D., & Jesse, R. (2008). Mystical-type experiences occasioned by psilocybin mediate the attribution of personal meaning and spiritual significance 14 months later. *Journal of Psychopharmacology, 22*, 621–632.

Guenther, M. (1992). *Holy listening: The art of spiritual direction.* Cambridge, MA: Cowley.

Hallfors, D., Cho, H., Sanchez, V., Khatapoush, S., Kim, H. M., & Bauer, D. (2006). Efficacy vs effectiveness trial results of an indicated "model" substance abuse program: Implications for public health. *American Journal of Public Health, 96*, 2254–2259.

Hamilton, E. (1999). *Mythology: Timeless tales of gods and heroes.* New York: Warner Books.

Hamilton, J. A., Kellogg, S., Kileen, T., Petry, N. M., Albright, L., Rosenfeld, R., et al. (2007). *Promoting awareness of motivational incentives (PAMI).* Bethesda, MD: National Institute on Drug Abuse.

Handelsman, L., Cochrane, K. J., Aronson, M. J., & Ness, R. (1987). Two new rating scales for opiate withdrawal. *American Journal of Drug and Alcohol Abuse, 13*(3), 293–308.

Hanson, J., & Emrick, C. D. (1983). Whom are we calling "alcoholic"? *Bulletin of the Society of Psychologists in Addictive Behaviors, 2*, 164–178.

Harris, K. B., & Miller, W. R. (1990). Behavioral self-control training for problem drinkers: Components of efficacy. *Psychology of Addictive Behaviors, 4*, 82–90.

Hart, C., Ksir, C., & Ray, O. (2008). *Drugs, society, and human behavior* (13th ed.). New York: McGraw Hill.

Hasin, D., Hartzenbuehler, M. L., Keyes, K., & Ogburn, E. (2006). Substance use disorders: Diagnostic and Statistical Manual of Mental Disorders, fourth edition (DSM-IV) and International Classification of Diseases, tenth edition (ICD-10). *Addiction, 101*(Suppl. 1), 59–75.

Hasin, D. S., Grant, B., & Endicott, J. (1990). The natural history of alcohol abuse:

Implications for definitions of alcohol use disorders. *The American Journal of Psychiatry, 147*(11), 1537–1541.

Hawkins, J. D., Catalano, R. F., & Miller, J. Y. (1992). Risk and protective factors for alcohol and other drug problems in adolescence and early adulthood: Implications for substance abuse prevention. *Psychological Bulletin, 112*, 64–105.

Hays, J. T., Croghan, I. T., Schroeder, D. R., Ebbert, J. O., & Hurt, R. D. (2011). Varenicline for tobacco dependence treatment in recovering alcohol-dependent smokers: An open-label pilot study. *Journal of Substance Abuse Treatment, 40*(1), 102–107.

Heath, A. C., Bucholz, K. K., Madden, P. A. F., Dinwiddie, S. H., Slutske, W. S., Bierut, L. J., et al. (1997). Genetic and environmental contributions to alcohol dependence risk in a national twin sample: Consistency of findings in women and men. *Psychological Medicine, 27*, 1381–1396.

Heather, N., Honekopp, J., Smailes, D., & UKATT Research Team. (2009). Progressive stage transition does mean getting better: A further test of the transtheoretical model in recovery from alcohol problems. *Addiction, 104*(6), 949–958.

Heather, N., & Robertson, I. (1984). *Controlled drinking.* London: Routledge.

Heffner, J. L., Tran, G. Q., Johnson, C. S., Barrett, S. W., Blom, T. J., Thompson, R. D., et al. (2010). Combining motivational interviewing with compliance enhancement therapy (MI-CET): Development and preliminary evaluation of a new manual-guided psychosocial adjunct to alcohol dependence pharmacotherapy. *Journal of Studies on Alcohol and Drugs, 71*, 61–70.

Henggeler, S. W., Melton, G. B., Brondino, M. J., & Scherer, D. G. (1997). Multisystemic therapy with violent and chronic juvenile offenders and their families: The role of treatment fidelity in successful dissemination. *Journal of Consulting and Clinical Psychology, 65*, 821–833.

Henggeler, S. W., Melton, G. B., & Smith, L. A. (1992). Family preservation using multisystemic therapy: An alternative to incarcerating serious juvenile offenders. *Journal of Consulting and Clinical Psychology, 60*, 953–961.

Henggeler, S. W., Schoenwald, S. K., Letourneau, J. G., & Edwards, D. L. (2002). Transporting efficacious treatments to field settings: The link between supervisory practices and therapist fidelity in MST programs. *Journal of Clinical Child and Adolescent Psychology, 31*, 155–167.

Henggeler, S. W., Schoenwald, S. K., Rowland, M. D., & Cunningham, P. B. (2002). *Serious emotional disturbance in children and adolescents: Multisystemic therapy.* New York: Guilford Press.

Hersen, M., & Turner, S. M. (Eds.). (2003). *Diagnostic interviewing* (3rd ed.). New York: Springer.

Hesse, M., Vanderplasschen, W., Rapp, R., Broekaert, E., & Fridell, M. (2007). Case management for persons with substance use disorders. *Cochrane Database of Systematic Reviews* (4).

Hester, R. K. (2003). Behavioral self-control training. In R. K. Hester & W. R. Miller (Eds.), *Handbook of alcoholism treatment approaches: Effective alternatives* (3rd ed., pp. 152–164). Boston: Allyn & Bacon.

Hester, R. K., & Delaney, H. D. (1997). Behavioral self-control program for Windows: Results of a controlled clinical trial. *Journal of Consulting and Clinical Psychology, 65,* 686–693.

Hester, R. K., Delaney, H. D., Campbell, W., & Handmaker, N. (2009). A web application for moderation training: Initial results of a randomized clinical trial. *Journal of Substance Abuse Treatment, 37,* 266–276.

Hester, R. K., Squires, D. D., & Delaney, H. D. (2005). The drinker's check-up: 12-month outcomes of a controlled clinical trial of a stand-alone software program for problem drinkers. *Journal of Substance Abuse, 28,* 159–169.

Hettema, J., Steele, J., & Miller, W. R. (2005). Motivational interviewing. *Annual Review of Clinical Psychology, 1,* 91–111.

Hibbert, L. J., & Best, D. W. (2011). Assessing recovery and functioning in former problem drinkers at different stages of their recovery journeys. *Drug and Alcohol Review, 30*(1), 12–30.

Higgins, S. T., & Abbott, P. J. (2001). CRA and treatment of cocaine and opioid dependence. In R. J. Meyers & W. R. Miller (Eds.), *A community reinforcement approach for addiction treatment* (pp. 123–146). Cambridge, UK: Cambridge University Press.

Higgins, S. T., Budney, A. J., Bickel, W. K., Foerg, F. E., Donham, R., & Badger, G. J. (1994). Incentives improve treatment retention and cocaine abstinence in ambulatory cocaine-dependent patients. *Archives of General Psychiatry, 51,* 568–576.

Higgins, S. T., Budney, A. J., Bickel, W. K., Foerg, F. E., Ogden, D., & Badger, G. J. (1995). Outpatient behavioral treatment for cocaine dependence: One-year outcome. *Experimental and Clinical Psychopharmacology, 3,* 205–212.

Higgins, S. T., Budney, A. J., Bickel, W. K., Hughes, J. R., Foerg, F., & Badger, G. (1993). Achieving cocaine abstinence with a behavioral approach. *American Journal of Psychiatry, 150,* 763–769.

Higgins, S. T., Delaney, D. D., Budney, A. J., Bickel, W. K., Hughes, J. R., Foerg, F., et al. (1991). A behavioral approach to achieving initial cocaine abstinence. *American Journal of Psychiatry, 148,* 1218–1224.

Higgins, S. T., & Katz, J. L. (Eds.). (1998). *Cocaine abuse: Behavior, pharmacology, and clinical applications.* San Diego: Academic Press.

Higgins, S. T., & Silverman, K. (Eds.). (1999). *Motivating behavior change among illicit-drug abusers: Research on contingency management interventions.* Washington, DC: American Psychological Association.

Higgins, S. T., Wong, C. J., Badger, G. J., Haug Ogden, D. E., & Dantona, R. L. (2000). Contingent reinforcement increases cocaine abstinence during outpatient treatment and one year of follow-up. *Journal of Consulting and Clinical Psychology, 68,* 64–72.

Hill, P. C., & Hood, R. W. Jr. (1999). *Measures of religious behavior.* Birmingham, AL: Religious Education Press.

Hill, P. C., & Pargament, K. I. (2003). Advances in the conceptualization and measurement of religion and spirituality. *American Psychologist, 58,* 64–74.

Hill, P. C., Pargament, K. I., Hood, R. W. Jr., McCullough, M. E., Swyers, J. P., Larson, D. B., et al. (2000). Conceptualizing religion and spirituality: Points of communality, points of departure. *Journal for the Theory of Social Behavior, 30,* 51–77.

Hilton, M. E. (1991). The demographic distribution of drinking problems in 1984. In W. B. Clark & M. E. Hilton (Eds.), *Alcohol in America: Drinking practices and problems* (pp. 87–101). Albany: State University of New York Press.

Hilton, M. E., Maisto, S. A., Conigliaro, J., McNiel, M., Kraemer, K., Kelley, M. E., et al. (2001). Improving alcoholism treatment across the spectrum of services. *Alcoholism—Clinical and Experimental Research, 25*(1), 128–135.

Hingson, R., Heeren, T., Winter, M., & Wechsler, H. (2005). Magnitude of alcohol-related mortality and morbidity among U.S. college students aged 18–24: Changes from 1998 to 2001. *Annual Review of Public Health, 26,* 259–279.

Hoffman, N. G., Halikas, J. A., & Mee-Lee, D. (1987). *The Cleveland admission, discharge and transfer criteria: Model for chemical dependence treatment programs.* Cleveland, OH: Northern Ohio Chemical Dependency Treatment Directors Association.

Hoffman, N. G., Halikas, J. A., Mee-Lee, D., & Weedman, R. (1991). *American Society of Addiction Medicine placement criteria for the treatment of psychoactive substance use disorders.* Washington, DC: American Society of Addiction Medicine.

Holdstock, L., & de Wit, H. (1998). Individual differences in biphasic effects of ethanol. *Alcoholism: Clinical and Experimental Research, 22,* 1903–1911.

Hood, R. W. Jr., Hill, P. C., & Spilka, B. (2009). *The psychology of religion: An empirical approach* (4th ed.). New York: Guilford Press.

Horsfall, J., Cleary, M., & Hunt, G. E. (2010). Acute inpatient units in a comprehensive (integrated) mental health system: A review of the literature. *Issues in Mental Health Nursing, 31*(4), 273–278.

Horsfall, J., Cleary, M., Hunt, G. E., & Walter, G. (2009). Psychosocial treatments for people with co-occurring severe mental illnesses and substance use disorders (dual diagnosis): A review of empirical evidence. *Harvard Review of Psychiatry, 17*(1), 24–34.

Horvath, A. T. (2000). SMART Recovery: Addiction recovery support from a cognitive-behavioral perspective. *Journal of Rational-Emotive and Cognitive Behavior Therapy, 18,* 181–191.

Hughes, J. R., Helzer, J. E., & Lindberg, S. A. (2006). Prevalence of DSM/ICD-defined nicotine dependence. *Drug and Alcohol Dependence, 85,* 91–102.

Hughes, R. (1987). *The fatal shore: The epic of Australia's founding.* New York: Knopf.

Hulse, G. K., & Tait, R. J. (2003). Five-year outcomes of a brief alcohol intervention for adult in-patients with psychiatric disorders. *Addiction, 98,* 1061–1068.

Humphreys, K. (1993). Psychotherapy and the twelve step approach for substance abusers: The limits of integration. *Psychotherapy, 30,* 207–213.

Humphreys, K. (2003). Alcohol and drug abuse: A research-based analysis of the Moderation Management controversy. *Psychiatric Services, 54,* 621–622.

Humphreys, K., & Klaw, E. (2001). Can targeting nondependent problem drinkers and providing Internet-based services expand access to assistance for alcohol problems?: A study of the Moderation Management self-help/mutual aid organization. *Journal of Studies on Alcohol, 62,* 528–532.

Humphreys, K., & Moos, R. (2001). Can encouraging substance abuse patients to participate in self-help groups reduce demand for health care?: A quasi-experimental study. *Alcoholism: Clinical and Experimental Research, 25,* 711–716.

Humphreys, K., Wing, S., McCarty, D., Chappel, J., Gallant, L., Haberle, B., et al. (2004). Self-help organizations for alcohol and drug problems: Toward evidence-based practice and policy. *Journal of Substance Abuse Treatment, 26,* 151–158.

Hunt, G. M., & Azrin, N. H. (1973). A community-reinforcement approach to alcoholism. *Behaviour Research and Therapy, 11,* 91–104.

Hunt, Y. M., Rash, C. L., Burke, R. S., & Parker, J. D. (2010). Smoking cessation in recovery: Comparing 2 different cognitive behavioral treatments. *Addictive Disorders and Their Treatment, 9*(2), 64–74.

Hunter-Reel, D., McCrady, B., & Hildebrandt, T. (2009). Emphasizing interpersonal factors: An extension of the Witkiewitz and Marlatt relapse model. *Addiction, 104*(8), 1281–1290.

Hurcom, C., Copello, A., & Orford, J. (2000). The family and alcohol: Effects of excessive drinking and conceptualizations of spouses over recent decades. *Substance Use and Misuse, 35*(4), 473–502.

Imel, Z. E., Wampold, B. E., & Miller, S. D. (2008). Distinctions without a difference: Direct comparisons of psychotherapies for alcohol use disorders. *Psychology of Addictive Behaviors, 22*(4), 533–543.

Inciardi, J. A., Martin, S. S., & Scarpitti, F. R. (1996). Appropriateness of assertive case management for drug-involved prison releasees. *Journal of Case Management, 3*(4), 145–149.

Ingersoll, K. S., Wagner, C. C., & Gharib, S. (2000). *Motivational groups for community substance abuse programs.* Richmond, VA: Mid-Atlantic Addiction Technology Transfer Center, Center for Substance Abuse Treatment (Mid-ATTC/CSAT).

Institute of Medicine. (1990). *Broadening the base of treatment for alcohol problems.* Washington, DC: National Academy Press.

Institute of Medicine. (1998). *Bridging the gap between practice and research: Forging partnerships with community-based drug and alcohol treatment.* Washington, DC: National Academy Press.

Jackson, J. K. (1954). The adjustment of the family to the crisis of alcoholism. *Quarterly Journal of Studies on Alcohol, 15,* 562–586.

James, W. (1902). *The varieties of religious experience.* New York: Longmans.

Janis, I. L., & Mann, L. (1977). *Decision making: A psychological analysis of conflict, choice, and commitment.* New York: Free Press.

Jellinek, E. M. (1960). *The disease concept of alcoholism.* Highland Park, NJ: Hillhouse Press.

Jennison, K. M. (2004). The short-term effects and unintended long-term consequences of binge drinking in college: A 10-year follow-up study. *American Journal of Drug and Alcohol Abuse, 30,* 659–684.

Jessor, R., & Jessor, S. L. (1977). *Problem behavior and psychosocial development: A longitudinal study of youth.* New York: Academic Press.

Johnson, B. A., Ait-Daoud, N., Bowden, C. L., DiClemente, C. C., Roache, J. D., Lawson, I., et al. (2003). Oral topiramate for treatment of alcohol dependence: A randomized controlled trial. *Lancet, 361,* 1677–1685.

Johnson, B. A., Rosenthal, N., Capece, J. A., Wiegand, F., Mao, L., Beyers, K., et al. (2007). Topiramate for treating alcohol dependence: A randomized controlled trial. *Journal of the American Medical Association, 298*, 1641–1651.

Johnson, E., & Herringer, L. G. (1993). A note on the utilization of common support activities and relapse following substance abuse treatment. *Journal of Psychology, 127*, 73–78.

Johnson, V. E. (1973). *I'll quit tomorrow*. New York: Harper & Row.

Jones, B. T., Corbin, W., & Fromme, K. (2001). A review of expectancy theory and alcohol consumption. *Addiction, 96*, 57–72.

Jones, B. T., & McMahon, J. (1994). Negative alcohol expectancy predicts posttreatment abstinence survivorship: The whether, when, and why of relapse to first drink. *Addiction, 89*, 1653–1665.

Jones, M. C. (1968). Personality correlated and antecedents of drinking patterns in adult males. *Journal of Consulting and Clinical Psychology, 32*, 2–12.

Joslyn, G., Ravindranathan, A., Busch, G., Schuckit, M. A., & White, R. L. (2010). Human variation in alcohol response is influenced by variation in neuronal signaling genes. *Alcoholism: Clinical and Experimental Research, 34*, 800–812.

Julian, R. M., Advokat, C. D., & Comaty, J. E. (2007). *A primer of drug action: A comprehensive guide to the actions, uses, and side effects of psychoactive drugs* (11th ed.). New York: Worth.

Jung, C. G. (1975). Letter to William G. Wilson, 30 January 1961. In G. Adler (Ed.), *Letters of Carl G. Jung* (Vol. 2, pp. 623–625). London: Routledge & Kegan Paul. (Original work published 1961)

Kabat-Zinn, J. (2006). *Mindfulness for beginners* [Audio book]. Louisville, CO: Sounds True.

Kadden, R., Carroll, K., Donovan, D., Cooney, N., Monti, P., Abrams, D., et al. (1992). *Cognitive-behavioral coping skills therapy manual* (Vol. 3). Rockville, MD: National Institute on Alcohol Abuse and Alcoholism.

Kalichman, S. C. (1999). Therapeutic jurisprudence and mandated reporting. In S. C. Kalichman (Ed.), *Mandated reporting of suspected child abuse: Ethics, law, and policy* (2nd ed., pp. 97–104). Washington, DC: American Psychological Association.

Kaminer, Y. (2001). Adolescent substance abuse treatment: Where do we go from here? *Psychiatric Services, 52*(2), 147–149.

Kampman, K. M., Dackis, C., Pettinati, H. M., Lynch, K. G., Sparkman, T., & O'Brien, C. P. (2011). A double-blind, placebo-controlled pilot trial of acamprosate for the treatment of cocaine dependence. *Addictive Behaviors, 36*(3), 217–221.

Kampman, K. M., Pettinati, H. M., Lynch, K. G., Dackis, C., Sparkman, T., Weigley, C., et al. (2004). A pilot trial of topiramate for the treatment of cocaine dependence. *Drug and Alcohol Dependence, 75*, 233–240.

Kampman, K. M., Volpicelli, J. R., McGinnis, D. E., Alterman, A. I., Weinrieb, R. M., D'Angelo, L., et al. (1998). Reliability and validity of the Cocaine Selective Severity Assessment. *Addictive Behaviors, 23*(4), 449–461.

Karno, M. P., & Longabaugh, R. (2003). Patient depressive symptoms and therapist focus on emotional material: A new look at Project MATCH. *Journal of Studies on Alcohol, 64*, 607–615.

Karno, M. P., & Longabaugh, R. (2005). An examination of how therapist directiveness interacts with patient anger and reactance to predict alcohol use. *Journal of Studies on Alcohol, 66*, 825–832.

Kaskutas, L. A. (1994). What do women get out of self-help?: Their reasons for attending Women for Sobriety and Alcoholics Anonymous. *Journal of Substance Abuse Treatment, 11*, 185–195.

Kaskutas, L. A. (1996). Pathways to self-help among Women for Sobriety. *American Journal of Drug and Alcohol Abuse, 22*, 259–280.

Keating, T. (2009a). *Divine therapy and addiction: Centering prayer and the twelve steps*. Brooklyn, NY: Lantern Books.

Keating, T. (2009b). *Intimacy with God: An introduction to centering prayer*. Brooklyn, NY: Crossroad.

Kelly, J. F., & Moos, R. (2003). Dropout from 12-step self-help groups: Prevalence, predictors, and counteracting treatment influences. *Journal of Substance Abuse Treatment, 24*, 241–250.

Kelly, J. F., Stout, R., Zywiak, W., & Schneider, R. (2006). A 3-year study of addiction mutual-help group participation following intensive outpatient treatment. *Alcoholism: Clinical and Experimental Research, 30*, 1381–1392.

Kelly, J. F., Stout, R. L., Magill, M., Tonigan, J. S., & Pagano, M. E. (2011). Spirituality in recovery: A lagged mediational analysis of Alcoholics Anonymous' principal theoretical mechanism of behavior change. *Alcoholism: Clinical and Experimental Research, 35*(3), 454–463.

Kelly, J. F., & Westerhoff, C. M. (2010). Does it matter how we refer to individuals with substance-related conditions?: A randomized study of two commonly used terms. *International Journal of Drug Policy, 21*(3), 202–207.

Kessler, R. C. (1995). The National Comorbidity Survey: Preliminary results and future directions. *International Journal of Methods in Psychiatric Research, 5*, 139–151.

Kessler, R. C., Berglund, P., Demler, O., Jin, R., Merikangus, K. R., & Walters, E. E. (2005). Lifetime prevalence and age-of-onset distributions of DSM-IV disorders in the National Comorbidity Survey replication. *Archives of General Psychiatry, 62*, 593–602.

Kessler, R. C., & Merikangas, K. R. (2004). The National Comorbidity Survey Replication (NCS-R): Background and aims. *International Journal of Methods in Psychiatric Research, 13*(2), 60–68.

Khantzian, E. J., Halliday, K. S., & McAuliffe, W. E. (1990). *Addiction and the vulnerable self: Modified dynamic group therapy for substance abusers*. New York: Guilford Press.

Kiefer, F., Jimenez-Arriero, M. A., Klein, O., Diehl, A., & Rubio, G. (2007). Cloninger's typology and treatment outcome in alcohol-dependent subjects during pharmacotherapy with naltrexone. *Addiction Biology, 13*, 124–129.

Killeen, T., Carter, R. E., Copersino, M. L., Petry, N. M., & Stitzer, M. L. (2007). Effectiveness of motivational incentives in stimulant abusing outpatients with different treatment histories. *American Journal of Drug and Alcohol Abuse, 33*, 129–137.

Kiluk, B. D., Nich, C., Babuscio, T., & Carroll, K. M. (2010). Quality versus quantity: Acquisition of coping skills following computerized cognitive-behavioral therapy for substance use disorders. *Addiction, 105*(12), 2120–2127.

Kirby, M. W., Braucht, G. N., Brown, E., Krane, S., McCann, M., & VanDeMark,

N. (1999). Dyadic case management as a strategy for prevention of homelessness among chronically debilitated men and women with alcohol and drug dependence. *Alcoholism Treatment Quarterly, 17*(1–2), 53–72.

Kirkpatrick, J. (1999). *Turnabout: New help for the woman alcoholic.* Fort Lee, NJ: Barricade Books.

Kishline, A. (1994). *Moderate drinking: The Moderation Management guide for people who want to reduce their drinking.* New York: Crown.

Kishline, A., & Maloy, S. (2007). *Face to face.* New York: Meredith Books.

Klaw, E., Horst, D., & Humphreys, K. (2006). Inquirers, triers, and buyers of an alcohol harm reduction self-help organization. *Addiction Research and Theory, 14*(5), 527–535.

Koenig, H. G., Larson, D. B., & Weaver, A. J. (1998). Research on religion and serious mental illness. *New Directions for Mental Health Services, 80,* 81–85.

Kogan, L. S. (1957). The short-term case in a family agency: Part II. Results of a study. *Social Casework, 38,* 296–302.

Koob, G. F. (2005). The neurobiology of addiction: A hedonic Calvinist view. In W. R. Miller & K. M. Carroll (Eds.), *Rethinking substance abuse: What the science shows, and what we should do about it* (pp. 25–45). New York: Guilford Press.

Kosok, A. (2006). The Moderation Management programme in 2004: What type of drinker seeks controlled drinking? *International Journal of Drug Policy, 17,* 295–303.

Kosten, T., & O'Connor, P. G. (2003). Management of drug and alcohol withdrawal. *New England Journal of Medicine, 348*(18), 1786–1795.

Kouimtsidis, C., Reynolds, M., Drummond, C., Davis, P., & Tarrier, N. (2007). *Cognitive-behavioral therapy in the treatment of addiction: A treatment planner for clinicians.* Chichester, UK: Wiley.

Koumans, A. J. R., & Muller, J. J. (1967). Use of letters to increase motivation for treatment in alcoholics. *Psychological Reports, 16,* 1152.

Koumans, A. J. R., Muller, J. J., & Miller, C. F. (1967). Use of telephone calls to increase motivation for treatment in alcoholics. *Psychological Reports, 21,* 327–328.

Kranzler, H. R., & Van Kirk, J. (2001). Efficacy of naltrexone and acamprosate for alcoholism treatment: A meta-analysis. *Alcoholism: Clinical and Experimental Research, 25,* 1335–1341.

Kristenson, H., Ohlin, H., Hulten-Nosslin, M., Hood, B., & Trell, E. (1983). Identification and intervention of heavy drinking middle aged men: Results and follow-up of 24–60 months on long-term studies with randomized centers. *Alcoholism: Clinical and Experimental Research, 7,* 203–209.

Krystal, J. H., Cramer, J. A., Krol, W. F., Kirk, G. F., Rosenbech, R. A., & Group, f. t. V. A. N. C. S. (2001). Naltrexone in the treatment of alcohol dependence. *New England Journal of Medicine, 345*(24), 1734–1739.

Kurtz, E. (1979). *Not-God: A history of Alcoholics Anonymous.* Center City, MN: Hazelden.

Kurtz, E. (1991). *Not-God: A history of Alcoholics Anonymous* (Expanded ed.). Center City, MN: Hazelden.

Kurtz, E., & Ketcham, K. (1992). *The spirituality of imperfection: Storytelling and the journey to wholeness.* New York: Bantam Books.

Lambert, M. J., Burlingame, G. M., Umphress, V., Hansen, N. B., Vermeersch, D. A., Clouse, G. C., & Yanchar, S. C. (1996). The reliability and validity of the Outcome Questionnaire. *Clinical Psychology and Psychotherapy, 3*, 249–258.

Lambert, M. J., Whipple, J., Smart, D., Vermeersch, D., Nielsen, S., & Hawkins, E. (2001). The effects of providing therapists with feedback on patient progress during psychotherapy: Are outcomes enhanced? *Psychotherapy Research, 11*(1), 49–68.

Lancaster, T., Stead, L., Silagy, C., Sowden, A., & Group, t. C. T. A. R. (2000). Effectiveness of interventions to help people stop smoking: Findings from the Cochrane Library. *British Medical Journal, 321*, 355–358.

Lapham, S., Forman, R., Alexander, M., Illeperuma, A., & Bohn, M. J. (2009). The effects of extended-release naltrexone on holiday drinking in alcohol-dependent patients. *Journal of Substance Abuse Treatment, 36*, 1–6.

Larson, D. B., & Wilson, W. P. (1980). Religious life of alcoholics. *Southern Medical Journal, 73*, 723–727.

Laslett, A. M., Dietze, P., Matthews, S. M., & Clemens, S. (2004). *The Victorian alcohol statistics handbook* (Vol. 6: Alcohol-related mortality). Fitzroy, Victoria, Australia: Turning Point Alcohol and Drug Centre.

Lawental, E. (2000). Ultra rapid opiate detoxification compared to 30-day inpatient detoxification program: A retrospective follow-up study. *Journal of Substance Abuse, 11*(2), 173–181.

Lawrence, E. C., & Sovik-Johnston, A. F. (2010). A competence approach to therapy with families with multiple problems. In D. A. Crenshaw (Ed.), *Reverence in healing: Honoring strengths without trivializing suffering* (pp. 137–149). Lanham, MD: Jason Aronson.

Leake, G. J., & King, A. S. (1977). Effect of counselor expectations on alcoholic recovery. *Alcohol Health and Research World, 11*(3), 16–22.

Lean, G. (1985). *Frank Buchman: A life*. London: Constable & Company.

Lee, J. D., Grossman, E., DiRicco, D., Truncali, A., Hanley, K., Stevens, D., et al. (2010). Extended-release naltrexone for treatment of alcohol dependence in primary care. *Journal of Substance Abuse Treatment, 39*, 14–21.

Leventhal, A. M., & Schmitz, J. M. (2006). The role of drug use outcome expectancies in substance abuse risk: An interactional-transformational model. *Addictive Behaviors, 31*, 2038–2062.

Levy, M. S. (2007). *Take control of your drinking ... and you may not need to quit*. Baltimore: Johns Hopkins University Press.

Lewinsohn, P. M., Muñoz, R. F., Youngren, M. A., & Zeiss, A. M. (1992). *Control your depression* (rev. ed.). New York: Fireside.

Lhuintre, J. P., Moore, N., Tran, G., Steru, L., Langrenon, S., Daoust, S., et al. (1990). Acamprosate appears to decrease alcohol intake in weaned alcoholics. *Alcohol and Alcoholism, 25*, 613–622.

Lichtenstein, E., Zhu, S.-H., & Tedeschi, G. J. (2010). Smoking cessation quitlines: An underrecognized intervention success story. *American Psychologist, 65*(4), 252–261.

Liddle, H. A. (2004). Family-based therapies for adolescent alcohol and drug use: Research contributions and future research needs. *Addiction, 99*(Suppl. 2), 76–92.

Liddle, H. A., Dakof, G. A., Turner, R. M., Henderson, C. E., & Greenbaum, P. E. (2008). Treating adolescent drug abuse: A randomized trial comparing multidimensional family therapy and cognitive behavior therapy. *Addiction, 103*(10), 1660–1670.

Liddle, H. A., Rodriguez, R. A., Dakof, G. A., Kanzki, E., & Marvel, F. A. (2005). Multidimensional family therapy: A science-based treatment for adolescent drug abuse. In J. L. Lebow (Ed.), *Handbook of clinical family therapy* (pp. 128–163). Hoboken, NJ: Wiley.

Liddle, H. A., Rowe, C. L., Dakof, G. A., Henderson, C. E., & Greenbaum, P. E. (2009). Multidimensional family therapy for young adolescent substance abuse: Twelve-month outcomes of a randomized controlled trial. *Journal of Consulting and Clinical Psychology, 77*(1), 12–25.

Lieberman, M. A., Yalom, I. D., & Miles, M. D. (1973). *Encounter groups: First facts.* New York: Basic Books.

Lisansky, E. S. G. (1999). Women. In B. McCrady & E. E. Epstein (Eds.), *Addictions: A comprehensive guidebook* (pp. 527–541). London: Oxford University Press.

Litman, G. K. (1986). Alcoholism survival: The prevention of relapse. In W. R. Miller & N. Heather (Eds.), *Treating addictive behaviors: Processes of change* (pp. 391–405). New York: Plenum Press.

Litt, M. D., Kadden, R. M., Cooney, N. L., & Kabela, E. (2003). Coping skills and treatment outcomes in cognitive-behavioral and interactional group therapy for alcoholism. *Journal of Consulting and Clinical Psychology, 71*(1), 118–128.

Logan, F. A. (1993). Animal learning and motivation and addictive drugs. *Psychological Reports, 73*, 291–306.

Longabaugh, R., Beattie, M., Noel, N., Stout, R., & Malloy, P. (1993). The effect of social investment on treatment outcome. *Journal of Studies on Alcohol, 54*, 465–478.

Longabaugh, R., & Wirtz, P. W. (Eds.). (2001). *Project MATCH hypotheses: Results and causal chain analyses* (Project MATCH Monograph Series, Vol. 8). Bethesda, MD: National Institute on Alcohol Abuse and Alcoholism.

Longabaugh, R., Wirtz, P. W., Zweben, A., & Stout, R. (2001). Network support for drinking. In R. Longabaugh & P. W. Wirtz (Eds.), *Project MATCH hypotheses: Results and causal chain analyses* (pp. 260–275). Bethesda, MD: National Institute on Alcohol Abuse and Alcoholism.

Longabaugh, R., Wirtz, P. W., Zweben, A., & Stout, R. L. (1998). Network support for drinking, Alcoholics Anonymous, and long-term matching effects. *Addiction, 93*, 1313–1333.

Longabaugh, R., Woolard, R. E., Nirenberg, T. D., Minugh, A. P., Becker, B., Clifford, P. R., et al. (2001). Evaluating the effects of a brief motivational intervention for injured drinkers in the emergency department. *Journal of Studies on Alcohol, 62*, 806–816.

Longabaugh, R., Zweben, A., LoCastro, J. S., & Miller, W. R. (2005). Origins, issues and options in the development of the Combined Behavioral Intervention. *Journal of Studies on Alcohol, Supplement No. 15*, 179–187.

Longshore, D., & Teruya, C. (2006). Treatment motivation in drug users: A theory-based analysis. *Drug and Alcohol Dependence, 81*(2), 179–188.

Lowman, C., Allen, J., & Miller, W. R. (1996). Perspectives on precipitants of relapse. *Addiction, 91*(Monograph suppl.).

Luborsky, L., McLellan, A. T., Diguer, L., Woody, G., & Seligman, D. A. (1997). The psychotherapist matters: Comparison of outcomes across twenty-two therapists and seven patient samples. *Clinical Psychology: Science and Practice, 4*, 53–65.

Luborsky, L., McLellan, A. T., Woody, G. E., O'Brien, C. P., & Auerbach, A. (1985). Therapist success and its determinants. *Archives of General Psychiatry, 42*, 602–611.

Luckie, L. F., White, R. F., Miller, W. R., Icenogle, M. V., & Lasoski, M. C. (1995). Prevalence estimates of alcohol problems in a V.A. outpatient population: AUDIT vs. MAST. *Journal of Clinical Psychology, 51*, 422–425.

Lundahl, B., & Burke, B. L. (2009). The effectiveness and applicability of motivational interviewing: A practice-friendly review of four meta-analyses. *Journal of Clinical Psychology, 65*, 1232–1245.

Lyne, J. P., O'Donoghue, B., Clancy, M., & O'Gara, C. (2011). Comorbid psychiatric diagnoses among individuals presenting to an addiction treatment program for alcohol dependence. *Substance Use & Misuse, 46*(4), 351–358.

MacDonough, T. S. (1976). Evaluation of the effectiveness of intensive confrontation in changing the behavior of alcohol and drug abusers. *Behavior Therapy, 7*, 408–409.

Madras, B. K., Compton, W. M., Avula, D., Stegbauer, T., Stein, J. B., & Clark, H. W. (2009). Screening, brief interventions, referral to treatment (SBIRT) for illicit drug and alcohol use at multiple healthcare sites: Comparison at intake and 6 months later. *Drug and Alcohol Dependence, 99*, 280–295.

Madsen, W. (1974). *The American alcoholic: The nature–nurture controversy in alcoholic research and therapy.* Springfield, IL: Thomas.

Madson, M. B., Loignon, A. C., & Lane, C. (2009). Training in motivational interviewing: A systematic review. *Journal of Substance Abuse Treatment, 36*, 101–109.

Magill, M., Barnett, N. P., Apodaca, T. R., Rohsenow, D. J., & Monti, P. M. (2009). The role of marijuana use in brief motivational intervention with young adult drinkers treated in an emergency department. *Journal of Studies on Alcohol and Drugs, 70*, 409–413.

Magill, M., Mastroleo, N. R., Apodaca, T. R., Barnett, N. P., Colby, S. M., & Monti, P. M. (2010). Motivational interviewing with significant other participation: Assessing therapeutic alliance and patient satisfaction and engagement. *Journal of Substance Abuse Treatment, 39*(4), 391–398.

Magura, S. (2008). Effectiveness of dual focus mutual aid for co-occurring substance use and mental health disorders: A review and synthesis of the "double trouble" in recovery evaluation. *Substance Use and Misuse, 43*(12–13), 1904–1926.

Magura, S., Staines, G., Kosanke, N., Rosenblum, A., Foote, J., DeLuca, A., et al. (2003). Predictive validity of the ASAP patient placement criteria for naturalistically matched vs. mismatched alcoholism patients. *American Journal on Addictions, 12*, 386–397.

Maisto, S. A., & McKay, J. R. (1995). Diagnosis. In J. P. Allen & M. Columbus (Eds.), *Assessing alcohol problems: A guide for clinicians and researchers* (pp. 41–54). Rockville, MD: National Institute on Alcohol Abuse and Alcoholism.

Maisto, S. A., O'Farrell, T. J., Connors, G. J., & McKay, J. R. (1988). Alcoholics' attributions of factors affecting their relapse to drinking and reasons for terminating relapse episodes. *Addictive Behaviors, 13*(1), 79–82.

Maltzman, I. (2008). *Alcoholism: Its treatments and mistreatments.* Singapore: World Scientific.

Mann, M. (1950). *Primer on alcoholism.* New York: Rinehart.

Mannuzza, S., Klein, R. G., Truong, N. L., Moulton, J. L., Roizen, E. R., Howell, K. H., et al. (2008). Age of methyphenidate treatment initiation in children with ADHD and later substance abuse: Prospective follow-up into adulthood. *American Journal of Psychiatry, 165,* 604–609.

Manohar, V. (1973). Training volunteers as alcoholism treatment counselors. *Quarterly Journal of Studies on Alcohol, 34,* 869–877.

Manuel, J. K., Austin, J. L., Miller, W. R., McCrady, B. S., Tonigan, J. S., Meyers, R. J., et al. (in press). Community reinforcement and family training: A comparison of group and self-delivery format. *Journal of Substance Abuse Treatment.*

Maremmani, I., Balestri, C., Sbrana, A., & Tagliamonte, A. (2003). Substance (ab)use during methadone and naltrexone treatment: Interest of adequate methadone dosage. *Journal of Maintenance in the Addictions, 2*(1–2), 19–36.

Margolese, H. C., Malchy, L., Negrete, J. C., Tempier, R., & Gill, K. (2004). Drug and alcohol use among patients with schizophrenia and related psychoses: Levels and consequences. *Schizophrenia Research, 67*(2–3), 157–166.

Margolis, R. D., & Zweben, J. E. (1998). *Treating patients with alcohol and other drug problems: An integrated approach.* Washington, DC: American Psychological Association.

Marijuana Treatment Project Research Group. (2004). Brief treatments for cannabis dependence: Findings from a randomized multisite trial. *Journal of Consulting and Clinical Psychology, 72,* 455–466.

Markland, D., Ryan, R. M., Tobin, V., & Rollnick, S. (2005). Motivational interviewing and self-determination theory. *Journal of Social and Clinical Psychology, 24,* 785–805.

Marlatt, G. A. (1996). Taxonomy of high-risk situations for alcohol relapse: Evolution and development of a cognitive-behavioral model. *Addiction, 91*(Suppl.), S37–S49.

Marlatt, G. A., & Donovan, D. M. (Eds.). (2005). *Relapse prevention: Maintenance strategies in the treatment of addictive behaviors* (2nd ed.). New York: Guilford Press.

Marlatt, G. A., & Marques, J. K. (1977). Meditation, self-control, and alcohol use. In R. B. Stuart (Ed.), *Behavioral self-management: Strategies, techniques, and outcome* (pp. 117–153). New York: Brunner/Mazel.

Marques, A. C. P. R., & Formigoni, M. L. c. O. S. (2001). Comparison of individual and group cognitive-behavioral therapy for alcohol and/or drug-dependent patients. *Addiction, 96*(6), 835–846.

Marsden, J., Stillwell, G., Barlow, H., Boys, A., Taylor, C., Hunt, N., et al. (2006). An evaluation of a brief motivational intervention among young ecstasy and cocaine users: No effect on substance and alcohol use outcomes. *Addiction,* *101*(7), 1014–1026.

Martin, C. S., Chung, T., & Langenbucher, J. W. (2008). How should we revise diagnostic criteria for substance use disorders in the DSM-V? *Journal of Abnormal Psychology, 117*(3), 561–575.

Martin, G., Copeland, J., & Swift, W. (2005). The adolescent cannabis check-up: Feasibility of a brief intervention for young cannabis users. *Journal of Substance Abuse Treatment, 29,* 207–213.

Martin, G. W. (1995). The core-shell model: An institutional experiment. The emergence of assessment/referral programs in Ontario: An experiment in changing treatment systems through community development. *Contemporary Drug Problems, 22,* 13–26.

Martin, J. (1980). Too few counselors effective. *U.S. Journal of Drug and Alcohol Dependence, 3*(12), 9.

Martino, S., Ball, S. A., Nich, C., Frankforter, T. C., & Carroll, K. M. (2009). Informal discussions in substance abuse treatment sessions. *Journal of Substance Abuse Treatment, 36,* 366–375.

Martins, R. K., & McNeil, D. W. (2009). Review of motivational interviewing in promoting health behaviors. *Clinical Psychology Review, 29,* 283–293.

Maslow, A. H. (1943). A theory of human motivation. *Psychological Review, 50,* 370–396.

Maslow, A. H. (1970). *Motivation and personality* (2nd ed.). New York: Harper & Row.

Mason, B. J., & Goodman, A. M. (1997). *Brief intervention and medication compliance procedures: Therapist's manual.* New York: Lipha Pharmaceuticals.

Mason, B. J., Goodman, A. M., Chabac, S., & Lehert, P. (2006). Effect of oral acamprosate in patients with alcohol dependence in a double-blind, placebo-controlled trial: The role of patient motivation. *Journal of Psychiatric Research, 40,* 383–393.

Mason, B. J., & Ownby, R. L. (2000). Acamprosate for the treatment of alcohol dependence: A review of double-blind, placebo-controlled trials. *CNS Spectrums, 5*(2), 58–69.

McCrady, B. S. (2006). Family and other close relationships. In W. R. Miller & K. M. Carroll (Eds.), *Rethinking substance abuse: What the science shows, and what we should do about it* (pp. 166–181). New York: Guilford Press.

McCrady, B. S., & Epstein, E. E. (1996). Theoretical bases of family approaches to substance abuse treatment. In F. Rotgers, D. S. Keller, & J. Morgenstern (Eds.), *Treating substance abuse: Theory and technique* (pp. 117–142). New York: Guilford Press.

McCrady, B. S., & Epstein, E. E. (Eds.). (1999). *Addictions: A comprehensive guidebook.* New York: Oxford University Press.

McCrady, B. S., & Epstein, E. E. (2009a). *A cognitive-behavioral treatment program for overcoming alcohol problems: Therapist guide.* Oxford, UK: Oxford University Press.

McCrady, B. S., & Epstein, E. E. (2009b). *Overcoming alcohol problems: A couples-focused program workbook.* New York: Oxford University Press.

McCrady, B. S., Epstein, E. E., Cook, S., Jensen, N., & Hildebrandt, T. (2009). A randomized trial of individual and couple behavioral alcohol treatment for women. *Journal of Consulting and Clinical Psychology, 77*(2), 243–256.

McCrady, B. S., Epstein, E. E., & Kahler, C. W. (2004). Alcoholics Anonymous and relapse prevention as maintenance strategies after conjoint behavioral alcohol treatment for men: 18-month outcomes. *Journal of Consulting and Clinical Psychology, 72*, 870–878.

McCrady, B. S., & Miller, W. R. (Eds.). (1993). *Research on Alcoholics Anonymous: Opportunities and alternatives.* New Brunswick, NJ: Rutgers Center of Alcohol Studies.

McDonald, H. P., Garg, A. X., & Haynes, R. B. (2002). Interventions to enhance patient adherence to medication prescriptions. *Journal of the American Medical Association, 288*(22), 2868–2879.

McGovern, M. P., Clark, R. E., & Samnaliev, M. (2007). Co-occurring psychiatric and substance use disorders: A multistate feasibility study of the quadrant model. *Psychiatric Services, 58*(7), 949–954.

McHugh, F., Lindsay, G. M., Hanlon, P., Hutton, I., Brown, M. R., Morrison, C., et al. (2001). Nurse led shared care for patients on the waiting list for coronary artery bypass surgery: A randomised controlled trial. *Heart, 86*(3), 317–323.

McKay, J. R., Alterman, A. I., McLellan, A. T., & Snider, E. C. (1994). Treatment goals, continuity of care, and outcome in a day hospital substance abuse rehabilitation program. *American Journal of Psychiatry, 151*, 254–259.

McKay, J. R., Cacciola, J. S., McLellan, A. T., Alterman, A. I., & Wirtz, P. W. (1997). An initial evaluation of the psychosocial dimensions of the American Society of Addiction Medicine criteria for inpatient versus outpatient substance abuse rehabilitation. *Journal of Studies on Alcohol, 58*, 239–252.

McKay, J. R., McLellan, A. T., & Alterman, A. I. (1992). An evaluation of the Cleveland criteria for inpatient substance abuse treatment. *American Journal of Psychiatry, 149*, 1212–1218.

McKee, M. (1999). Alcohol in Russia. *Alcohol and Alcoholism, 34*, 824–829.

McKellar, J., Stewart, E., & Humphreys, K. (2003). Alcoholics Anonymous involvement and positive alcohol-related outcomes: Cause, consequence, or just a correlate? A prospective 2-year study of 2,319 alcohol-dependent men. *Journal of Consulting and Clinical Psychology, 71*, 302–308.

McKetin, R., Hickey, K., Devlin, K., & Lawrence, K. (2010). The risk of psychotic symptoms associated with recreational methamphetamine use. *Drug and Alcohol Review, 29*, 358–363.

McLachlan, J. F. C. (1972). Benefit from group therapy as a funciton of patient–therapists match on conceptual level. *Psychotherapy: Theory, Research and Practice, 9*, 317–323.

McLellan, A. T. (2006). What we need is a system: Creating a responsive and effective substance abuse treatment system. In W. R. Miller & K. M. Carroll (Eds.), *Rethinking substance abuse: What the science shows, and what we should do about it* (pp. 275–292). New York: Guilford Press.

McLellan, A. T., Grisson, G. R., Zanis, D., Randall, M., Brill, P., & O'Brien, C. P. (1997). Problem–service matching in addiction treatment. *Archives of General Psychiatry, 54*, 730–735.

McLellan, A. T., Hagan, T. A., Levine, M., Gould, F., Meyers, K., Bencivengo, M., et al. (1998). Supplemental social services improve outcomes in public addiction treatment. *Addiction, 93,* 1489–1499.

McLellan, A. T., Hagan, T. A., Levine, M., Meyers, K., Gould, F., Bencivengo, M., et al. (1999). Does clinical case management improve outpatient addiction treatment? *Drug and Alcohol Dependence, 55,* 91–103.

McLellan, A. T., Kushner, H., Metzger, D., & Peters, R. (1992). The fifth edition of the Addiction Severity Index. *Journal of Substance Abuse Treatment, 9*(3), 199–213.

McLellan, A. T., Lewis, D. C., O'Brien, C. P., & Kleber, H. D. (2000). Drug dependence, a chronic medical illness: Implications for treatment, insurance, and outcomes evaluation. *Journal of the American Medical Association, 284,* 1689–1695.

McLellan, A. T., Luborsky, L., Woody, G. E., O'Brien, C. P., & Druley, K. (1983). Predicting response to alcohol and drug abuse treatments: Role of psychiatric severity. *Archives of General Psychiatry, 40,* 620–625.

McLellan, A. T., McKay, J. R., Forman, R., Cacciola, J., & Kemp, J. (2010). Reconsidering the evaluation of addiction treatment: From retrospective follow-up to concurrent recovery monitoring. *Addiction, 100,* 447–458.

McLellan, A. T., Parikh, G., Bragg, A., Cacciola, J., Fureman, B., & Incmikofki, R. (1990). *Addiction Severity Index administration manual.* Philadelphia: Penn-VA Center for Studies of Addiction.

McLellan, A. T., Woody, G. E., Luborsky, L., & Goehl, L. (1988). Is the counselor an "active ingredient" in substance abuse rehabilitation?: An examination of treatment success among four counselors. *Journal of Nervous and Mental Disease, 176,* 423–430.

Merrall, E. L. C., Kariminia, A., Binswanger, I. A., Hobbs, M. S., Farrell, M., Marsden, J., et al. (2010). Meta-analysis of drug-related deaths soon after release from prison. *Addiction, 105*(9), 1545–1554.

Merton, T. (1986). *Spiritual direction and meditation.* Collegeville, MN: Liturgical Press.

Mewton, L., Slade, T., McBride, O., Grove, R., & Teesson, M. (2011). An evaluation of the proposed DSM-5 alcohol use disorder criteria using Australian national data. *Addiction, 106*(5), 941–950.

Meyers, R. J., & Miller, W. R. (Eds.). (2001). *A community reinforcement approach to addiction treatment.* Cambridge, UK: Cambridge University Press.

Meyers, R. J., Miller, W. R., Hill, D. E., & Tonigan, J. S. (1999). Community reinforcement and family training (CRAFT): Engaging unmotivated drug users in treatment. *Journal of Substance Abuse, 10*(3), 1–18.

Meyers, R. J., Miller, W. R., Smith, J. E., & Tonigan, J. S. (2002). A randomized trial of two methods for engaging treatment-refusing drug users through concerned significant others. *Journal of Consulting and Clinical Psychology, 70,* 1182–1185.

Meyers, R. J., & Smith, J. E. (1995). *Clinical guide to alcohol treatment: The community reinforcement approach.* New York: Guilford Press.

Meyers, R. J., & Wolfe, B. L. (2004). *Get your loved one sober: Alternatives to nagging, pleading and threatening.* Center City, MN: Hazelden.

Milam, J. R., & Ketcham, K. (1984). *Under the influence: A guide to the myths and realities of alcoholism.* New York: Bantam.

Miller, N. S., & Kipnis, S. S. (Eds.). (2006). *Detoxification and substance abuse treatment (Treatment Improvement Protocol 45)*. Rockville, MD: Center for Substance Abuse Treatment.

Miller, P. G., & Sønderlund, A. L. (2010). Using the Internet to research hidden populations of illicit drug users: A review. *Addiction, 105*(9), 1557–1567.

Miller, S. D., Duncan, B. L., Brown, J., Sparks, J., & Claud, D. (2003). The Outcome Rating Scale: A preliminary study of the reliability, validity, and feasibility of a brief visual analog measure. *Journal of Brief Therapy, 2*(2), 91–100.

Miller, S. D., Duncan, B. L., Sorrell, R., & Brown, G. S. (2005). The Partners for Change outcome management system. *Journal of Clinical Psychology, 61*(2), 199–208.

Miller, S. D., Duncan, B. L., Brown, J., Sorrell, R., & Chalk, M. B. (2006). Using formal client feedback to improve retention and outcome: Making ongoing real-time assessment feasible. *Journal of Brief Therapy, 5*(1), 5–22.

Miller, W. R. (1976). Alcoholism scales and objective assessment methods: A review. *Psychological Bulletin, 83*, 649–674.

Miller, W. R. (1983). Motivational interviewing with problem drinkers. *Behavioural Psychotherapy, 11*, 147–172.

Miller, W. R. (1985). Motivation for treatment: A review with special emphasis on alcoholism. *Psychological Bulletin, 98*, 84–107.

Miller, W. R. (1996a). *Form 90: A structured assessment interview for drinking and related behaviors* (Vol. 5). Bethesda, MD: National Institute on Alcohol Abuse and Alcoholism.

Miller, W. R. (1996b). What is a relapse?: Fifty ways to leave the wagon. *Addiction, 91*(Suppl.), S15–S27.

Miller, W. R. (1998). Researching the spiritual dimensions of alcohol and other drug problems. *Addiction, 93*, 979–990.

Miller, W. R. (1999a). Diversity training in spiritual and religious issues. In W. R. Miller (Ed.), *Integrating spirituality into treatment: Resources for practitioners* (pp. 253–263). Washington, DC: American Psychological Association.

Miller, W. R. (Ed.). (1999b). *Integrating spirituality into treatment: Resources for practitioners*. Washington, DC: American Psychological Association.

Miller, W. R. (2000). Rediscovering fire: Small interventions, large effects. *Psychology of Addictive Behaviors, 14*, 6–18.

Miller, W. R. (2003). Spirituality, treatment, and recovery. In M. Galanter (Ed.), *Recent developments in alcoholism* (Vol. 16: Research on Alcoholism Treatment, pp. 391–404). New York: Plenum Press.

Miller, W. R. (Ed.). (2004). *Combined behavioral intervention manual: A clinical research guide for therapists treating people with alcohol abuse and dependence* (Vol. 1). Bethesda, MD: National Institute on Alcohol Abuse and Alcoholism.

Miller, W. R. (2008a). The ethics of harm reduction. In C. M. A. Geppert & L. W. Roberts (Eds.), *The book of ethics: Expert guidance for professionals who treat addiction* (pp. 41–53). Center City, MN: Hazelden.

Miller, W. R. (2008b). *Living as if: Your road, your life*. Carson City, NV: The Change Companies.

Miller, W. R., & Baca, L. M. (1983). Two-year follow-up of bibliotherapy and therapist-directed controlled drinking training for problem drinkers. *Behavior Therapy, 14*, 441–448.

Miller, W. R., Benefield, R. G., & Tonigan, J. S. (1993). Enhancing motivation for change in problem drinking: A controlled comparison of two therapist styles. *Journal of Consulting and Clinical Psychology, 61*, 455–461.

Miller, W. R., & Brown, J. M. (1991). Self-regulation as a conceptual basis for the prevention and treatment of addictive behaviours. In N. Heather, W. R. Miller, & J. Greeley (Eds.), *Self-control and the addictive behaviours* (pp. 3–79). Sydney: Maxwell Macmillan Publishing Australia.

Miller, W. R., & Brown, S. A. (1997). Why psychologists should treat alcohol and drug problems. *American Psychologist, 52*, 1269–1272.

Miller, W. R., & C'de Baca, J. (2001). *Quantum change: When epiphanies and sudden insights transform ordinary lives*. New York: Guilford Press.

Miller, W. R., & Caddy, G. R. (1977). Abstinence and controlled drinking in the treatment of problem drinkers. *Journal of Studies on Alcohol, 38*, 986–1003.

Miller, W. R., & Carroll, K. M. (Eds.). (2006). *Rethinking substance abuse: What the science shows and what we should do about it*. New York: Guilford Press.

Miller, W. R., & Cooney, N. L. (1994). Designing studies to investigate client/treatment matching. *Journal of Studies on Alcohol, Supplement No. 12*, 38–45.

Miller, W. R., Forcehimes, A., O'Leary, M., & LaNoue, M. (2008). Spiritual direction in addiction treatment: Two clinical trials. *Journal of Substance Abuse Treatment, 35*, 434–442.

Miller, W. R., Gribskov, C. J., & Mortell, R. L. (1981). Effectiveness of a self-control manual for problem drinkers with and without therapist contact. *International Journal of the Addictions, 16*, 1247–1254.

Miller, W. R., & Heather, N. (Eds.). (1998). *Treating addictive behaviors* (2nd ed.). New York: Plenum Press.

Miller, W. R., Hedrick, K. E., & Taylor, C. A. (1983). Addictive behaviors and life problems before and after behavioral treatment of problem drinkers. *Addictive Behaviors, 8*(4), 403–412.

Miller, W. R., & Hester, R. K. (1986). Inpatient alcoholism treatment: Who benefits? *American Psychologist, 41*, 794–805.

Miller, W. R., & Hester, R. K. (1986). Matching problem drinkers with optimal treatments. In W. R. Miller & N. Heather (Eds.), *Treating addictive behaviors: Processes of change* (pp. 175–203). New York: Plenum Press.

Miller, W. R., & Johnson, W. R. (2008). A natural language screening measure for motivation to change. *Addictive Behaviors, 33*, 1177–1182.

Miller, W. R., & Kurtz, E. (1994). Models of alcoholism used in treatment: Contrasting A.A. and other perspectives with which it is often confused. *Journal of Studies on Alcohol, 55*, 159–166.

Miller, W. R., Leckman, A. L., Delaney, H. D., & Tinkcom, M. (1992). Long-term follow-up of behavioral self-control training. *Journal of Studies on Alcohol, 53*, 249–261.

Miller, W. R., & Mee-Lee, D. (2010a). *Self-management: A guide to your feelings, motivation, and positive mental health.* Carson City, NV: The Change Companies.

Miller, W. R., & Mee-Lee, D. (2010b). *Facilitator guide for self-management: A guide to your feelings, motivations, and positive mental health.* Carson City, NV: The Change Companies.

Miller, W. R., Meyers, R. J., & Hiller-Sturmhofel, S. (1999). The community-reinforcement approach. *Alcohol Research and Health, 23*(2), 116–121.

Miller, W. R., Meyers, R. J., & Tonigan, J. S. (1999). Engaging the unmotivated in treatment for alcohol problems: A comparison of three strategies for intervention through family members. *Journal of Consulting and Clinical Psychology, 67*(5), 688–697.

Miller, W. R., Meyers, R. J., Tonigan, J. S., & Grant, K. A. (2001). Community reinforcement and traditional approaches: Findings of a controlled trial. In R. J. Meyers & W. R. Miller (Eds.), *A community reinforcement approach to addiction treatment* (pp. 79–103). Cambridge, UK: Cambridge University Press.

Miller, W. R., & Mount, K. A. (2001). A small study of training in motivational interviewing: Does one workshop change clinician and client behavior? *Behavioural and Cognitive Psychotherapy, 29*, 457–471.

Miller, W. R., Moyers, T. B., Arciniega, L. T., Ernst, D., & Forcehimes, A. (2005). Training, supervision and quality monitoring of the COMBINE study behavioral interventions. *Journal of Studies on Alcohol*(Suppl. 15), 188–195.

Miller, W. R., & Muñoz, R. F. (2005). *Controlling your drinking: Tools to make moderation work for you.* New York: Guilford Press.

Miller, W. R., & Page, A. (1991). Warm turkey: Other routes to abstinence. *Journal of Substance Abuse Treatment, 8*, 227–232.

Miller, W. R., & Pechacek, T. F. (1987). New roads: Assessing and treating psychological dependence. *Journal of Substance Abuse Treatment, 4*, 73–77.

Miller, W. R., & Rollnick, S. (1991). *Motivational interviewing: Preparing people to change addictive behavior.* New York: Guilford Press.

Miller, W. R., & Rollnick, S. (2002). *Motivational interviewing: Preparing people for change* (2nd ed.). New York: Guilford Press.

Miller, W. R., & Rose, G. S. (2009). Toward a theory of motivational interviewing. *American Psychologist, 64*, 527–537.

Miller, W. R., & Sanchez, V. C. (1994). Motivating young adults for treatment and lifestyle change. In G. Howard (Ed.), *Issues in alcohol use and misuse by young adults* (pp. 55–82). Notre Dame, IN: University of Notre Dame Press.

Miller, W. R., Sorensen, J. L., Selzer, J., & Brigham, G. (2006). Disseminating evidence-based practices in substance abuse treatment: A review with suggestions. *Journal of Substance Abuse Treatment, 31*, 25–39.

Miller, W. R., & Sovereign, R. G. (1989). The check-up: A model for early intervention in addictive behaviors. In T. Løberg, W. R. Miller, P. E. Nathan, & G. A. Marlatt (Eds.), *Addictive behaviors: Prevention and early intervention* (pp. 219–231). Amsterdam: Swets & Zeitlinger.

Miller, W. R., Sovereign, R. G., & Krege, B. (1988). Motivational interviewing with problem drinkers: II. The Drinker's Check-up as a preventive intervention. *Behavioural Psychotherapy, 16*, 251–268.

Miller, W. R., & Taylor, C. A. (1980). Relative effectiveness of bibliotherapy, individual and group self-control training in the treatment of problem drinkers. *Addictive Behaviors, 5*, 13–24.

Miller, W. R., Taylor, C. A., & West, J. C. (1980). Focused versus broad spectrum behavior therapy for problem drinkers. *Journal of Consulting and Clinical Psychology, 48*, 590–601.

Miller, W. R., & Thoresen, C. E. (1999). Spirituality and health. In *Integrating spirituality into treatment: Resources for practitioners* (pp. 3–18). Washington, DC: American Psychological Association.

Miller, W. R., & Thoresen, C. E. (2003). Spirituality, religion, and health: An emerging research field. *American Psychologist, 58*, 24–35.

Miller, W. R., & Tonigan, J. S. (1996). Assessing drinkers' motivation for change: The Stages of Change Readiness and Treatment Eagerness Scale (SOCRATES). *Psychology of Addictive Behaviors, 10*(2), 81–89.

Miller, W. R., Tonigan, J. S., & Longabaugh, R. (1995). *The Drinker Inventory of Consequences (DrInC): An instrument for assessing adverse consequences of alcohol abuse* (Vol. 4). Bethesda, MD: National Institute on Alcohol Abuse and Alcoholism.

Miller, W. R., Villanueva, M., Tonigan, J. S., & Cuzmar, I. (2007). Are special treatments needed for special populations? *Alcoholism Treatment Quarterly, 25*(4), 63–78.

Miller, W. R., Walters, S. T., & Bennett, M. E. (2001). How effective is alcoholism treatment in the United States? *Journal of Studies on Alcohol, 62*, 211–220.

Miller, W. R., & Weisner, C. (Eds.). (2002). *Changing substance abuse through health and social systems.* New York: Kluwer/Plenum.

Miller, W. R., Westerberg, V. S., Harris, R. J., & Tonigan, J. S. (1996). What predicts relapse? Prospective testing of antecedent models. *Addiction, 91*(Suppl.), S155–S171.

Miller, W. R., Westerberg, V. S., & Waldron, H. B. (2003). Evaluating alcohol problems in adults and adolescents. In R. K. Hester & W. R. Miller (Eds.), *Handbook of alcoholism treatment approaches: Effective alternatives* (3rd ed., pp. 78–112). Boston: Allyn & Bacon.

Miller, W. R., & Wilbourne, P. L. (2002). Mesa Grande: A methodological analysis of clinical trials of treatment for alcohol use disorders. *Addiction, 97*(3), 265–277.

Miller, W. R., Wilbourne, P. L., & Hettema, J. (2003). What works?: A summary of alcohol treatment outcome research. In R. K. Hester & W. R. Miller (Eds.), *Handbook of alcoholism treatment approaches: Effective alternatives* (3rd ed., pp. 13–63). Boston: Allyn & Bacon.

Miller, W. R., Yahne, C. E., Moyers, T. B., Martinez, J., & Pirritano, M. (2004). A randomized trial of methods to help clinicians learn motivational interviewing. *Journal of Consulting and Clinical Psychology, 72*, 1050–1062.

Miller, W. R., Yahne, C. E., & Tonigan, J. S. (2003). Motivational interviewing in drug abuse services: A randomized trial. *Journal of Consulting and Clinical Psychology, 71*, 754–763.

Miller, W. R., Zweben, A., DiClemente, C. C., & Rychtarik, R. C. (1992). *Motivational Enhancement Therapy manual: A clinical research guide for therapists treating individuals with alcohol abuse and dependence* (Project MATCH

Monograph Series, Vol. 2). Rockville, MD: National Institute on Alcohol Abuse and Alcoholism.

Miller, W. R., Zweben, J. E., & Johnson, W. (2005). Evidence-based treatment: Why, what, where, when, and how? *Journal of Substance Abuse Treatment, 29,* 267–276.

Milmoe, S., Rosenthal, R., Blane, H. T., Chafetz, M. E., & Wolf, I. (1967). The doctor's voice: Postdictor of successful referral of alcoholic patients. *Journal of Abnormal Psychology, 72,* 78–84.

Miranda, R., Meyerson, L. A., Myers, R. R., & Lovallo, W. R. (2003). Altered affective modulation of the startle reflex in alcoholics with antisocial personality disorder. *Alcoholism: Clinical and Experimental Research, 27,* 1901–1911.

Mitcheson, L., Bhavsar, K., & McCambridge, J. (2009). Randomized trial of training and supervision in motivational interviewing with adolescent drug treatment providers. *Journal of Substance Abuse Treatment, 37,* 73–78.

Montgomery, H. A., Miller, W. R., & Tonigan, J. S. (1993). Differences among AA groups: Implications for research. *Journal of Studies on Alcohol, 54,* 502–504.

Montgomery, H. A., Miller, W. R., & Tonigan, J. S. (1995). Does Alcoholics Anonymous involvement predict treatment outcome? *Journal of Substance Abuse Treatment, 12,* 241–246.

Monti, P. M., Abrams, D. B., Kadden, R. M., & Cooney, N. L. (1989). *Treating alcohol dependence: A coping skills training guide.* New York: Guilford Press.

Monti, P. M., Colby, S. M., Barnett, N. P., Spirito, A., Rohsenow, D. J., Myers, M., et al. (1999). Brief intervention for harm reduction with alcohol-positive older adolescents in a hospital emergency department. *Journal of Consulting and Clinical Psychology, 67(6),* 989–994.

Monti, P. M., Colby, S. M., & O'Leary, T. A. (2001). *Adolescents, alcohol, and substance abuse: Reaching teens through brief interventions.* New York: Guilford Press.

Monti, P. M., Kadden, R. M., Rohsenow, D. J., Cooney, N. L., & Abrams, D. B. (2002). *Treating alcohol dependence: A coping skills training guide* (2nd ed.). New York: Guilford Press.

Moore, T. (1994). *Care of the soul: A guide for cultivating depth and sacredness in everyday life.* New York: HarperCollins.

Moos, R. (1993). *Coping Responses Inventory (CRI): Adult form manual.* Odessa, FL: Psychological Assessment Resources.

Moos, R., Finney, J. W., & Maude-Griffin, P. (1993). The social climate of self-help and mutual support groups: Assessing group implementation, process, and outcome. In B. S. McCrady & W. R. Miller (Eds.), *Research on Alcoholics Anonymous: Opportunities and alternatives* (pp. 251–274). Piscataway, NJ: Rutgers University, Center of Studies on Alcohol.

Moos, R. H., Finney, J. W., & Cronkite, R. C. (1990). *Alcoholism treatment: Context, process, and outcome.* New York: Oxford University Press.

Moos, R. H., & Moos, B. S. (2005). Paths of entry into Alcoholics Anonymous: Consequences for participation and remission. *Alcoholism: Clinical and Experimental Research, 29,* 1858–1868.

Moos, R. H., & Moos, B. S. (2006). Participation in treatment and Alcoholics Anonymous: A 16-year follow-up of initially untreated individuals. *Journal of Clinical Psychology, 62*, 735–750.

Morgenstern, J., Blanchard, K. A., Kahler, C., Barbosa, K. M., McCrady, B. S., & McVeigh, K. H. (2008). Testing mechanisms of action for intensive case management. *Addiction, 103*(3), 469–477.

Morgenstern, J., Hogue, A., Dauber, S., Dasaro, C., & McKay, J. R. (2009). A practical clinical trial of coordinated care management to treat substance use disorders among public assistance beneficiaries. *Journal of Consulting and Clinical Psychology, 77*(2), 257–269.

Morgenstern, J., Kahler, C., Frey, R. M., & Lavouvie, E. (1996). Modeling therapeutic response to 12-step treatment: Optimal responders, nonresponders, and partial responders. *Journal of Substance Abuse, 8*, 45–59.

Morgenstern, J., & Longabaugh, R. (2000). Cognitive-behavioral treatment for alcohol dependence: A review of evidence for its hypothesized mechanisms of action. *Addiction, 95*, 1475–1490.

Morini, L. P., & Polettini, A. (2009). Ethyl glucuronide in hair: A sensitive and specific marker of chronic heavy drinking. *Addiction, 104*(6), 915–920.

Moyer, A., Finney, J. W., Swearingen, C. E., & Vergun, P. (2002). Brief interventions for alcohol problems: A meta-analytic review of controlled investigations in treatment-seeking and non-treatment-seeking populations. *Addiction, 97*(3), 279–292.

Moyers, T. B., & Martin, T. (2006). Therapist influence on client language during motivational interviewing sessions. *Journal of Substance Abuse Treatment, 30*, 245–252.

Moyers, T. B., Martin, T., Christopher, P. J., Houck, J. M., Tonigan, J. S., & Amrhein, P. C. (2007). Client language as a mediator of motivational interviewing efficacy: Where is the evidence? *Alcoholism: Clinical and Experimental Research, 31*(Suppl.), 40S–47S.

Moyers, T. B., & Miller, W. R. (1993). Therapists' conceptualizations of alcoholism: Measurement and implications for treatment. *Psychology of Addictive Behaviors, 7*, 238–245.

Moyers, T. B., Miller, W. R., & Hendrickson, S. M. L. (2005). How does motivational interviewing work?: Therapist interpersonal skill predicts client involvement within motivational interviewing sessions. *Journal of Consulting and Clinical Psychology, 73*, 590–598.

Mueller, T. I., Goldenberg, I. M., Gordon, A. L., Keller, M. B., & Warshaw, M. G. (1996). Benzodiazepine use in anxiety disordered patients with and without a history of alcoholism. *Journal of Clinical Psychiatry, 57*(2), 83–89.

Mueser, K. T. (2004). Clinical interventions for severe mental illness and co-occurring substance use disorder. *Acta Neuropsychiatrica, 16*(1), 26–35.

Mueser, K. T., & Drake, R. E. (2007). Comorbidity: What have we learned and where are we going? *Clinical Psychology: Science and Practice, 14*(1), 64–69.

Mueser, K. T., Drake, R. E., Turner, W., & McGovern, M. (2006). Comorbid substance use disorders and psychiatric disorders. In W. R. Miller & K. M. Carroll (Eds.), *Rethinking substance abuse: What the science shows, and what we should do about it* (pp. 115–133). New York: Guilford Press.

Mulligan, D. H. (Ed.). (1995). *The tuberculosis epidemic: Legal and ethical issues for alcohol and other drug abuse treatment providers* (Treatment Improvement Protocol 18). Rockville, MD: Center for Substance Abuse Treatment.

Muñoz, R. F., Le, H.-N., Clarke, G. N., Barrera, A. Z., & Torres, L. D. (2009). Preventing first onset and recurrence of major depressive episodes. In I. H. Gotlib & C. L. Hammen (Eds.), *Handbook of depression* (2nd ed., pp. 533–553). New York: Guilford Press.

Naar-King, S., & Suarez, M. (2011). *Motivational interviewing with adolescents and young adults.* New York: Guilford Press.

Najavits, L. M. (2002). *Seeking safety: A treatment manual for PTSD and substance abuse.* New York: Guilford Press.

Najavits, L. M., Crits-Christoph, P., & Dierberger, A. (2000). Clinicians' impact on the quality of substance use disorder treatment. *Substance Use & Misuse, 35*(12–14), 2161–2190. doi: 10.3109/10826080009148253

Najavits, L. M., & Weiss, R. D. (1994). Variations in therapist effectiveness in the treatment of patients with substance use disorders: An empirical review. *Addiction, 89,* 679–688.

Najavits, L. M., Weiss, R. D., Shaw, S. R., & Muenz, L. (1998). Seeking safety: Outcome of a new cognitive-behavioral psychotherapy for women with posttraumatic stress disorder and substance dependence. *Journal of Traumatic Stress, 11,* 437–456.

National Institute on Alcohol Abuse and Alcoholism. (1996). *How to cut down on your drinking.* Retrieved May 28, 2001, from *pubs.niaaa.nih.gov/publications/handout.htm.*

National Institute on Alcohol Abuse and Alcoholism. (2005). *Helping patients who drink too much: A clinician's guide.* Bethesda, MD: National Institutes of Health.

National Institute on Drug Abuse. (2003). *Preventing drug use among children and adolescents* (2nd ed.). Bethesda, MD: National Institutes of Health.

National Institute on Drug Abuse. (2005). *NIDA junior scientists program: Brain power! Module 3: Neurotransmission.* Bethesda, MD: Author. Available at *www.drugabuse.gov/JSP3/MOD3/Mod3.pdf.*

National Institute on Drug Abuse. (2010). *Screening for drug use in general medical settings.* Bethesda, MD: National Institutes of Health.

Nay, W. N. (2004). *Taking charge of anger: How to resolve conflict, sustain relationships, and express yourself without losing control.* New York: Guilford Press.

Nirenberg, T. D., Sobell, L. C., & Sobell, M. B. (1980). Effective and inexpensive procedures for decreasing client attrition in an outpatient alcohol treatment program. *Journal of Drug and Alcohol Abuse, 7,* 73–82.

Noel, N. E., & McCrady, B. S. (1993). Alcohol-focused spouse involvement with behavioral marital therapy. In T. J. O'Farrell (Ed.), *Treating alcohol problems: Marital and family interventions* (pp. 210–235). New York: Guilford Press.

Noel, P. E. (2006). The impact of therapeutic case management on participation in adolescent substance abuse treatment. *American Journal of Drug and Alcohol Abuse, 32*(3), 311–327.

Norcross, J. C. (Ed.). (2002). *Psychotherapy relationships that work: Therapist contributions and responsiveness to patients.* New York: Oxford University Press.

Nowinski, J. (1999). Self-help groups for addictions. In B. McCrady & B. Epstein (Eds.), *Addictions: A comprehensive guidebook* (pp. 328–346). New York: Oxford University Press.

Nowinski, J., & Baker, S. (1998). *The twelve-step facilitation handbook: A systematic approach to early recovery from alcoholism and addiction.* San Francisco: Jossey Bass.

Nowinski, J., Baker, S., & Carroll, K. M. (1992). *Twelve step facilitation therapy manual: A clinical research guide for therapists treating individuals with alcohol abuse and dependence.* Rockville, MD: National Institute on Alcohol Abuse and Alcoholism.

O'Connell, D. F., & Alexander, C. N. (Eds.). (1994). *Self-recovery: Treating addictions using transcendental meditation and Maharishi Ayur-Veda.* Binghamton, NY: Hayworth Press.

O'Farrell, T. J., & Fals-Stewart, W. (2006). *Behavioral couples therapy for alcoholism and drug abuse.* New York: Guilford Press.

O'Farrell, T. J., Murphy, C. M., Stephan, S. H., Fals-Stewart, W., & Murphy, M. (2004). Partner violence before and after couples-based alcoholism treatment for male alcoholic patients: The role of treatment involvement and abstinence. *Journal of Consulting and Clinical Psychology, 72*(2), 202–217.

O'Farrell, T. J., Murphy, M., Alter, J., & Fals-Stewart, W. (2010). Behavioral family counseling for substance abuse: A treatment development pilot study. *Addictive Behaviors, 35*(1), 1–6.

Oliveto, A., Poling, J., Mancino, M. J., Feldman, Z., Cubells, J. F., Pruzinsky, R., et al. (2010). Randomized, double blind, placebo-controlled trial of disulfiram for the treatment of cocaine dependence in methadone-stabilized patients. *Drug and Alcohol Dependence, 113*(2–3), 184–191.

O'Malley, S. S., & Kosten, T. R. (2006). Pharmacotherapy of addictive disorders. In W. R. Miller & K. M. Carroll (Eds.), *Rethinking substance abuse: What the science shows and what we should do about it* (pp. 240–256). New York: Guilford Press.

O'Malley, S. S., Rounsaville, B. J., Farren, C., Namkoong, K., Wu, R., Robinson, J., et al. (2003). Initial and maintenance naltrexone treatment for alcohol dependence using primary care vs. specialty care: A nested sequence of three randomized trials. *Archives of Internal Medicine, 163*, 1695–1704.

O'Toole, T. P., Polling, R. A., Ford, D., & Bigelow, G. (2006). Physical health as a motivator for substance abuse treatment among medically ill adults: Is it enough to keep them in treatment? *Journal of Substance Abuse Treatment, 31*, 143–150.

Ogle, R. L., & Miller, W. R. (2004). The effects of alcohol intoxication and gender on the social information processing of hostile provocations involving male and female provocateurs. *Journal of Studies on Alcohol, 65*, 54–62.

Oslin, D. W., Lynch, K. G., Pettinati, H. M., Kampman, K. M., Gariti, P., Gelfand, L., et al. (2008). A placebo-controlled randomized clinical trial of naltrexone in the context of different levels of psychosocial intervention. *Alcoholism: Clinical and Experimental Research, 32*, 1299–1308.

Ouimette, P. C., Finney, J. W., & Moos, R. H. (1997). Twelve-step and cognitive-behavioral treatment for substance abuse: A comparison of treatment effectiveness. *Journal of Consulting and Clinical Psychology, 65,* 230–240.

Ouimette, P. C., Gima, K., Moos, R. H., & Finney, J. W. (1999). A comparative evaluation of substance abuse treatment, IV: The effect of comorbid psychiatric diagnoses on amount of treatment, continuing care, and 1-year outcomes. *Alcoholism: Clinical and Experimental Research, 23*(3), 552–557.

Palfai, T. P., Zisserson, R., & Saitz, R. (2011). Using personalized feedback to reduce alcohol use among hazardous drinking college students: The moderating effect of alcohol-related negative consequences. *Addictive Behaviors, 36*(5), 539–542.

Palmateer, N., Kimber, J., Hickman, M., Hutchinson, S., Rhodes, T., & Goldberg, D. (2010). Evidence for the effectiveness of sterile injecting equipment provision in preventing hepatitis C and human immunodeficiency virus transmission among injecting drug users: A review of reviews. *Addiction, 105*(5), 844–859.

Palola, E. G., Jackson, J. K., & Kelleher, D. (1961). Defensiveness in alcoholics: Measures based on the Minnesota Multiphasic Personality Inventory. *Journal of Health and Human Behavior, 2*(3), 185–189.

Panepinto, W. C., & Higgins, M. J. (1969). Keeping alcoholics in treatment: Effective follow-through procedures. *Quarterly Journal of Studies on Alcohol, 30,* 414–419.

Paolino, T. J., McCrady, B. S., & Kogan, K. B. (1978). Alcoholic marriages: A longitudinal empirical assessment of alternative theories. *British Journal of Addiction, 73*(2), 129–138.

Pargament, K. I., Murray-Swank, N., Magyar, G. M., & Ano, G. G. (2005). Spiritual struggle: A phenomenon of interest to psychology and religion. In W. R. Miller & H. D. Delaney (Eds.), *Judeo-Christian perspectives on psychology: Human nature, motivation, and change* (pp. 245–268). Washington, DC: American Psychological Association.

Parsons, J. T., Rosof, E., Punzalan, J. C., & DiMaria, I. (2005). Integration of motivational interviewing and cognitive behavioral therapy to improve HIV medication adherence and reduce substance use among HIV-positive men and women: Results of a pilot project. *AIDS Patient Care and STDs, 19,* 31–39.

Patterson, G. R., & Forgatch, M. S. (1985). Therapist behavior as a determinant for client noncompliance: A paradox for the behavior modifier. *Journal of Consulting and Clinical Psychology, 53,* 846–851.

Peele, S. (2000). What addiction is and is not: The impact of mistaken notions of addiction. *Addiction Research, 8*(6), 599–607.

Pérez-Maña, C., Castells, X., Vidal, X., Casas, M., & Capella, D. (2011). Efficacy of indirect dopamine agonists for psychostimulant dependence: A systematic review and meta-analysis of randomized clinical trials. *Journal of Substance Abuse Treatment, 40*(2), 109–122.

Peteet, J. R. (1993). A closer look at the role of a spiritual approach in the addictions treatment. *Journal of Substance Abuse Treatment, 10,* 263–267.

Peterson, C., & Seligman, M. E. P. (2004). *Character strengths and virtues: A handbook and classification.* New York: Oxford University Press.

Petry, N. M., & Armentano, C. (1999). Prevalence, assessment, and treatment of pathological gambling: A review. *Psychiatric Services, 50*(8), 1021–1027.

Petry, N. M., Martin, B., Cooney, J. L., & Kranzler, H. R. (2000). Give them prizes and they will come: Contingency management for treatment of alcohol dependence. *Journal of Consulting and Clinical Psychology, 68*(2), 250–257.

Petry, N. M., Peirce, J. M., Stitzer, M. L., Blaine, J., Roll, J. M., Cohen, A., et al. (2005). Effect of prize-based incentives on outcomes in stimulant abusers in outpatient psychosocial treatment programs. *Archives of General Psychiatry, 62*, 1148–1156.

Petry, N. M., Weinstock, J., Ledgerwood, D. M., & Morasco, B. (2008). A randomized trial of brief interventions for problem and pathological gamblers. *Journal of Consulting and Clinical Psychology, 76*, 318–328.

Pettinati, H. M., Volpicelli, J. R., Pierce, J. D. J., & O'Brien, C. P. (2000). Improving naltrexone response: An intervention for medical practioners to enhance medication compliance in alcohol dependent patients. *Journal of Addictive Diseases, 19*, 71–83.

Pettinati, H. M., Weiss, R. D., Dundon, W., Miller, W. R., Donovan, D. M., Ernst, D. B., et al. (2005). A structured approach to medical management: A psychosocial intervention to support pharmacotherapy in the treatment of alcohol dependence. *Journal of Studies on Alcohol and Drugs (Suppl. 15), 170–178.*

Pettinati, H. M., Weiss, R. D., Miller, W. R., Donovan, D. M., Ernst, D. B., & Rounsaville, B. J. (2004). *Medical management (MM) treatment manual: A clinical research guide for medically trained clinicians providing pharmacotherapy as part of the treatment for alcohol dependence* (Vol. 2). Bethesda, MD: National Institute on Alcohol Abuse and Alcoholism.

Pollack, K. I., Alexander, S. C., Coffman, C., Tulsky, J. A., Luna, P., Dolor, R. J., et al. (2010). Physician communication techniques and weight loss in adults: Project CHAT. *American Journal of Preventive Medicine, 39*(4), 321–328.

Pope, K. S., & Vasquez, M. J. T. (2007). *Ethics in psychotherapy and counseling: A practical guide* (3rd ed.). San Francisco: Jossey-Bass.

Posternak, M. A., & Mueller, T. I. (2001). Assessing the risks and benefits of benzodiazepines for anxiety disorders in patients with a history of substance abuse or dependence. *American Journal on Addictions, 10*, 48–68.

Powers, M. B., Vedel, E., & Emmelkamp, P. M. G. (2008). Behavioral couples therapy (BCT) for alcohol and drug use disorders: A meta-analysis. *Clinical Psychology Review, 28*(6), 952–962.

Preston, J. D., & Johnson, J. (2009). *Clinical psychopharmacology made ridiculously simple* (6th ed.). Miami, FL: Medmaster.

Prochaska, J. O. (1994). Strong and weak principles for progressing from precontemplation to action on the basis of twelve problem behaviors. *Health Psychology, 13*, 47–51.

Prochaska, J. O., & DiClemente, C. C. (1984). *The transtheoretical approach: Crossing traditional boundaries of therapy.* Homewood, IL: Dow/Jones Irwin.

Prochaska, J. O., & DiClemente, C. C. (1992). Stages of change in the modification of problem behaviors. In M. Hersen, R. M. Eisler, & P. M. Miller (Eds.), *Progress in behavior modification* (pp. 184–212). Sycamore, IL: Sycamore Publishing.

Prochaska, J. O., & Norcross, J. C. (2009). *Systems of psychotherapy: A transtheoretical analysis* (7th ed.). Belmont, CA: Brooks-Cole.

Project MATCH Research Group. (1993). Project MATCH: Rationale and methods for a multisite clinical trial matching patients to alcoholism treatment. *Alcoholism: Clinical and Experimental Research, 17*, 1130–1145.

Project MATCH Research Group. (1997a). Matching alcoholism treatments to client heterogeneity: Project MATCH posttreatment drinking outcomes. *Journal of Studies on Alcohol, 58*, 7–29.

Project MATCH Research Group. (1997b). Project MATCH secondary *a priori* hypotheses. *Addiction, 92*, 1671–1698.

Project MATCH Research Group. (1998a). Matching alcoholism treatment to client heterogeneity: Treatment main effects and matching effects on within-treatment drinking. *Journal of Mental Health, 7*(6), 589–602.

Project MATCH Research Group. (1998b). Matching alcoholism treatments to client heterogeneity: Project MATCH three-year drinking outcomes. *Alcoholism: Clinical and Experimental Research, 22*, 1300–1311.

Project MATCH Research Group. (1998c). Matching alcoholism treatments to client heterogeneity: Treatment main effects and matching effects on drinking during treatment. *Journal of Studies on Alcohol, 59*, 631–639.

Project MATCH Research Group. (1998d). Therapist effects in three treatments for alcohol problems. *Psychotherapy Research, 8*, 455–474.

Prue, D. M., Keane, T. M., Cornell, J. E., & Foy, D. W. (1979). An analysis of distance variables that affect aftercare attendance. *Community Mental Health Journal, 15*, 149–154.

Pruyser, P. W. (1976). *The minister as diagnostician: Personal problems in pastoral perspective*. Philadelphia: Westminster Press.

Rabinowitz, J., Cohen, H., & Atias, S. (2002). Outcomes of naltrexone maintenance following ultra rapid opiate detoxification versus intensive inpatient detoxification. *American Journal on Addictions, 11*(1), 52–56.

Rabinowitz, J., Cohen, H., Tarrasch, R., & Kotler, M. (1997). Compliance to naltrexone treatment after ultra-rapid opiate detoxification: An open label naturalistic study. *Drug and Alcohol Dependence, 47*(2), 77–86.

Rachman, A. W. (1990). Judicious self-disclosure in group analysis. *Group, 14*(3), 132–144.

Randall, J., Henggeler, S. W., Cunningham, P. B., Rowland, M. D., & Swenson, C. C. (2001). Adapting multisystemic therapy to treat adolescent substance abuse more effectively. *Cognitive and Behavioral Practice, 8*(4), 359–366.

Rapp, R. (2002). Strengths-based case management: Enhancing treatment for persons with substance abuse problems. In D. Saleebey (Ed.), *The strengths perspective in social work practice* (3rd ed., pp. 124–142). New York: Allyn & Bacon.

Rapp, R. C., Kelliher, C. W., Fisher, J. H., & Hall, F. J. (1996). Strengths-based case management: A role in addressing denial in substance abuse treatment. In H. A. Siegal & R. C. Rapp (Eds.), *Case management and substance abuse treatment: Practice and experience* (pp. 21–36). New York: Springer.

Rapp, R. C., Otto, A. L., Lane, D. T., Redko, C., McGatha, S., & Carlson, R. G. (2008). Improving linkage with substance abuse treatment using brief case management and motivational interviewing. *Drug and Alcohol Dependence, 94*(1–3), 172–182.

Rawls, J. (1999). *A theory of justice.* Boston: Belknap Press of Harvard University Press. (Original work published 1971)

Regier, D. A., Farmer, M. E., Rae, D. S., Locke, B. Z., Keith, S. J., & Judd, L. L. (1990). Combordity of mental disorders with alcohol and other drug abuse: Results from the Epidemiologic Catchment Area (ECA) Study. *JAMA: Journal of the American Medical Association, 264*, 2511–2518.

Rehm, J., Baliunas, D., Borges, G. L. G., Graham, K., Irving, H., Kehoe, T., et al. (2010). The relation between different dimensions of alcohol consumption and burden of disease: An overview. *Addiction, 105*(5), 817–843.

Richards, S. P., & Bergin, A. E. (1997). *A spiritual strategy for counseling and psychotherapy.* Washington, DC: American Psychological Association.

Ridgely, M. S. (1996). Practical issues in the application of case management to substance abuse treatment. In H. A. Siegal & C. A. Rapp (Eds.), *Case management and substance abuse treatment: Practice and experience* (pp. 1–20). New York: Springer.

Roberts, M. (2001). *Horse sense for people.* Toronto, ON: Knopf of Canada.

Robbins, M. S., Szapocznik, J., & Horigian, V. E. (2009). Brief strategic family therapy™ for adolescents with behavior problems. In J. H. Bray & M. Stanton (Eds.), *The Wiley-Blackwell handbook of family psychology* (pp. 416–430). Malden, MA: Wiley-Blackwell.

Robins, L. N., Cottler, L. B., Bucholz, K. K., Compton, W. M., North, C. S., & Rourke, K. M. (2000). Diagnostic interview schedule for the DSM-IV (DIS-IV). St. Louis, MO: Washington University School of Medicine.

Robins, L. N., & Przybeck, T. R. (1985). Etiology of drug abuse: Implications for prevention. In C. L. Jones & R. J. Battjes (Eds.), *Etiology of drug abuse: Implications for prevention* (pp. 178–192). Rockville, MD: National Institute on Drug Abuse.

Robinson, E. A. R., Cranford, J. A., Webb, J. R., & Brower, K. J. (2007). Six-month changes in spirituality, religiousness, and heavy drinking in a treatment-seeking sample. *Journal of Studies on Alcohol and Drugs, 68*, 282–290.

Rogers, C. R. (1959). A theory of therapy, personality, and interpersonal relationships as developed in the client-centered framework. In S. Koch (Ed.), *Psychology: The study of a science. Vol. 3. Formulations of the person and the social contexts* (pp. 184–256). New York: McGraw-Hill.

Rogers, C. R. (1980). *A way of being.* Boston: Houghton Mifflin.

Rogers, E. M. (1995). *Diffusion of innovations* (4th ed.). New York: Free Press.

Rogers, E. M. (2002). Diffusion of preventive innovations. *Addictive Behaviors, 27*, 989–993.

Rohsenow, D. J. (1983). Drinking habits and expectancies about effects for self versus others. *Journal of Consulting and Clinical Psychology, 51*(5), 752–756.

Rokeach, M. (1973). *The nature of human values.* New York: Free Press.

Rollnick, S. (1998). Readiness, importance, and confidence: Critical conditions of change in treatment. In W. R. Miller & N. Heather (Eds.), *Treating addictive behaviors* (2nd ed., pp. 49–60). New York: Plenum Press.

Rollnick, S., Heather, N., Gold, R., & Hall, W. (1992). Development of a short "readiness to change" questionnaire for use in brief, opportunistic interventions among excessive drinkers. *British Journal of Addiction, 87,* 743–754.

Rollnick, S., Miller, W. R., & Butler, C. C. (2008). *Motivational interviewing in health care: Helping patients change behavior.* New York: Guilford Press.

Room, R., & Greenfield, T. (1993). Alcoholics Anonymous, other 12-step movements, and psychotherapy in the US population, 1990. *Addiction, 88,* 555–562.

Rose, S., & Zweben, A. (2003). Interrelationship of substance abuse and social problems. In W. R. Miller & C. Weisner (Eds.), *Addressing addictions through health and social systems* (pp. 145–156). New York: Plenum Press.

Rose, S., Zweben, A., & Stoffel, V. (1999). Interface between substance abuse treatment and other health and social systems. In B. S. McCrady & E. E. Epstein (Eds.), *Addiction: A comprehensive guidebook for practitioners* (pp. 421–436). New York: Guilford Press.

Rose, S. J., Brondino, M. J., & Barnack, J. L. (2009). Screening for problem substance use in community-based agencies. *Journal of Social Work Practice in the Addictions, 9*(1), 41–54.

Rosenbaum, D. P., & Hanson, G. S. (1998). Assessing the effects of school-based drug education: A six-year multi-level analysis of Project D.A.R.E. *Journal of Research in Crime and Delinquency, 35,* 381–412.

Rosengren, D. B. (2009). *Building motivational interviewing skills: A practitioner workbook.* New York: Guilford Press.

Rothman, J. (2003). An overview of case management. In A. R. Roberts & G. J. Greene (Eds.), *Social worker's desk reference* (pp. 467–480). Washington, DC: National Association of Social Workers.

Rotunda, R. J., West, L., & O'Farrell, T. J. (2004). Enabling behavior in a clinical sample of alcohol-dependent clients and their partners. *Journal of Substance Abuse Treatment, 26*(4), 269–276.

Ruether, R. R. (1998). *Women and redemption: A theological history.* Minneapolis, MN: Augsburg Fortress.

Rukowski, B. A., Gallon, S., Rawson, R. A., Freese, T. E., Bruehl, A., Crevecoeur-MacPhail, D., et al. (2010). Improving client engagement and retention in treatment: The Los Angeles County experience. *Journal of Substance Abuse Treatment, 39,* 78–86.

Russell, M., Martier, S. S., & Sokol, R. J. (1994). Screening for pregnancy risk-drinking: TWEAKING the tests. *Alcoholism: Clinical and Experimental Research, 18,* 1156–1161.

Rychtarik, R. G., Connors, G. J., Dermen, K. H., & Stasiewicz, P. R. (2000). Alcoholics Anonymous and the use of medications to prevent relapse: An anonymous survey of member attitudes. *Journal of Studies on Alcohol, 61,* 134–138.

Sacks, S., & Ries, R. K. (Eds.). (2005). *Substance abuse treatment for persons with co-occurring disorders (Treatment Improvement Protocol 42).* Rockville, MD: Substance Abuse and Mental Health Services Administration.

Safren, S. A., Sprich, S., Perlman, C. A., & Otto, M. W. (2005). *Mastering your adult ADHD: A cognitive-behavioral treatment program client workbook.* New York: Oxford University Press.

Saitz, R. (2005). Unhealthy alcohol use. *New England Journal of Medicine, 352*, 596–607.

Saitz, R., Horton, N. J., Larson, M. J., Winter, M., & Samet, J. H. (2005). Primary medical care and reductions in addiction severity: A prospective cohort study. *Addiction, 100*, 70–78.

Salvendy, J. T. (1999). Ethnocultural considerations in group psychotherapy. *International Journal of Group Psychotherapy, 49*, 429–464.

Samet, J. H., Friedmann, P., & Saitz, R. (2002). Benefits of linking primary medical care and substance abuse services. *Archives of Internal Medicine, 161*, 85–91.

Sanchez-Craig, M. (1980). Random assignment to abstinence or controlled drinking in a cognitive-behavioral program: Short-term effects on drinking behavior. *Addictive Behaviors, 5*, 35–39.

Sanchez-Craig, M. (1996). *A therapist's manual: Secondary prevention of alcohol problems*. Toronto, ON: Addiction Research Foundation.

Sanchez-Craig, M., Davila, R., & Cooper, G. (1996). A self-help approach for high-risk drinking: Effect of an initial assessment. *Journal of Consulting and Clinical Psychology, 64*, 694–700.

Santisteban, D. A., Perez-Vidal, A., Coatsworth, J. D., Kurtines, W. M., Schwartz, S. J., LaPerriere, A., et al. (2003). Efficacy of brief strategic family therapy in modifying Hispanic adolescent behavior problems and substance use. *Journal of Family Psychology, 17*(1), 121–133.

Sartor, C. E., Lynskey, M. T., Heath, A. C., Jacob, T., & True, W. (2007). The role of childhood risk factors in initiation of alcohol use and progression to alcohol dependence. *Addiction, 102*(2), 216–225. doi: 10.1111/j.1360-0443.2006.01661.x

Sass, H., Soyka, M., Mann, K., & Zieglgansberger, W. (1996). Relapse prevention by acamprosate: Results from a placebo-controlled study on alcohol dependence. *Archives of General Psychiatry, 53*, 673–680.

Saunders, B., Wilkinson, C., & Phillips, M. (1995). The impact of a brief motivational intervention with opiate users attending a methadone programme. *Addiction, 90*, 415–424.

Sayers, S. L., Kohn, C. S., & Heavey, C. (1998). Prevention of marital dysfunction: Behavioral approaches and beyond. *Clinical Psychology Review, 18*(6), 713–744.

Schaef, A. W. (1986). *Co-dependence: Misunderstood-mistreated*. San Francisco: Harper & Row.

Schmidt, E. A., Carns, A., & Chandler, C. (2001). Assessing the efficacy of Rational Recovery in the treatment of alcohol/drug dependency. *Alcoholism Treatment Quarterly, 19*, 97–10.

Schomerus, G., Corrigan, P. W., Klauer, T., Kuwert, P., Freyberger, H. J., & Lucht, M. (2011). Self-stigma in alcohol dependence: Consequences for drinking-refusal self-efficacy. *Drug and Alcohol Dependence, 114*(1), 12–17.

Schomerus, G., Lucht, M., Holzinger, A., Matschinger, H., Carta, M. G., & Angermeyer, M. C. (2011). The stigma of alcohol dependence compared with other mental disorders: A review of population studies. *Alcohol & Alcoholism, 46*(2), 105–112.

Schuckit, M. A. (2009). An overview of genetic influences in alcoholism. *Journal of Substance Abuse Treatment, 36*(1), S5–S14.

Schuckit, M. A., Mazzanti, C., Smith, T. L., Ahmed, U., Radel, M., Iwata, N., et al. (1999). Selective genotyping for the role of 5–HT2A, 5–HT2C, and GABAa6 receptors and the serotonin transporter in the level of response to alcohol: A pilot study. *Biological Psychiatry, 45*, 647–651.

Schuckit, M. A., & Smith, T. L. (2010). Onset and course of alcoholism over 25 years in middle class men. *Drug and Alcohol Dependence, 113*(1), 21–28.

Schumm, J. A., O'Farrell, T. J., Murphy, C. M., & Fals-Stewart, W. (2009). Partner violence before and after couples-based alcoholism treatment for female alcoholic patients. *Journal of Consulting and Clinical Psychology, 77*(6), 1136–1146.

Schunk, D. H. (1991). Self-efficacy and academic motivation. *Educational Psychologist, 26*, 207–231.

Schwab, M., Gmel, G., Annaheim, B., Mueller, M., & Schwappach, D. (2010). Leisure time activities that predict initiation, progression and reduction of cannabis use: A prospective, population-based panel survey. *Drug and Alcohol Review, 29*, 378–384.

Scott, C. K., & Dennis, M. L. (2009). Results from two randomized clinical trials evaluating the impact of quarterly recovery management checkups with adult chronic substance users. *Addiction, 104*(6), 959–971.

Secretary of Health and Human Services. (2000). *10th special report to the U.S. Congress on alcohol and health.* Bethesda, MD: National Institute on Alcohol Abuse and Alcoholism.

Selzer, M. L. (1971). The Michigan Alcoholism Screening Test: The quest for a new diagnostic instrument. *American Journal of Psychiatry, 127*, 1653–1658.

Semaan, S., Neumann, M. S., Hutchins, K., D'Anna, L. H., & Kamb, M. L. (2010). Brief counseling for reducing sexual risk and bacterial STIs among drug users—Results from project RESPECT. *Drug and Alcohol Dependence, 106*(1), 7–15.

Sharon, E., Krebs, C., Turner, W., Desai, N., Binus, G., & Penk, W. (2004). Predictive validity of the ASAM patient placement criteria for hospital utilization. *Journal of Addictive Diseases, 22*, 79–93.

Shavelson, L. (2001). *Hooked: Five addicts challenge our misguided rehab system.* New York: Norton.

Shorkey, C. T., & Rosen, W. (1993). Alcohol addiction and codependency. In E. M. Freeman (Ed.), *Substance abuse treatment: A family systems perspective.* (pp. 100–122). Thousand Oaks, CA: Sage.

Siegal, H. A., Fisher, J. H., Kelliher, C. W., Wagner, J. H., O'Brien, W. F., & Cole, P. A. (1996). Enhancing substance abuse treatment with case management. *Journal of Substance Abuse Treatment, 13*, 93–98.

Siegal, H. A., Li, L., & Rapp, R. C. (2002). Case management as a therapeutic enhancement impact on post-treatment criminality. *Journal of Addictive Diseases, 21*, 37–46.

Siegal, H. A., Rapp, R. C., Kelliher, C. W., Fisher, J. H., Wagner, J. H., & Cole, P. A. (1995). The strengths perspective of case management: A promising inpatient substance abuse treatment enhancement. *Journal of Psychoactive Drugs, 27*, 67–72.

Siegal, H. A., Rapp, R. C., Li, L., Saha, P., & Kirk, K. D. (1997). The role of case management in retaining clients in substance abuse treatment: An exploratory analysis. *Journal of Drug Issues, 27*, 821–831.

Simon, S. B., Howe, L. W., & Kirschenbaum, H. (1995). *Values clarification: A practical, action-directed workbook*. New York: Warner Books.

Simoni-Wastila, L. (2004). The use of abusable prescription drugs: The role of gender. *Journal of Women's Health and Gender-Based Medicine, 9*, 289–297.

Simpson, T. L., & Miller, W. R. (2002). Concomitance between childhood sexual and physical abuse and substance use disorders. *Clinical Psychology Review, 22*, 27–77.

Sindelar, J. L., Olmstead, T. A., & Peirce, J. M. (2007). Cost-effectiveness of prize-based contingency management in methadone maintenance treatment programs. *Addiction, 102*, 1463–1471.

Singh, J., & Basu, D. (2010). Ultra-rapid opioid detoxification: Current status and controversies. *Journal of Postgraduate Medicine, 50*(3), 227–232.

Singleton, C. K., & Martin, P. R. (2001). Molecular mechanisms of thiamine utilization. *Current Molecular Medicine, 1*(2), 197–207.

Sisson, R. W., & Azrin, N. H. (1993). Community reinforcement training for families: A method to get alcoholics into treatment. In T. J. O'Farrell (Ed.), *Treating alcohol problems: Marital and family interventions* (pp. 242–258). New York: Guilford Press.

Sisson, R. W., & Mallams, J. H. (1981). The use of systematic encouragement and community access procedures to increase attendance at Alcoholics Anonymous and Al-Anon meetings. *American Journal of Drug and Alcohol Abuse, 8*, 371–376.

Skinner, H. A. (1982). The Drug Abuse Screening Test. *Addictive Behaviors, 7*(4), 363–371.

Skinner, H. A., & Horn, J. L. (1984). *Alcohol Dependence Scale: Users guide*. Toronto, ON: Addiction Research Foundation.

Slavert, J. D., Stein, L. A. R., Klein, J. L., Colby, S. M., Barnett, N. P., & Monti, P. M. (2005). Piloting the family check-up with incarcerated adolescents and their parents. *Psychological Services, 2*, 123–132.

Slesnick, N., Meyers, R. J., Mead, M., & Segelken, D. H. (2000). Bleak and hopeless no more: Engagement of runaway substance abusing youth and their families. *Journal of Substance Abuse Treatment, 19*, 215–222.

Slesnick, N., & Prestopnik, J. L. (2009). Comparison of family therapy outcome with alcohol-abusing, runaway adolescents. *Journal of Marital and Family Therapy, 35*(3), 255–277.

Slesnick, N., Prestopnik, J. L., Meyers, R. J., & Glassman, M. (2007). Treatment outcome for street-living, homeless youth. *Addictive Behaviors, 32*, 1237–1251.

Smelson, D. A., Dixon, L., Craig, T., Remolina, S., Batki, S. L., Niv, N., et al. (2008). Pharmacological treatment of schizophrenia and co-occurring substance use disorders. *CNS Drugs, 22*(11), 903–916.

Smith, J. E., & Meyers, R. J. (2004). *Motivating substance abusers to enter treatment: Working with family members*. New York: Guilford Press.

Smith, J. E., Meyers, R. J., & Delaney, H. D. (1998). The community reinforcement approach with homeless alcohol-dependent individuals. *Journal of Consulting and Clinical Psychology, 66,* 541–548.

Smith, P. C., Schmidt, S. M., Allensworth-Davies, D., & Saitz, R. (2010). A single question screening test for drug use in primary care. *Archives of Internal Medicine, 170*(13), 1155–1160.

Smith, P. F., & Darlington, C. L. (1996). The development of psychosis in epilepsy: A reexamination of the kindling hypothesis. *Behavioural Brain Research, 75*(1–2), 59–66.

Smith, S. S., Jorenby, D. E., Fiore, M. C., Anderson, J. E., Mielke, M. M., Beach, K. E., et al. (2001). Strike while the iron is hot: Can stepped-care treatments resurrect relapsing smokers? *Journal of Consulting and Clinical Psychology, 69,* 429–439.

Sobell, L. C., & Sobell, M. B. (1992). Timeline follow-back: A technique for assessing self-reported alcohol consumption. In R. A. Litten & J. P. Allen (Eds.), *Measuring alcohol consumption: Psychosocial and biological methods.* Totowa, NJ: Humana Press.

Sobell, L. C., & Sobell, M. B. (1996). *Timeline follow back: A calendar method for assessing alcohol and drug use (user's guide)* (pp. 41–72). Toronto, ON: Addiction Research Foundation.

Sobell, L. C., & Sobell, M. B. (2011). *Group therapy for substance use disorders: A motivational cognitive-behavioral approach.* New York: Guilford Press.

Sobell, M. B., & Sobell, L. C. (2000). Stepped care as a heuristic approach to the treatment of alcohol problems. *Journal of Consulting and Clinical Psychology, 68,* 573–579.

Solomon, K. E., & Annis, H. M. (1990). Outcome and efficacy expectancy in the prediction of post-treatment drinking behaviour. *British Journal of Addiction, 85,* 659–665.

Somers, J. M., Goldner, E. M., Waraich, P., & Hsu, L. (2004). Prevalence studies of substance-related disorders: A systematic review of the literature. *Canadian Journal of Psychiatry, 49,* 373–384.

Sournia, J. C. (1990). *A history of alcoholism* [English translation]. Cambridge, MA: Basic Blackwell.

Soyez, V., DeLeon, G., Broekaert, E., & Rosseel, Y. (2006). The impact of a social network intervention on retention in Belgian therapeutic communities: A quasi-experimental study. *Addiction, 101,* 1027–1034.

Spirito, A., Monti, P. M., Barnett, N. P., Colby, S. M., Sindelar, H., Rohsenow, D. J., et al. (2004). A randomized clinical trial of a brief motivational intervention for alcohol-positive adolescents treated in an emergency department. *Journal of Pediatrics, 145*(3), 396–402.

Stahl, S. M. (2009). *Stahl's essential psychopharmacology: The prescriber's guide.* New York: Cambridge University Press.

Steiner, C. M. (1984). *Games alcoholics play.* New York: Ballantine Books.

Stephens, R. S., Roffman, R. A., & Curtin, L. (2000). Comparison of extended versus brief treatments for marijuana use. *Journal of Consulting and Clinical Psychology, 68,* 898–908.

Stevens, S., Arbiter, N., & Glider, P. (1989). Women residents: Expanding their role to increase treatment effectiveness in substance abuse programs. *International Journal of the Addictions, 24*(5), 425–434.

Stinson, F. S., & DeBakey, S. F. (1992). Alcohol-related mortality in the United States: 1979–1988. *British Journal of Addiction, 87,* 777–783.

Stitzer, M. L., Petry, N., Peirce, J., Kirby, K., Killeen, T., Roll, J., et al. (2007). Effectiveness of abstinence-based incentives: Interaction with intake stimulant test results. *Journal of Consulting and Clinical Psychology, 75,* 805–811.

Stitzer, M. L., Petry, N. M., & Peirce, J. (2010). Motivational incentives research in the National Drug Abuse Treatment Clinical Trials Network. *Journal of Substance Abuse Treatment, 38*(Suppl. 1), S61–S69.

Stockwell, T., Sitarthan, T., McGrath, D., & Lang, E. (1994). The measurement of alcohol dependence and impaired control in community samples. *Addiction, 89,* 167–174.

Stout, R. L., Rubin, A., Zwick, W., Zywiak, W., & Bellino, L. (1999). Optimizing the cost-effectiveness of alcohol treatment: A rationale for extended case monitoring. *Addictive Behaviors, 24*(1), 17–35.

Strain, E. C. (2009). *Incorporating alcohol pharmacotherapies into medical practice* (Treatment Improvement Protocol [TIP] Series, Vol. 49). Rockville, MD: Center for Substance Abuse Treatment.

Substance Abuse and Mental Health Services Administration. (1998). *Comprehensive case management for substance abuse treatment. Center for Substance Abuse Treatment: Treatment Improvement Protocol (TIP) Series,* Vol. 27. Rockville, MD: U.S. Department of Health and Human Services.

Substance Abuse and Mental Health Services Administration. (2009). *Results from the 2008 National Survey on Drug Use and Health: National findings.* Rockville, MD: U.S. Department of Health and Human Services.

Sullivan, J. T., Sykora, K., Schneiderman, J., Naranjo, C. A., & Sellers, E. M. (1989). Assessment of alcohol withdrawal: The Revised Clinical Institute Withdrawal Assessment for Alcohol Scale (CIWA-Ar). *British Journal of Addiction, 84,* 1353–1357.

Sullivan, W. P. (2003). Case management with substance-abusing clients. In A. R. Roberts & G. J. Greene (Eds.), *Social worker's desk reference* (pp. 492–496). Washington, DC: National Association of Social Workers.

Sullivan, W. P., Wolk, J., & Hartman, D. (1992). Case management in alcohol and drug treatment: Improving client outcomes. *Families in Society, 73,* 195–203.

Swann, A. C. (2010). The strong relationship between bipolar and substance-use disorder. *Annals of the New York Academy of Sciences, 1187,* 276–293.

Swartz, M. S., Wagner, H. R., Swanson, J. W., Stroup, T. S., McEvoy, J. P., McGee, M., et al. (2006). Substance use and psychosocial functioning in schizophrenia among new enrollees in the NIMH CATIE Study. *Psychiatric Services, 57*(8), 1110–1116.

Swift, J. K., & Callahan, J. L. (2010). A comparison of client preferences for intervention empirical support versus common therapy variables. *Journal of Clinical Psychology, 66*(12), 1217–1231.

Swift, J. K., Callahan, J. L., & Vollmer, B. M. (2011). Preferences. *Journal of Clinical Psychology: In Session, 67*(2), 155–165.

Swift, R. M. (2003). Medications. In R. K. Hester & W. R. Miller (Eds.), *Handbook of alcoholism treatment approaches: Effective alternatives* (3rd ed., pp. 259–281). Boston: Allyn & Bacon.

Szapocznik, J., Hervis, O., & Schwartz, S. (2003). *Brief strategic family therapy for adolescent drug abuse.* Bethesda, MD: National Institute on Drug Abuse.

Szapocznik, J., & Williams, R. A. (2000). Brief strategic family therapy: Twenty-five years of interplay among theory, research, and practice in adolescent behavior problems and drug abuse. *Clinical Child and Family Psychology Review, 3*(2), 117–134.

Talamo, A., Centorrino, F., Tondo, L., Dimitri, A., Hennen, J., & Baldessarini, R. J. (2006). Comorbid substance-use in schizophrenia: Relation to positive and negative symptoms. *Schizophrenia Research, 86*(1–3), 251–255.

Taleff, M. J. (2009). *Advanced ethics for addiction professionals.* New York: Springer.

Tarter, R. E., Kirisci, L., Mezzich, A., Cornelius, J. R., Pajer, K., Vanyukov, M., et al. (2003). Neurobehavioral disinhibition in childhood predicts early age at onset of substance use disorder. *American Journal of Psychiatry, 160*(6), 1078–1085.

Test, M. A. (2003). Guidelines for assertive community treatment teams. In A. R. Roberts & G. J. Greene (Eds.), *Social worker's desk reference* (pp. 511–513). Washington, DC: National Association of Social Workers.

Thomas, E. J., Santa, C., Bronson, D., & Oyserman, D. (1987). Unilateral family therapy with spouses of alcoholics. *Journal of Social Service Research, 10,* 145–163.

Thompson, M. J. (2005). *Soul feast: An invitation to the Christian spiritual life.* Louisville, KY: Westminster John Knox Press.

Thorne, B. (1998). *Person-centered counselling and Christian spirituality: The secular and the holy.* London: Whurr.

Tillich, P. (1973). *Systematic theology* (Vol. 1). Chicago: University of Chicago Press.

Timko, C., Moos, R. H., Finney, J. W., & Lesar, M. D. (2000). Long-term outcomes of alcohol use disorders: Comparing untreated individuals with those in Alcoholics Anonymous and formal treatment. *Journal of Studies on Alcohol, 61,* 529–540.

Tomlin, K. M., & Richardson, H. (2004). *Motivational interviewing and stages of change: Integrating best practices for the substance abuse professional.* Center City, MN: Hazelden.

Tonigan, J. S. (2001). Benefits of Alcoholics Anonymous attendance: Replication of findings between clinical research sites in Project MATCH. *Alcoholism Treatment Quarterly, 19,* 67–66.

Tonigan, J. S. (2003). Spirituality and AA practices three and ten years after Project MATCH. *Alcoholism: Clinical and Experimental Research, 26*(5, Suppl.), 660A.

Tonigan, J. S., Ashcroft, F., & Miller, W. R. (1995). A.A. group dynamics and 12-step activity. *Journal of Studies on Alcohol, 56,* 616–621.

Tonigan, J. S., Connors, G. J., & Miller, W. R. (1996). The Alcoholics Anonymous Involvement Scale (AAI): Reliability and norms. *Psychology of Addictive Behaviors, 10,* 75–80.

Tonigan, J. S., Connors, G. J., & Miller, W. R. (2003). Participation and involvement in Alcoholics Anonymous. In T. F. Babor & F. K. Del Boca (Eds.), *Treat-*

ment matching in alcoholism (pp. 184–204). Cambridge, UK: Cambridge University Press.

Tonigan, J. S., & Kelly, J. F. (2004). Beliefs about AA and the use of medications: A comparison of three groups of AA-exposed alcohol dependent persons. *Alcoholism Treatment Quarterly, 22*, 67–78.

Tonigan, J. S., & Miller, W. R. (2002). The Inventory of Drug Use Consequences (InDUC): Test–retest stability and sensitivity to detect change. *Psychology of Addictive Behaviors, 16*, 165–168.

Tonigan, J. S., Miller, W. R., & Brown, J. M. (1994). The reliability of Form 90: An instrument for assessing alcohol treatment outcome. *Journal of Studies on Alcohol, 58*, 358–364.

Tonigan, J. S., Miller, W. R., & Connors, G. J. (2001). The search for meaning in life as a predictor of alcoholism treatment outcome. In R. Longabaugh & P. W. Wirtz (Eds.), *Project MATCH hypotheses: Results and causal chain analyses* (Vol. 8, pp. 154–165). Bethesda, MD: National Institute on Alcohol Abuse and Alcoholism.

Tonigan, J. S., Miller, W. R., & Schermer, C. (2002). Atheists, agnostics and Alcoholics Anonymous. *Journal of Studies on Alcohol, 63*, 534–541.

Tonigan, J. S., & Rice, S. L. (2010). Is it beneficial to have an Alcoholics Anonymous sponsor? *Psychology of Addictive Behaviors, 24*(3), 397–403.

Tornay, C. B., Favrat, B., Monnat, M., Daeppen, J. B., Schnyder, C., Bertschy, G., et al. (2003). Ultra-rapid opiate detoxification using deep sedation and prior oral buprenorphine preparation: Long-term results. *Drug and Alcohol Dependence, 69*(3), 283–288.

Toumbourou, J. W., Hamilton, M., U'Ren, A., Stevens-Jones, P., & Storey, G. (2002). Narcotics Anonymous participation and changes in substance use and social support. *Journal of Substance Abuse Treatment, 23*, 61–66.

Trimpey, J., Velten, E., & Dain, R. (1993). Rational recovery from addictions. In W. Dryden & L. K. Hill (Eds.), *Innovations in rational-emotive therapy* (pp. 253–271). Thousand Oaks, CA: Sage.

Tross, S., Campbell, A. N. C., Cohen, L. R., Calsyn, D., Pavlicova, M., Miele, G., et al. (2008). Effectiveness of HIV-STD sexual risk reduction groups for women in substance abuse treatment programs: Results of a NIDA Clinical Trials Network trial. *Journal of Acquired Immune Deficiency Syndrome, 48*(5), 581–589.

UKATT Research Team. (2005). Effectiveness of treatment for alcohol problems: Findings of the randomized UK Alcohol Treatment Trial (UKATT). *British Medical Journal, 331*, 541–544.

U.S. Department of Health and Human Services. (1999). *Mental health: A report of the surgeon general.* Washington, DC: U.S. Government Printing Office.

Vaillant, G. E. (1993). *The wisdom of the ego.* Cambridge, MA: Harvard University Press.

Vaillant, G. E. (1995). *The natural history of alcoholism revisited* (Updated ed.). Cambridge, MA: Harvard University Press.

Vaillant, G. E. (1996). A long-term follow-up of male alcohol abuse. *Archives of General Psychiatry, 53*, 243–249.

Valle, S. K. (1981). Interpersonal functioning of alcoholism counselors and treatment outcome. *Journal of Studies on Alcohol, 42*, 783–790.

Van Staden, C. W., & Krüger, C. (2003). Incapacity to give informed consent owing to mental disorder. *Journal of Medical Ethics, 29*, 41–43.

Vanderplasschen, W., Rapp, R. C., Wolf, J. R., & Broekaert, E. (2004). The development and implementation of case management for substance use disorders in North America and Europe. *Psychiatric Services, 55*(8), 913–922.

Vanderplasschen, W., Wolf, J., Rapp, R. C., & Broekaert, E. (2007). Effectiveness of different models of case management for substance-abusing populations. *Journal of Psychoactive Drugs, 39*(1), 81–95.

Velasquez, M., Maurer, G. G., Crouch, C., & Diclemente, C. C. (2001). *Group treatment for substance abuse: A stages-of-change therapy manual.* New York: Guilford Press.

Velicer, W. F., Prochaska, J. O., & Redding, C. A. (2006). Tailored communications for smoking cessation: Past successes and future directions. *Drug and Alcohol Review, 25*(1), 49–57.

Venner, K. L., Feldstein, S. W., & Tafoya, N. (2006). *Adapting helpful treatments for Native Americans: A manual for using motivational interviewing with Native Americans.* Albuquerque: University of New Mexico, Center on Alcoholism, Substance Abuse and Addictions.

Venner, K. L., & Miller, W. R. (2001). Progression of alcohol problems in a Navajo sample. *Journal of Studies on Alcohol, 62*, 158–165.

Villanueva, M., Tonigan, J. S., & Miller, W. R. (2007). Response of Native American clients to three treatment methods for alcohol dependence. *Journal of Ethnicity in Substance Abuse, 6*(2), 41–48.

Viner, R. M., Christie, D., Taylor, V., & Hey, S. (2003). Motivational/solution-focused intervention improves HbA_{1c} in adolescents with Type 1 diabetes: A pilot study. *Diabetic Medicine, 20*(9), 739–742.

Vlasova, N., Schumacher, J. E., Oryschhuk, O., Dumchev, K. V., Slobodyanyuk, P., Moroz, V. M., et al. (2011). STEPS outpatient program improves alcohol treatment outcomes in Ukranian regional narcologic dispensary. *Addictive Disorders and Their Treatment, 10*(1), 6–13.

Voegtlin, W. L., & Lemere, F. (1942). The treatment of alcohol addiction: A review of the literature. *Quarterly Journal of Studies on Alcohol, 2*, 717–803.

Vohs, K. D., & Baumeister, R. F. (2010). *Handbook of self-regulation: Research, theory, and applications* (2nd ed.). New York: Guilford Press.

Volpicelli, J. R., Pettinati, H. M., McLellan, A. T., & O'Brien, C. P. (2001). *Combining medication and psychosocial treatments for addictions: The BRENDA approach.* New York: Guilford Press.

Vuchinich, R. E., & Heather, N. (Eds.). (2003). *Choice, behavioural economics and addiction.* New York: Pergamon.

W., W. (1949). The society of Alcoholics Anonymous. *American Journal of Psychiatry, 106*, 370–375.

Waldron, H. B., Kern-Jones, S., Turner, C. W., Peterson, T. R., & Ozechowski, T. J. (2007). Engaging resistant adolescents in drug abuse treatment. *Journal of Substance Abuse Treatment, 32*, 133–142.

Waldron, H. B., Miller, W. R., & Tonigan, J. S. (2001). Client anger as a predictor of differential response to treatment. In R. Longabaugh & P. W. Wirtz (Eds.), *Project MATCH hypotheses: Results and causal chain analyses* (Vol.

8, pp. 134–148). Bethesda, MD: National Institute on Alcohol Abuse and Alcoholism.

Waldron, H. B., & Turner, C. W. (2008). Evidence-based psychosocial treatments for adolescent substance abuse. *Journal of Clinical Child and Adolescent Psychology, 37*(1), 238–261.

Walitzer, K. S., Dermen, K. H., & Connors, G. J. (1999). Strategies for preparing clients for treatment: A review. *Behavior Modification, 23*(1), 129–151.

Wallace, P., Cutler, S., & Haines, A. (1988). Randomized controlled trial of general practitioner intervention in clients with excessive alcohol consumption. *British Medical Journal, 297,* 663–668.

Walsh, D. C., Hingson, R. W., Merrigan, D. M., Morelock Levenson, S., Cupples, A., Heeren, T., et al. (1991). A randomized trial of treatment options for alcohol-abusing workers. *New England Journal of Medicine, 325,* 775–782.

Walsh, J. (2003). Clinical case management. In A. R. Roberts & G. J. Greene (Eds.), *Social worker's desk reference* (pp. 472–476). Washington, DC: National Association of Social Workers.

Walters, O. S. (1957). The religious background of 50 alcoholics. *Quarterly Journal of Studies on Alcohol, 18,* 405–413.

Walters, S. T., Bennett, M. E., & Miller, J. H. (2000). Reducing alcohol use in college students: A controlled trial of two brief interventions. *Journal of Drug Education, 30,* 361–372.

Walters, S. T., Miller, J. E., & Chiauzzi, E. (2005). Wired for wellness: E-interventions for addressing college drinking. *Journal of Substance Abuse Treatment, 29,* 139–145.

Walters, S. T., Vader, A. M., & Harris, T. R. (2007). A controlled trial of web-based feedback for heavy drinking college students. *Prevention Science, 8*(2), 83–88.

Webb, J. R., & Trautman, R. P. (2010). Forgiveness and alcohol use: Applying a specific spiritual principle to substance abuse problems. *Addictive Disorders and Their Treatment, 9*(1), 8–17.

Wegscheider-Cruse, S. (1990). Co-dependency and dysfunctional family systems. In R. C. Engs (Ed.), *Women: Alcohol and other drugs* (pp. 157–163). Dubuque, IA: Kendall/Hunt.

Weisner, C. (1995). The core-shell model: Implications for treatment assessment and community work. The emergence of assessment/referral programs in Ontario: An experiment in changing treatment systems through community development. *Contemporary Drug Problems, 22,* 151–158.

Weisner, C. (2002). What is the scope of the problem and its impact on health and social systems? In W. R. Miller & C. Weisner (Eds.), *Changing substance abuse through health and social systems* (pp. 3–14). New York: Kluwer Academic/Plenum Press.

Weisner, C., Mertens, J., Parthasarathy, S., Moore, C., & Lu, Y. (2001). Integrating primary medical care with addiction treatment: A randomized controlled trial. *Journal of the American Medical Association, 286,* 1715–1723.

Weiss, B., Caron, A., Ball, S., Tapp, J., Johnson, M., & Weisz, J. R. (2005). Iatrogenic effects of group treatment for antisocial youths. *Journal of Consulting and Clinical Psychology, 73*(6), 1036–1044.

Weiss, R. D. (2004). Adherence to pharmacotherapy in patients with alcohol and opioid dependence. *Addiction, 99*, 1382–1392.

Weiss, R. D., & Connery, H. S. (2011). *Integrated group therapy for bipolar disorder and substance abuse.* New York: Guilford Press.

Weissman, M. M., Markowitz, J. C., & Klerman, G. (2000). *Comprehensive guide to interpersonal psychotherapy.* New York: Basic Books.

Welfel, E. R., Danzinger, P. R., & Santoro, S. (2000). Mandated reporting of abuse/maltreatment of older adults: A primer for counselors. *Journal of Counseling and Development, 78*(3), 284–292.

Wells, E. A., Peterson, P. L., Gainey, R. R., Hawkins, J. D., & Catalano, R. F. (1994). Outpatient treatment for cocaine abuse: A controlled comparison of relapse prevention and twelve-step approaches. *American Journal of Drug and Alcohol Abuse, 20*, 1–17.

Westerberg, V. S., Tonigan, J. S., & Miller, W. R. (1998). Reliability of Form 90D: An instrument for quantifying drug use. *Substance Abuse, 19*, 179–189.

White, W. L. (1998). *Slaying the dragon: The history of addiction treatment and recovery in America.* Bloomington, IL: Chestnut Health Systems.

White, W. L. (2004). Transformational change: A historical review. *Journal of Clinical Psychology, 60*, 461–470.

White, W. L., & Miller, W. R. (2007). The use of confrontation in addiction treatment: History, science, and time for a change. *The Counselor, 8*(4), 12–30.

Whitworth, A., Oberbauer, H., Fleischhacker, W. W., Lesch, O., Walter, H., Nimmerrichter, A., et al. (1996). Comparison of acamprosate and placebo in long-term treatment of alcohol dependence. *The Lancet, 347*, 1438–1442.

WHO ASSIST Working Group. (2002). The Alcohol, Smoking and Substance Involvement Screen Test (ASSIST): Development, reliability and feasibility. *Addiction, 97*, 1183–1194.

Wiggins, J. S. (1973). *Personality and prediction.* Reading, MA: Addison-Wesley.

Wild, T. C., Cunningham, J. A., & Ryan, R. M. (2006). Social pressure, coercion, and client engagement at treatment entry. *Addictive Behaviors, 31*, 1858–1872.

Wilens, T. E., Faraone, S. V., Biederman, J., & Gunawardene, S. (2003). Does stimulant therapy of attention-deficit/hyperactivity disorder beget later substance abuse?: A meta-analytic review of the literature. *Pediatrics, 111*, 179–185.

Willenbring, M. L. (1994). Case management applications in substance use disorders. *Journal of Case Management, 3*(4), 150–157.

Willenbring, M. L. (1996). Case management applications in substance use disorders. In H. A. Siegal & R. C. Rapp (Eds.), *Case management and substance abuse treatment: Practice and experience* (pp. 51–76). New York: Springer.

Willenbring, M. L., & Olson, D. H. (1999). A randomized trial of integrated outpatient treatment for medically ill alcoholic men. *Archives of Internal Medicine, 159*, 1946–1952.

Williams, R., & Vinson, D. C. (2001). Validation of a single screening question for problem drinking. *Journal of Family Practice, 50*, 307–312.

Wilsnack, S. (1973). The needs of the female drinker: Dependency, power or what? In M. E. Chafetz (Ed.), *Proceedings of the Second Annual Alcoholism Conference of the National Institute on Alcohol Abuse and Alcoholism* (pp. 65–83). Washington, DC: U.S. Government Printing Office.

Winhusen, T., Kropp, F., Babcock, D., Hague, D., Erickson, S. J., Renz, C., et al. (2008). Motivational enhancement therapy to improve treatment utilization and outcome in pregnant substance users. *Journal of Substance Abuse Treatment, 35*, 161–173.

Witkiewitz, K., Hartzler, B., & Donovan, D. (2010). Matching motivation enhancement treatment to client motivation: Re-examining the Project MATCH motivation matching hypothesis. *Addiction, 105*, 1403–1413.

Woititz, J. G. (1984). Adult children of alcoholics. *Alcoholism Treatment Quarterly, 1*(1), 71–99.

World Health Organization. (1990). *International classification of diseases and related health problems* (10th ed.). Geneva: Author.

Xie, H., Drake, R. E., McHugo, G. J., Xie, L., & Mohandas, A. (2010). The 10-year course of remission, abstinence, and recovery in dual diagnosis. *Journal of Substance Abuse Treatment, 39*(2), 132–140.

Yablonsky, L. (1965). *Synanon: The tunnel back*. Baltimore: Penguin Books.

Yahne, C. E., & Miller, W. R. (1999). Evoking hope. In W. R. Miller (Ed.), *Integrating spirituality into treatment: Resources for practitioners* (pp. 217–233). Washington, DC: American Psychological Association.

Yalom, I. D. (1995). *The theory and practice of group psychotherapy*. New York: Basic Books.

Yalom, I. D., & Leszcz, M. (2005). *The theory and practice of group psychotherapy* (5th ed.). New York: Basic Books.

Zuroff, D. C., Kelly, A. C., Leybman, M. J., Blatt, S. J., & Wampold, B. E. (2010). Between-therapist and within-therapist differences in the quality of the therapeutic relationship: Effects on maladjustment and self-critical perfectionism. *Journal of Clinical Psychology, 66*, 681–697.

Zweben, A. (1991). Motivational counseling with alcoholic couples. In W. R. Miller & S. Rollnick (Eds.), *Motivational interviewing: Preparing people to change addictive behavior* (pp. 225–235). New York: Guilford Press.

Zweben, A., & Barrett, D. (1993). Brief couples treatment for alcohol problems. In T. J. O'Farrell (Ed.), *Treating alcohol problems: Marital and family interventions* (pp. 353–380). New York: Guilford Press.

Zweben, A., & Barrett, D. (1997). Facilitating compliance in alcoholism treatment. In B. Blackwell (Ed.), *Compliance and treatment alliance in serious mental illness* (pp. 277–293). Newark, NJ: Gordon & Breach.

Zweben, A., Bonner, M., Chaim, G., & Santon, P. (1988). Facilitative strategies for retaining the alcohol-dependent client in outpatient treatment. *Alcoholism Treatment Quarterly, 5*(1–2), 3–24.

Zweben, A., & Li, S. (1981). The efficacy of role induction in preventing early dropout from outpatient treatment of drug dependency. *American Journal of Drug and Alcohol Abuse, 8*(2), 171–183.

Zweben, A., Pettinati, H., Weiss, R., Youngblood, M., Cox, C., Mattson, M., et al. (2008). Relationship between patient adherence and treatment outcomes:

The COMBINE study. *Alcoholism: Clinical and Experimental Research, 32,* 1661–1669.

Zweben, A., Rose, S. J., Stout, R. L., & Zywiak, W. H. (2003). Case monitoring and motivational style brief interventions. In R. K. Hester & W. R. Miller (Eds.), *Handbook of alcoholism treatment approaches: Effective alternatives* (3rd ed., pp. 113–130). Boston: Allyn & Bacon.

Zweben, A., & Zuckoff, A. (2002). Motivational interviewing and treatment adherence. In W. R. Miller & S. Rollnick (Eds.), *Motivational interviewing: Preparing people for change* (2nd ed., pp. 299–319). New York: Guilford Press.

Index